Inclusive Leisure Services: Responding to the Rights of People with Disabilities

Inclusive Leisure Services: Responding to the Rights of People with Disabilities

John Dattilo, Ph.D.
University of Georgia

Venture Publishing, Inc.
State College, PA

Production and Manuscript Editing: Richard Yocum
Additional Editing: Michele L. Barbin
Cover Design: Sandra Sikorski

Library of Congress Catalogue Card Number 94-61217
ISBN 0-910251-68-1

For Dad

Acknowledgments

My appreciation is extended to the many people I have come to know in my personal and professional life. I am especially indebted to those who, among many other characteristics, happen to have a disability. Their comments helped to enrich this book and have greatly influenced my ideas.

This book has evolved over the past decade while I taught and conducted research on leisure for people with disabilities. While the book carries with it a 1994 publication date, and much of the refinement and piloting of the text occurred in 1993, the book really took shape in 1992. The year of 1992, more than any other year in my life, was one of transition. In the early portion of the year I spent time with my father during the last months of his life. In the later part of the same year my son was born. As a result of these events, I spent considerable time with my family; however, when not spending time with my family, I attended to this book.

I would like to thank my father who has given me so much support over my life and whose memories continue to inspire me. He taught me through his example to have a strong commitment to family and compassion for others. My mother continues to motivate me with her positive ways; to her, as well, I am indebted. Although my son, David, is too young to recognize his contribution, his constant smiles and first words of "Dada" and "book" have been a joyous incentive. In addition, I would like to acknowledge my wife, Anne, who unselfishly encouraged me to write this book and continues to help me keep an optimistic perspective on life.

Students enrolled in my courses about recreation for people with disabilities at the University of Nebraska, Penn State University and the University of Georgia have been most helpful in the compilation of this book. Their suggestions and feedback concerning the material I presented in class helped shape the content of this text. Most recently, I thank the University of Georgia students who worked through earlier drafts of this text and took time to complete helpful evaluations.

Many people associated with the University of Georgia deserve special recognition. I thank Dr. Douglas Kleiber, Chair of the Department of Recreation and Leisure Studies, for his contributions to chapters 6 and 8, and for helping me to better understand leisure behavior; I am grateful for his continuous professional and personal support. I acknowledge Robin Yaffe for her valuable assistance in piloting and reviewing a draft of the book, her contributions to Section III of the text, and her help with the glossary. I recognize the efforts of Kathleen Sheldon for her contribution to Section III, and especially her work on Chapter 17. I credit Diane Groff for her meticulous work on ensuring the citations and references were accurate. I appreciate Mary Ann Devine's input concerning recent topics in the literature. I value the important efforts of Brenda Arnold who typed many portions of this book, Roger Nielsen who helped with copyediting, Marlee Stewart who generated the graphics, and Lynda Greer who took the photographs presented in Chapters 14-17. I recognize the contributions by Bonnie Godbey, Richard Yocum, Michele L. Barbin, and the entire Venture staff for publishing the book.

Several professionals across the country have made helpful contributions to different chapters in this text. Appreciation, in alphabetical order, is extended to the following people: George Alderson who motivated me with his talks and writings on accessibility and terminology and helped shape Chapters 4 and 10; Attorney John McGovern who was kind enough to take the time to review Chapter 7 that featured many of his writings on the Americans with Disabilities Act; Dr. William Murphy for his assistance in Chapter 12, a revised version of the material on adaptations we originally prepared for our text Leisure Education Program Planning; Dr. Stuart Schleien whose many writings are featured throughout this text; Dr. Ralph Smith for his help in shaping the initial draft of a paper devoted to the use of sensitive terminology as presented in Chapter 4; Dr. Susan St. Peter for her help in conceptualizing the leisure education model presented in Chapter 9; and to Mary Ulrich whose experiences and insights as a parent helped me address family issues reflected in Chapter 5.

It is my goal that this text will assist readers in understanding the importance of inclusive leisure services. I am hopeful that this knowledge is applied to systematic service delivery so that enjoyment and leisure can be experienced by people who, among many other characteristics, happen to have a disability.

—J. D.

Table of Contents

An Introduction

"If we are to achieve a culture, rich in contrasting values,
we must recognize the whole gamut of human potentialities,
and so we are a less arbitrary social fabric,
one in which each diverse human gift will find a fitting place."
—Margaret Mead

The intent of this book is to encourage providers of leisure services to promote inclusion of people with disabilities into their programs. Throughout the book you are encouraged to facilitate opportunities for people with and without disabilities to engage in leisure pursuits together. Hopefully, by working through this book, you will become more relaxed in your interactions with people having disabilities. It is my intent to assist you in understanding the value of coming into contact with people with disabilities and getting to know them. To this end, Karen Mihalyi stated the following as reported by Bogdan and Taylor (1992, p. 6):

> It's difficult at first when you are not familiar with a group you have a stereotype about. If you are not used to relating to people with disabilities, you are not sure how to. You don't want to make a mistake, do something that might offend them. So you hold back. Now I dive right in and hope that people know I am trying my hardest. I am really losing my self-consciousness around people with disabilities. At first I think I listened mostly. I listened to people and read some—mainly by people who had disabilities. But my ease mostly came by getting close with people, hearing their stories and loving them.

As a current or future leisure services provider, you are in an excellent position to enhance the lives of people with disabilities. The very services you design often are structured to enhance participants' sense of competence and self-determination. The ability to make choices and take control of one's life can permit all individuals to effectively match their skills to the challenges presented in community recreation opportunities. When this "match" is achieved, people experience enjoyment. The opportunities we have as professionals were identified by Wallach (1991, p. 53):

> The one community agency that provides a means of communication and contact across a broad front is the recreation provider . . . (P)ark and recreation facilities are natural meeting places for all elements of a community.

Once recreation professionals recognize their ability to enhance the quality of life for people with disabilities, it is then time to develop strategies to promote inclusive leisure services. Mount and Zwernik (1988) encouraged professionals to build on people's capacities and opportunities in networks and communities and consider that all people bring important gifts to community life. Stereotypes limit the ability of community members both to see people's capacities and to identify the presence of (or potential to develop) skills and abilities (Mount & Zwernik, 1988).

According to Murphy (1975), the fundamental consideration for all human beings is that individuals should have a measure of **freedom**, autonomy, choice and self-determination. And if you consider Bregha's (1985) position that leisure is the most precious expression of our freedom, it becomes clear that leisure is an inalienable human right. Therefore, every effort must be made to help people with disabilities become involved in active leisure participation. The challenge lies in finding ways to remove barriers to participation while providing opportunities to develop the skills, awareness, and understanding needed to freely choose participation in various leisure experiences. The goal in providing leisure services to people with disabilities, then, is to help individuals develop the skills and opportunities needed to feel free to participate in such chosen experiences (Dattilo, 1991).

Kelly (1983; 1987) and Kleiber and Kelly (1980) reported that leisure is important to the well-being of people by virtue of the opportunity to make personal choices, the opportunity to interact with others in noncoercive ways, and the emotional value of enjoyment. A mission statement developed by the Community Recreation Department of Nova Scotia entitled "Recreation for People with a Disability: The Value of Leisure," illustrates the value of leisure for all people, including people with disabilities:

> The value of leisure experience in enhancing the quality of life for people with a disability should not be underestimated. Recreation offers most people with a disability the same fun and challenge it does all participants. For some people, the recreation environment is a safe, nonthreatening setting in which to experience decision making, risk taking, and community involvement. It can also provide an ideal opportunity for people with a disability to develop basic social and

motor skills. The chance to independently choose activities in which to become involved, or even to decide whether or not to participate, can be a significant learning experience. Satisfying leisure experiences can contribute to a sense of self-worth, contribution, and belonging to the community that may otherwise be missing.

What is a Disability?

To understand issues surrounding people with disabilities and actions that can be taken to promote inclusion, it is often useful to clarify our identification of people with disabilities. According to the Americans with Disabilities Act (ADA), a person with a disability is anyone who has a physical or mental impairment that substantially limits one or more major life activity. Major life activities include seeing, hearing, speaking, walking, dressing, feeding oneself, working, learning, recreating, and other daily physical or mental activities. This broad definition incorporates many people, including individuals with:

(a) sensory impairments (e.g., visual and hearing impairments);
(b) communication disorders (e.g., speech impairments);
(c) cognitive disabilities (e.g., mental retardation, traumatic brain injury);
(d) physical disabilities (e.g., cerebral palsy, multiple sclerosis);
(e) chronic health disorders (e.g., cardiac, pulmonary);
(f) impaired mental health (e.g., depression, schizophrenia);
(g) chemical dependence; and
(h) HIV infection.

People who are covered by ADA also include people who have a record of a disability. Examples include people with histories of alcoholism or chemical dependence, mental or emotional illness, heart disease or cancer who are currently free of disease or impairment and are not limited in major life activities, or people who have been misclassified as having a disability when they, in fact, did not (people who have been misclassified as having mental retardation or mental illness).

In addition, people who are regarded as having a disability are covered by the ADA. An example of a person regarded as having a disability is an individual who has a significant facial deformity which does not limit major life activities. While the person is not physically or mentally restricted in his or her activities, public reaction to the person's appearance may result in discrimination. Another example is a person rumored to be, but who is not, infected with HIV.

In summary, a person with a disability is anyone who:

(a) has a physical or mental impairment substantially limiting one or more major life activities;
(b) has a record of such impairment; or
(c) is regarded as having such an impairment.

This book is designed to provide assistance to leisure services providers in accommodating individuals identified as having a disability. Shapiro (1993, p. 5) identified the diversity associated with people who have disabilities with the following description:

> There are hundreds of different disabilities. Some are congenital; most come later in life. Some are progressive, like muscular dystrophy, cystic fibrosis, and some forms of vision and hearing loss. Others, like seizure conditions, are episodic. Multiple sclerosis is episodic and progressive. Some conditions are static, like the loss of a limb. Still others, like cancer and occasionally paralysis, can even go away. Some disabilities are "hidden," like epilepsy or diabetes. Disability law also applies to people with perceived disabilities such as obesity or stuttering, which are not disabling but create prejudice and discrimination. Each disability comes in differing degrees of severity. Hearing aids can amplify sounds for most deaf and hard-of-hearing people but do nothing for others. Some people with autism spend their lives in institutions; others graduate from Ivy League schools or reach the top of their professions.

What is Leisure?

Although there is continuing debate over the definitions of the terms "recreation," "free time," and "leisure," there appears to be consensus regarding the meanings of these terms among consumers, practitioners, researchers and theorists about their meanings. This section presents definitions of these terms.

Typically, **recreation** is defined as an activity developed by a society that is designed for the primary reasons of fun, enjoyment, and satisfaction (e.g., swimming, table games, dance). The notion of recreation, therefore, relates directly to the activity and is independent of the participant's feelings and experiences. People who participate in recreational activities may experience enjoyment and satisfaction or may encounter failure, rejection, and feelings of helplessness.

The phrase **free time** is often used to describe an individual's unobligated time; time when daily tasks—such as responsibilities associated with family, work, or home maintenance—are not being attended to. So, when people are not busy performing specific required tasks, they possess free time. And, although many people experience enjoyment and satisfaction during their free time, this free time may trigger feelings of boredom, anxiety, and despair in others.

The third term, **leisure**, integrates elements of activity and time, but more importantly emphasizes the importance of a person's perception that he or she is free to choose to participate in meaningful, enjoyable, and satisfying experiences. As individuals get in touch with the positive feelings—control, competence, relaxation, excitement—associated with the leisure experience, they will be intrinsically motivated to participate. That is, they will participate in leisure simply to be involved in the experience, not for some tangible outcome or external reward. Leisure, then, is an experience, a process, a subjective state of mind born of psychological involvement. As a state-of-mind, leisure transcends time, environments, and situations. To fully partake in leisure is to express talents, demonstrate capabilities, achieve one's potential and experience a variety of positive emotions.

The practical value of knowing what contributes to experiencing leisure is clear and direct. It leads us to concentrate on facilitating the leisure experience. In addition, learning how to facilitate leisure makes it possible for us to reduce or eliminate constraints and barriers to leisure participation.

Psychological theories of leisure (e.g., Neulinger, 1974), have emphasized the "state-of-mind" of the person as the key to the leisure experience (Shamir, 1992). Goodale (1992) reported that two principal components of a subjective state of leisure are that the people perceive themselves to have freely chosen the activity engaged in, and they engage in the activity purely because doing so is meaningful and enjoyable. Shamir (1992) described these two related aspects of a leisure state-of-mind as **intrinsic motivation** and **perceived freedom**. He stated that intrinsic motivation commonly refers to doing the activity because of the expected pleasure of participation in the activity itself, not because of expected results or external rewards. Perceived freedom commonly refers to **self-determination** or the feeling of being the origin of the activity. Some theorists (de Charms, 1968; Deci, 1980) regard self-determination as the basis of intrinsic motivation.

Shamir (1988) identified two other aspects of perceived freedom that deserve some attention. He reported that the feeling of perceived control over the activity as opposed to being controlled or being restricted in the activity is important to the leisure experience. In addition, to experience leisure it is important for individuals to feel that they are free to discontinue participation when they desire to do so (Shamir, 1988).

In discussing positive ways to view ourselves and others, Fulghum (1988) illustrated the role leisure can play in defining our identities:

> Making a living and having a life are not the same thing. Making a living and making a life that's worthwhile are not the same thing. Living *the* good life and living *a* good life are not the same thing. A job title doesn't even come close to answering the question "What do you do?" But suppose that instead of answering that question with what we do to get money, we replied with what we do that gives us great pleasure or makes us feel useful to the human enterprise? (p. 65).

What is Inclusion?

> The time has come to adapt a new way of thinking, one founded on the premise that the community belongs to everyone, and everyone—regardless of level and type of ability—belongs to the community. Inclusive community leisure services can be powerful vehicles for promoting this ideal (Schleien, 1993, p. 67).

Inclusion is about ensuring choices, having support, having connections, and being valued (Moss, 1993). To illustrate these characteristics, Moss (1993) presented the following examples: "I can make many of the choices I do because I have friends and family and community to support me in those choices" (Moss, 1993, p. 1). The need for connections becomes obvious when you consider that every reference ever given for a job, credit application or housing application has been a person you have connected with. Many houses and apartments lived in, restaurants dined at, and stores shopped at have been identified by the people in my circle of support. People have connections and support from others because they are valued. Though people may lack many talents, people who know them have found qualities in them they like. For example, one friend values another because she can tell her friend anything and knows that her friend will not share the information with others. Another person values a friend because he will not quit working at something until it is done. Others may value a friend because she is an optimist. None of these traits are dependent on a high IQ or great physical ability.

Inclusion examines each person and determines how best that person can be fully included by determining what supports are necessary, what skills that person needs, what input the staff and students require, and how that support generalizes to other environments (Berger, 1994). To emphasize the importance of support Hutchison and McGill (1992, p. 9) stated that support involves:

> . . . encouraging someone to strengthen an existing interest. Other times, it involves supporting someone to develop an entirely new interest that could someday become a leisure identity. Encouragement and support takes many forms: from helping someone sign up for a recreation program; assisting someone to buy the equipment for an activity; introducing someone to other people who enjoy the activity; to recognizing a person's expertise and asking for advice and assistance. Supporting people in developing leisure identities contributes to helping them find the "essence of community."

Ferguson, Meyer, Jeanchild, Juniper, and Zingo (1992) called for "inclusion" for people with disabilities, with all its implications of being socially connected, exchanging and sharing responsibilities. If inclusion is to mean anything, it must mean that people with disabilities become full, active, learning members of the community (Ferguson et al., 1992). Remembering the words of Dr. Martin Luther King, Jr., Bullock (1993, p. 4) shared these words of inspiration:

> I have a dream! I have a dream that one day all people will be recognized as people, celebrated for who they are, and not recognized by their limitations. I challenge you to learn new ideas and new ways of being inclusive.

Inclusion infers that we decide that "diversity is valuable—not just a reality to be tolerated, accepted, or accommodated, but a reality to be valued (York, 1994, p. 11). According to York (1994), if we expect diversity and decide it is good, maybe it would be easier to:

(a) focus on capacities of people;
(b) recognize there is an array of contributions to be made;
(c) believe that all people are inherently worthy; and
(d) understand that doing one's best and helping others do the same is what is most important.

What is the Problem?

The findings of the U.S. Congress reported in "Findings and Purposes," Section 2 of the Americans With Disabilities Act (Public Law 101-336), July 26, 1990, (ADA, pp. 3-5), clearly illustrates the problems faced by people with disabilities.

Some 43 million Americans have one or more physical or mental disabilities, and this number is increasing as the population as a whole is growing older. Disability was ranked by the 1991 Institute of Medicine as the largest public-health problem in the United States that affects individuals with disabilities, their families and all of society.

Historically, society has tended to isolate and segregate individuals with disabilities and, despite some improvements, such forms of discrimination against individuals with disabilities continue to be a serious and pervasive social problem. Discrimination against individuals with disabilities persists in critical areas, such as recreation. Unlike individuals who have experienced discrimination on the basis of race, color, sex, national origin, religion, or age, individuals who have experienced discrimination on the basis of disability have often had no legal recourse to redress such discrimination. Individuals with disabilities continually encounter various forms of discrimination, including outright intentional exclusion, the discriminatory effects of architectural, transportation, and communication barriers, overprotective rules and policies, failure to make modifications to existing facilities and practices, exclusionary qualification standards and criteria, segregation, and relegation to lesser services, programs, activities, benefits, jobs, or other opportunities.

Census data, national polls, and other studies have documented that people with disabilities, as a group, occupy an inferior status in our society, and are severely disadvantaged socially, vocationally, economically, and educationally. Individuals with disabilities are a discrete and insular minority who have been faced with restrictions and limitations, subjected to a history of purposeful unequal treatment, and relegated to a position of political powerlessness in our society, based on characteristics that are beyond the control of such individuals and resulting from stereotypic assumptions not truly indicative of the individual ability of such individuals to participate in, and contribute to, society.

The nation's proper goals regarding individuals with disabilities are to assure equality of opportunity, full participation, independent living, and economic self-sufficiency. The continuing existence of unfair and unnecessary discrimination and prejudice denies people with disabilities the opportunity to compete on an equal basis and to pursue those opportunities for which our free society is justifiably famous, and costs the United States billions of dollars in unnecessary expenses resulting from dependency and nonproductivity.

What is in This Book?

Just as Terrill (1992, p. 8) identified the Americans with Disabilities Act as a springboard for "inclusion, independence, and the recognition that all people have the opportunity to be contributing members of society," this book is designed to bring the spirit of ADA to the field of recreation and leisure. The book attempts to provide current and future professionals with strategies that will facilitate meaningful leisure participation by all participants, while respecting the rights of people with disabilities.

To achieve this end, this book contains three distinct sections. The first section is devoted to awareness of important concepts. The second section presents readers with the Americans with Disabilities Act and specific strategies to facilitate compliance with the spirit of the Act. The final section introduces readers to people with disabilities, their characteristics, and methods for including them in community leisure services.

As an introduction to the first section, Chapter 1 provides information to increase awareness of attitude formation and to clarify the impact of negative attitudes. Chapter 2 supplies readers with information and opportunities on how to explore their attitudes. Strategies for enhancing positive attitude formation are presented in Chapter 3. Sensitivity to appropriate terminology and family issues is encouraged in Chapters 4 and 5. Chapter 6 concludes the awareness section of the book with the identification of barriers to leisure participation experienced by people with disabilities.

Chapter 7, the first chapter in the second section, provides information on the Americans with Disabilities Act and sets the tone for this section. The following six chapters provide specific suggestions to help professionals provide inclusive leisure services. Suggestions to encourage enhancement of self-determination are provided in Chapter 8. Guidelines for the development of comprehensive leisure education programs are presented in Chapter 9. In Chapter 10, accessibility issues are addressed. Chapter 11 is devoted to procedures for integration. Chapter 12 presents recommendations for making necessary accommodations and suggestions for advocacy are presented in Chapter 13.

The final section of the book introduces the reader to several people with disabilities. The information presented in Chapters 14-17 is intended to have the reader meet people with disabilities through pictures and written text, and develop an appreciation for the need for leisure in their lives. The specific descriptions and pictures of the people were chosen to provide a diverse introduction to people with disabilities who are living within their communities. However, after examining the broad definition of disability as defined by ADA, it became clear that an overview of each disabling condition presented within the confines of this text would be an unmanageable task. Therefore, a sampling of disabilities were chosen to be included in this book that are presented within the following major categories: physical limitations, cognitive limitations, and sensory limitations. In addition, the final chapter of the book introduces you to some people with disabilities who use assistive technology.

The chapters in this text are organized in a similar manner and contain segments designed to enhance learning. Each chapter begins with an orientation activity to familiarize the reader with the content presented in the chapter and to provide an opportunity to interact with others about the topic. The orientation activities provide an experiential preview of what is to come in the chapter and are designed to set the educational climate (Dattilo & Murphy, 1991). These orientation activities are immediately followed by debriefings to maximize learning associated with the activities. The debriefings consist of a brief discussion about the orientation activity and a few questions requiring the reader to reflect on the activity. Next, each chapter contains an introduction designed to briefly acquaint the reader with the topics to be covered in the chapter. The content of each chapter follows the introduction and comprises the majority of the chapter. A conclusion is provided at the end of each chapter in an attempt to make sense of the entire chapter by recapitulating the major points (Dattilo & Murphy, 1991). The chapters finish with several discussion questions to encourage the reader to review the material, identify important aspects of the content and engage in problem solving.

People associated with the disability rights movement believe that people with disabilities are not helpless "cripples," nor are they courageous or heroic "super-achievers." Most people with disabilities are just regular people trying to lead meaningful lives, not to inspire, nor to be pitied. Hopefully, by getting to know some people with disabilities through this book, the reader will avoid creating stereotypes and see the value in providing inclusive leisure services.

Section A

Develop an Awareness

Chapter 1

Understand Attitude Development

"Injustice anywhere is a threat to justice everywhere."
—Martin Luther King, Jr.

Orientation Activity: Examine Differences and Similarities

Directions. On a blank sheet of paper record the following headings at the top of the page: name, difference, and similarity. After the sheet is prepared, move about the room and attempt to talk with each person who is present. Ask a person what his or her name is and record the information in the space provided. Together, attempt to identify something about the two of you that is different and record this characteristic. Once you have determined one difference, identify something the two of you share or have in common. As you complete the information with each person, thank them, and continue moving about the room finding new people to interview.

Debriefing

You have spoken with a variety of people and were able to identify both differences and similarities between you and each person you encountered. According to Dattilo (1992), the unique qualities of people are what often makes them interesting. Why we like some people or why we respect other people is not necessarily that they are the same as us but frequently because they possess unique characteristics. However, it is helpful to begin relationships with the basic belief that we all share common characteristics. We must develop a bond with people so that we can accept their differences. Therefore, if we encounter people who happen to have a disability and are able to identify and focus on similarities with those individuals, we will increase the likelihood that we will include that person (i.e., in our lives, in community activities, in the services we provide) and accept their differences. Respond to the following questions related to the orientation activity:

1. What was the most difficult aspect of the orientation activity for you?
2. How did you feel when you talked about similarities with another person as compared with differences?

3. How do you feel when you meet people and they primarily focus their attention on how you are different from them?

Introduction

The focus of this chapter is on the development of attitudes toward people with disabilities. Since the goal of the book is to encourage the reader to accept diversity, especially in relationship to individuals with disabilities, examples that promote positive attitudes of acceptance will be provided. The attitude of professionals providing leisure services plays a critical role in supporting equal access to their programs. According to the Project LIFE Staff (1988), attitudes have the power of creating positive forces for change or can create major barriers. The intent of this chapter, and the entire book, is to encourage the removal of barriers to leisure and stimulate the development of approaches that facilitate meaningful leisure participation for all people.

Formation and Expression of Attitudes

To consider the impact of attitudes on our interactions with others, it may be helpful to examine how attitudes relate to our beliefs, our intentions, and our behaviors. Fishbein and Ajzen (1975) provided a frequently cited description of the relationship between antecedents to beliefs, beliefs, attitudes, intentions, and behaviors. **Antecedents to beliefs** are those conditions that "set the stage" for beliefs to develop. The community in which people reside, their past experiences, their families and friends, their individual characteristics, and a variety of circumstances can influence the development of attitudes. These various conditions are considered antecedents to the development of beliefs.

People's **beliefs** involve what they perceive to be true. These beliefs are composed of an individual's perception of information that has been available in the form of antecedent conditions. Beliefs result in the person acquiring knowledge and understanding and developing opinions. The beliefs that are acquired may or may not be correct. The convictions people obtain, based on their beliefs, influence the development of attitudes. According to Brown (1992, p. 27), "'beliefs' refer to generally accepted tenets of society that imply that people with disabilities are somehow 'less able' than people who are not disabled."

Fishbein and Ajzen (1975) described an **attitude** as a learned predisposition to respond in a consistently favorable or unfavorable manner with respect to a given object. That is to say, once people develop an attitude about a group of people, when they encounter a person affiliated with this group they will tend to respond to this person, or any other person, with the same group association, in a similar manner. Petty and Cacioppo (1981, p. 7) stated that "attitudes are the enduring positive or negative feeling about some person, object, or issue."

Rosenberg and Houland (1960) described attitudes as having cognitive, affective, and behavioral components. These three components were further articulated by Yuker in the Report to the White House Conference on People with Disabilities (1977). **Cognitive predispositions** involve a consistent way that people think or develop ideas. For example, some people have an attitude that people with disabilities are courageous. They will then have a tendency to think that any person they meet who happens to have a disability is heroic. **Affective predispositions** result in people feeling or having emotions that are fairly consistent. For example, some people have an attitude that tends to result in them being sad when they see a person with a disability. **Behavioral predispositions** involve a consistent desire to act in a particular way. For example, some people have a tendency to consider donating money when the topic of disability arises. Understanding the predispositions of cognition, affect, and behavior as they relate to attitude formation and expression may provide some insight into the complex nature of attitudes.

Intentions are those behavioral plans individuals make with respect to the presence of another person. Ajzen and Driver (1991) reported that intentions reflect motivations that influence behavior; intentions are indications of how much of an effort people plan to exert to perform the behavior. People anticipate behaving a given way based on the information they have acquired throughout their lives and the attitudes they have formed. However, what people intend to do is not always what they actually do. It has been said that the road to a not so desirable location is paved with good intentions.

The impact of attitudes is reflected in people's behaviors. **Behaviors** are any observable and measurable act, response, or movement by an individual (Dattilo & Murphy, 1987). According to Dattilo and Murphy, behavior can be detected with the five senses and, when described, generally means the same thing to different people.

As seen in Figure 1.1 (page 16), antecedents, beliefs, attitudes, intentions, and behaviors are interrelated in a dynamic process of attitude development and expression. Each component of the process is influenced by another. Therefore, when one component of the process is altered, frequently the other components change accordingly.

Because many individuals within our society possess negative attitudes toward people with disabilities, the next section of this chapter will focus on the problems associated with the development of negative attitudes toward individuals with disabilities. The Americans with Disabilities Act of 1990 stated that:

Individuals with disabilities are a discrete and insular minority who have been faced with restrictions and limitations, subjected to a history of purposeful unequal treatment, and relegated to a position of political powerlessness in our society, based on characteristics that are beyond the control of such individuals and resulting from stereotypic assumptions not truly indicative of the individual ability of such individuals to participate in, and contribute to, society.

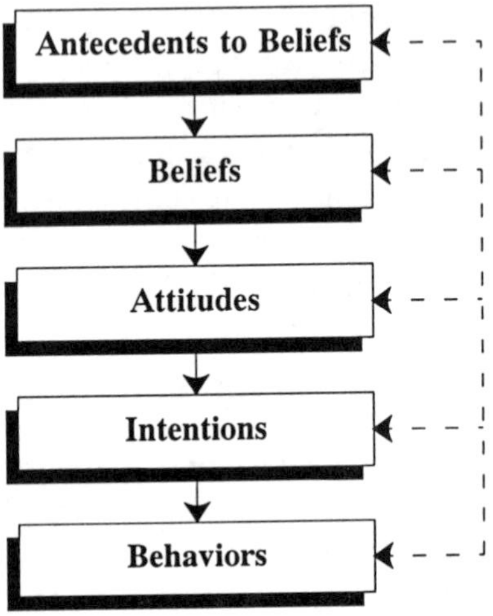

Figure 1.1 The dynamic process of attitude development and expression.

Development of Negative Attitudes

Only when we fully acknowledge the unacceptability of discrimination on the basis of disability and its resulting segregation of people with severe disabilities from the ordinary spheres of society—only then will we stop the devaluing and wasting of many people's lives and hasten the development of positive attitudes on the part of everyone (Bray, 1989, p. 7).

People with and without disabilities can experience stress when interacting with one another. Based on a literature review by Kleck and colleagues (Kleck, 1966, 1968; Kleck, Ono, & Hastorf, 1966), Makas (1988) noted that people without disabilities reported greater emotional distress, exhibited higher physiological arousal, showed less motor activity, displayed less variability in their verbal behavior, expressed opinions that were less representative of their previously reported beliefs, and terminated interactions sooner when interacting with a person who appeared disabled than when interacting with a person without disabilities.

Kelley, Hastorf, Jones, Thibaut, and Usdane (1960) and Goffman (1963) suggested that tension between people may result because neither person knows what the other expects. The perception of a person with a disability as being "different" results in personal stress, which can cause a strain in interactions followed by such emotions as fear and anxiety and such actions as avoidance and segregation (Howe-Murphy & Charboneau, 1987). During an interview with our research staff, Wanda illustrated this point when she said:

> People don't talk to me because of the way I am . . . They just kind of look at me and not really know what to say because they feel uncomfortable maybe, but I don't feel uncomfortable.

The stress many people without disabilities experience when interacting with people with disabilities can be traced to perceptions of people with disabilities as being different, generalized attitudes of people with disabilities, and generalized actions toward those individuals (see Figure 1.2, page 18). Perceptions of "differentness" can stem from concepts such as stigma and deviancy. Generalized attitudes include the development of stereotypes and prejudice while generalized actions involve segregation and discrimination. Often these concepts are used interchangeably without a clear understanding of their meaning and interactions. This section of the chapter is intended to alleviate some of the confusion surrounding the development of negative attitudes by defining some important concepts. In addition to the definitions provided in this section, information illustrating the relationship of the concepts will be presented.

Perceptions of Being Different

Stigma. Goffman (1963) defined stigma as an undesired differentness which separates the person from others in a society. Therefore, a stigma is not merely a difference, but a characteristic that deeply discredits a person's moral character (Goffman, 1963). In a later writing, Goffman (1974) reported that the person with a stigma is perceived as not quite human. A disabling condition may be so negatively valued that an individual is defined by that single attribute and devalued as a total person (Tripp & Sherrill, 1991).

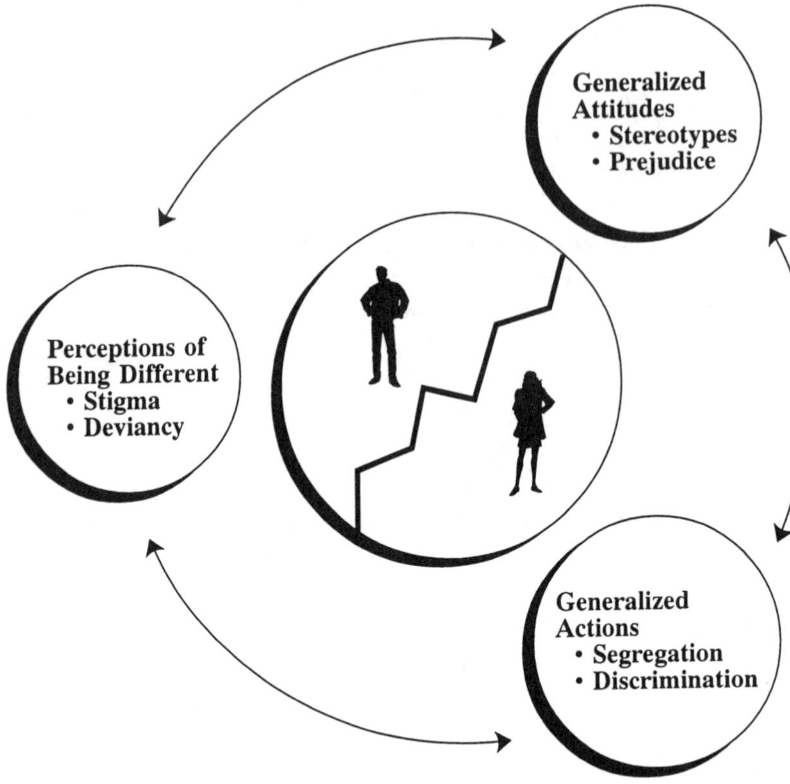

Figure 1.2 Concepts contributing to stressful interactions.

Personal and social identity come into question because of a disability. Goffman (1963) illustrated how the marginal social position of persons who have socially devalued physical characteristics pervades everyday life and the self-perceptions of such persons. Living with stigmatized characteristics transforms ordinary social concerns such as shopping and meeting strangers into socially demanding tasks (Brooks & Matson, 1987). Brooks and Matson (1987) reported that when this social strain is combined with the burden of caring for physical needs, disability and chronic illness becomes a cycle of never-ending *work*.

Tripp and Sherrill (1991) stated that stigma involves a negative valuation of a person because of an attribute possessed by the individual that deviates from the norm. The authors observed that an attribute that is perceived as negative will interfere with people's perceptions of positive attributes and create a perception of undesired difference from what was anticipated. Once people with disabilities become aware of their stigmatized label, their self-perceptions are affected (Eisenberg, 1982).

Deviancy. When an individual is stigmatized, the person is often identified as being deviant. Similar to stigma, deviancy infers that an individual has strayed away from the majority of society, an established standard, or a highly regarded principle. Therefore, deviant behavior is defined by societal norms (Edgar, 1992).

Wolfensberger (1972) stated that a person is considered deviant if he or she is perceived to be significantly different from others in some important characteristic and if this difference is negatively valued. The negative evaluation comes from the segment of society that constitutes the majority, which defines social norms (Wolfensberger & Thomas, 1983). Deviance requires the exhibition of behavior that violates people's expectations and departs from societal norms (Gibbons & Jones, 1975).

Since skill development is valued in our culture and people with disabilities are considered to have less skills than people without disabilities, these individuals have been identified by some people as being deviant. Safilios-Rothschild (1970) explained that people with disabilities are not deviant because of their disability, they are deviant because people label them as "deviant" because they possess an undesirable difference.

Generalized Attitudes

Stereotype. Most professionals and people with disabilities agree that one of the biggest problems facing people with disabilities is stereotypes. A stereotype is a standardized mental picture held in common by members of a group and represents an oversimplified opinion, attitude, or judgment. Our society may have developed stereotypes of people that result in a narrow view of them. For example, some people believe that individuals receiving psychiatric services are a threat to society. This response is based on a stereotype frequently presented in the media. In truth, an extremely small minority of people experiencing mental health problems (less than 3 percent) pose a threat to anyone.

Blaxter (1976) reported that stereotypes of people with disabilities tend to result in evaluating them as a category, rather than as individuals. In an effort to explain why stereotypes exist, Allport (1954, pp. 20-21) reported the following:

> We like to solve problems easily. We can do best if we can fit them rapidly into a satisfactory category and use this category as a means of prejudicing the solution. So long as we can get away with coarse overgeneralizations, we tend to do so. Why? Well, it takes less effort . . .

Prejudice. A major problem occurs when the distinctions created by stereotypes result in prejudicial outlooks toward individuals. Prejudice involves the development of a judgment in disregard of a person's rights, resulting in that individual being injured or damaged in some way. The word "prejudice" is composed of a prefix "pre," meaning beforehand, and the root word, "judic," meaning to judge. Prejudice and the rejection of people with disabilities may occur because of the tendency for people to respond differentially to difference (Thurman & Lewis, 1979).

Even though swift progress is being made that enhances the quality of life for people with disabilities, barriers persist. According to Shapiro (1993, p. 4):

> Rapid advances in technology, new civil rights protections, a generation of better-educated disabled students out of "mainstreamed" classrooms, a new group consciousness, and political activism mean more disabled people are seeking jobs and greater daily participation in American life. But prejudice, society's low expectations, and an antiquated welfare and social service system frustrate these burgeoning attempts at independence. As a result, the new aspirations of people with disabilities have gone unnoticed and misunderstood by mainstream America.

Generalized Actions

Segregation. If people are stigmatized and identified as deviant, the practice of segregation may occur. Segregation requires the separation or isolation of a group or individual in a restricted area by discriminatory means. Such segregation results in members of the group, or an individual, receiving treatment that is different from other people. In discussing segregation Hutchison and McGill (1992, pp. 18-19) reported that:

> Segregation is based on the belief that people who have been given similar labels have the same needs and that they can best be served together in a congregated environment. Segregation and congregation lead to further stigmatization and ostracization of the person by accentuating differences.

Educated by the Civil Rights movement in the United States during the 1960s, we are aware that different services resulting from segregation are clearly not equal. Howe-Murphy and Charboneau (1987) suggested that when people with disabilities are segregated from their peers who do not have disabilities they may not learn a full range of behaviors; rather, they may only model those behaviors exhibited by people with whom they have the most contact (i.e., other people with similar disabilities).

Anderson (1981) related segregation to the notion of **exclusion** which she defined as the barring of another person from oneself, resulting in the disregard of that person as a human presence in a face-to-face situation. The negative consequences of exclusion hinder the quantity and quality of interpersonal relationships and also affect a person's development (Howe-Murphy & Charboneau, 1987). Howe-Murphy and Charboneau (1987) provided a helpful presentation of the difference between exclusion and seclusion. As previously mentioned, exclusion involves ignoring someone's physical and social presence. Seclusion, on the other hand, involves individuals being left alone but being able to maintain verification of their value. Being left alone, or being able to seclude oneself is desirable, but being excluded results in people perceiving that they are not wanted.

Hutchison and McGill (1992) reported that when people with disabilities are congregated and served together it is difficult, if not impossible, for each person to be viewed and treated as an individual because of the tendency of other people to generalize and use stereotypes to describe them. Wolfensberger and Thomas (1983) also commented on congregation when they described the occurrence of deviancy transference. The authors presented the example of when people with physical disabilities are grouped together with people with mental disabilities, it is likely that all the individuals will be suspected of having both mental and physical limitations.

Discrimination. According to the president of the Disability Rights Education and Defense Fund, all people with disabilities share one common experience . . . discrimination. A frequent use of the word "discrimination" involves a person making a distinction categorically rather than individually about another person, then acting towards that person differently than another person. With discrimination, people make judgments about people based on the affiliation with a group rather than on who they are as an individual.

As an example of discrimination, a recreation professional may see an individual who is blind. The professional may automatically think that the individual with a visual impairment is musically talented. The inaccurate distinction was based on the category of blindness rather than on the person's individual abilities. Following that inaccurate distinction, the recreation professional may follow this by only offering programs that are musical in nature to this person.

An example of the possible effects of negative attitudes was reported in a pamphlet entitled "Fair Play" published by the Regional Rehabilitation Research Institute on Attitudinal, Legal, and Leisure Barriers. A young woman, Gloria, who is blind, went to an amusement park with a group of friends. Although her friends were required to pay admission, she was given free admission to the park. When stopping for lunch, a waitress asked her friends what Gloria wanted to eat. Ride attendants asked her friends if they thought she was capable of holding on properly during the ride. Gloria was refused admittance to the merry-go-round because the attendants were concerned that she might injure herself when riding alone. The attitudes that Gloria experienced occurred, in part, because people focused on her disability rather than her ability. Gloria's enjoyment and fun was reduced by the attitudes of the park personnel. She was treated "differently" by having been given free admission, not being spoken to directly, and the assumption that she was not capable of riding alone. By being overly protected, much of Gloria's excitement associated with park rides was lost.

Shapiro (1993, p. 25) clearly articulated the problems people with disabilities experience as a result of the many forms of discrimination in the following statement:

> Often the discrimination is crude bigotry, such as that of a private New Jersey zoo owner who refused to admit children with retardation to the monkey house, claiming they scared his chimpanzees. It may be intolerance that permitted a New Jersey restaurant owner to ask a woman with cerebral palsy to leave because her different appearance was disturbing other diners. Resentment may have led an airline employee in New York to throw a 66-year-old double amputee on a baggage dolly—"like a sack of potatoes," his daughter complained—rather than help him into a wheelchair and aid him in boarding a jetliner. Others may feel that disabled people are somewhat less than human and therefore fair game for victimization, as when a gang of New Jersey high school athletes raped a mildly retarded classmate with a baseball bat in 1989.

Labels and Expectations

As people without disabilities develop negative attitudes toward people with disabilities they begin to develop expectations of people with disabilities that can be destructive. Three possible reactions can occur that result in the person with a disability being stifled. These three reactions are the self-fulfilling prophecy, the spread phenomenon, and the overexaggeration assumption.

Self-fulfilling Prophecy

The steps by which the self-fulfilling prophecy occurs have been delineated in several writings (e.g., Darley & Fazio, 1980). Basically, professionals agree that the self-fulfilling prophecy requires interaction of two people. Initially, a person becomes aware of an expectation of another person. This first individual comprehends this expectation and retains the information. Next, this person must communicate the expectancy to the other person. As indicated in Figure 1.3, once this communication has occurred, the other person then must attend to this communication, comprehend, and act upon the expectancy (Barber et al., 1969).

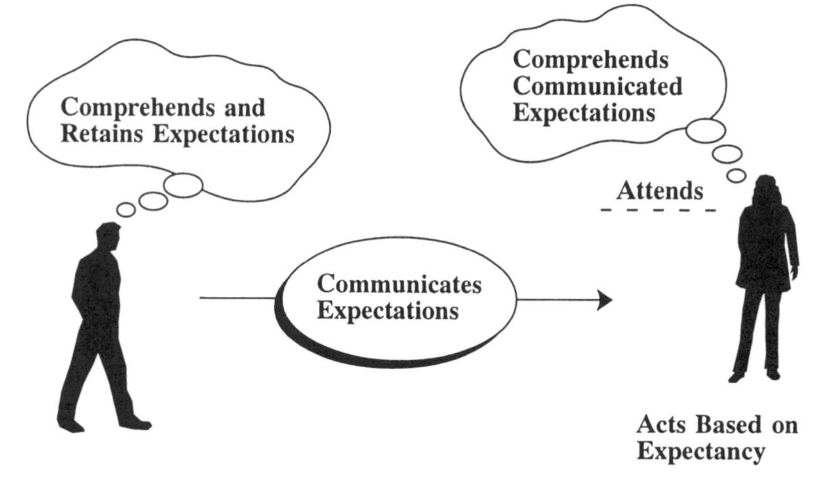

Figure 1.3 Aspects of the self-fulfilling prophesy.

The self-fulfilling prophecy can be described as how a person's expectation for another person's behavior can become an accurate prediction of the person's behaviors simply because it exists (Rosenthal & Jacobson, 1968). Labeling a person "disabled" reduces many people's expectancy for the person to succeed (Dunn, 1968). Some labels used for people with disabilities imply deficiencies which produce expectations that interfere with the person's development (Jones, 1972).

Often people have preconceived stereotypical expectancies about people with disabilities. Labeling a person "disabled" brings to mind stereotypes that influence perceptions of that person's behaviors (Ferguson, Ferguson, &

Taylor, 1992). This labeling of a person may result in the person's behavior being consistent with the label. People with disabilities are rewarded for behavior that conforms to social expectations associated with the disability role and punished for behavior that departs from these expectations (Bogdan & Taylor, 1982).

The rationale for not labeling people with disabilities is that the labels themselves can act as stigmas. The mere identification of a person who needs assistance from professionals can instill the belief that the person is not quite human (Blatt, 1982). Siperstein, Budoff, and Bak (1980) reported that among some young children, labels had the power to stigmatize children with disabilities.

Disability labels may generate negative expectations when compared to labels that imply "normalcy" (Algozzine, Mercer, & Countermine, 1977). For example, Foster, Ysseldyke, and Reese (1975) reported that children who were labeled "emotionally disturbed" were perceived more negatively than those labeled as "normal." Similar results have been demonstrated for the label "learning disabilities" (Foster, Schmidt, & Sabatino, 1976). According to Algozzine and colleagues (1977), an individual bearing a deviancy-related label, such as a person with a disability, is expected to behave in a consistent fashion that is negative. Kennedy, Austin, and Smith (1987) reported that the self-fulfilling prophecy may make it difficult for people with disabilities to develop a positive self-concept.

Although these examples demonstrate how the self-fulfilling prophecy can have negative impacts on the lives of individuals with disabilities, positive results also are possible. For example, when Rosenthal and Jacobson (1968) led teachers to believe that randomly selected students would improve substantially during the next school year, the students did achieve more than their classmates. Unfortunately, when the self-fulfilling prophecy is applied to people with disabilities, the results typically involve lowered expectations and lower participation and performance. As seen in Figure 1.4, the intent of this book is to help the reader contribute to a self-fulfilling prophecy that raises expectations and performance of people with disabilities.

Brown (1992) reported that people with disabilities often accept as truth what they experience or have been told. The tendency of individuals with disabilities to accept negative stereotyping about themselves is often referred to as **internalized oppression.** "Internalized oppression occurs when an individual comes to accept these stereotypical beliefs as truths and acts upon them." (Brown, 1992, p. 27). For example, one negative belief held by some members of society is that people with disabilities are not capable of participating in community recreation programs. As a consequence, people with disabilities might not try to enroll in existing integrated programs, or they may

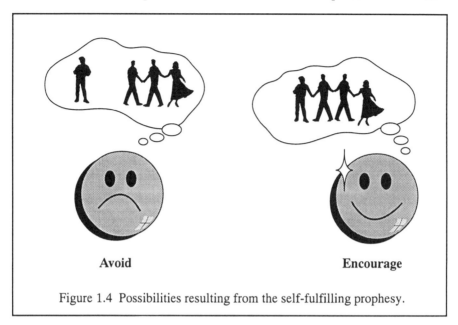

Figure 1.4 Possibilities resulting from the self-fulfilling prophesy.

feel excessively thankful to be even given a chance to participate. Individuals who feel grateful might not feel comfortable in asking for reasonable accommodations to enable them to participate effectively (Brown, 1992).

Spread Phenomenon

Tripp and Sherrill (1991) identified the occurrence of the spread phenomenon in relationship to people with disabilities. They reported that sometimes there is an association of additional imperfection to a person on the basis of the actual disabling condition. For example, there may be a tendency to speak loudly to an individual who can not see, or to develop a belief that an individual with a mental impairment lacks physical skills, or that a person with a speech impairment is not mentally alert.

The spread phenomenon further "handicaps" a person with a disability. Although people with disabilities may be limited in only one aspect of their life, many people believe that these people are "handicapped" in all situations. This generalization of the disability to all aspects of a person's life is extremely detrimental and a result of the spread phenomenon. During an interview with our research staff, Lori illustrated the occurrence of the spread phenomenon:

> One thing that really does perturb me is, uh, a lot of times people will, they act like, you know, something is wrong with your mind because

> you're in a chair. They, you know, they'll come up and they'll ask somebody else what happened to her, like I can't talk for myself, you know, and they'll talk to whoever I'm with instead of talking to me . . . I don't like that, I don't appreciate that at all.

An example of the spread phenomenon was reported in the pamphlet "Beyond the Sound Barrier" published by the Regional Rehabilitation Research Institute on Attitudinal, Legal and Leisure Barriers (RRRI). A woman, Maria, is approached by a person who knows she is deaf. The person hands her a note which says: "Can you read?" Maria writes back: "No!" Maria's sarcastic reply to the note clearly indicates her ability to read. It appears that the person assumed that one sensory impairment affected Maria's other senses. The person may have assumed that because Maria is deaf she also could not read.

In another example, a similar RRRI pamphlet entitled "The Invisible Battle: Attitudes Toward Disability" described a situation where Anthony, who uses a wheelchair, is seated in a restaurant with his wife and a waitress asks his wife if she would like to order for him. The waitress may have assumed that because Anthony was in a wheelchair he was helpless, unable to talk, or order dinner for himself. If the waitress feels uncomfortable with Anthony and his chair, she may limit communication with him by talking with his wife, who does not have an observable disability. In this situation, the waitress's reaction could have created discomfort for Anthony and his wife and reduced their enjoyment of the intended leisure experience.

Overexaggeration Assumption

If people overestimate or "overexaggerate" the extent to which being disabled affects the mental status of people with disabilities, they can experience difficulty developing relationships and providing useful services. Some people assume that people with disabilities think about their disability almost all the time. Therefore, when some people encounter a person with a disability they wrongly assume that "the disability" should be the focus of the discussion rather than other more relevant topics.

Some people may avoid interaction with people with disabilities either to prevent potentially embarrassing social comparison (Brickman & Bulman, 1977) or simply to avoid having to respond to what they expect are extremes of happiness or despair (Brickman, Coates, & Janoff-Bulman, 1978). This tendency for others to reduce interaction can make it more difficult on people with disabilities to develop relationships and necessary supports within their communities. Brickman and colleagues (1978) suggested that if members of society could be made aware that having a disability does not have as great an impact as might be expected, as the results of their study demonstrated, they might find it less threatening to interact with people with disabilities.

Conclusion

The development of attitudes is intertwined with antecedents, beliefs, intentions, and behaviors in a dynamic process. Unfortunately, negative attitudes may arise when people are confronted by people with disabilities. If having a disability results in the person being stigmatized, perceived as deviant, segregated from others, excluded from participation, discriminated against, viewed in a stereotypical way, and the recipient of prejudicial acts, the result can be the devaluation of individuals. Devaluation can result in abuse, neglect, and people receiving far less than their fair share of the things that make life pleasurable (Edgar, 1992). Edgar explained that, unfortunately, some people even consider these individuals to be less human than those with more skills.

Although behaviors that reflect negative attitudes can limit opportunities for people with disabilities, these negative attitudes, and subsequent behaviors, can be changed. Recreation professionals can play an important role in moving people's attitudes about people with disabilities from those that are negative to attitudes that reflect acceptance and understanding of diversity. The next chapter will present various strategies that can be employed to cultivate positive attitudes.

Discussion Questions

1. How do antecedents to beliefs and beliefs influence the development of people's attitudes?

2. What is an attitude?

3. How do cognitive, affective, and behavioral predispositions relate to the expression of attitudes?

4. How do people's intentions relate to their attitudes?

5. How are attitudes manifested in a way that other people are influenced by these attitudes?

6. What is the relationship between stress and the development of negative attitudes toward people with disabilities?

7. What is meant by the words "stigma," "deviancy," "discrimination," "stereotype," and "prejudice?"

8. What is the relationship between segregation and exclusion?

9. How does the self-fulfilling prophecy occur, and what is its impact on people with disabilities?

10. What is meant by the "spread phenomenon" and how does it influence people's feelings about people with disabilities?

Chapter 2

Enhance Your Attitude

"Things do not change, we do."
—Henry David Thoreau

Orientation Activity: Identify Significant Experiences

Directions When Alone. Read each of the following questions. On a blank sheet of paper record a brief answer for each question. Write any questions you might have as you are completing the exercise.

Directions With Others. After dividing into small groups, your group will be assigned specific questions to discuss. After a specified time, discuss your responses with the entire group.

1. What was your first experience with a person with a disability?
2. How do you feel about the experience?
3. How do your parent(s) view people with disabilities?
4. What events do you think had an impact on your parent(s') attitudes?
5. In what ways have your parent(s') attitudes affected yours?
6. How were their attitudes communicated to you?
7. How do you think your peers view people with disabilities?
8. What events do you think had an impact on their attitudes?
9. In what ways have your peers' attitudes affected yours?
10. How were your peers' attitudes communicated to you?
11. What indirect exposure to people with disabilities have you experienced (e.g., books, films, jokes, television)?
12. Has this exposure been generally positive or negative?
13. How would you describe your reactions to the exposure?
14. What direct contact to people with disabilities have you experienced?
15. Has this contact been generally positive or negative?
16. How would you describe your reactions to the direct contact?
17. How would you summarize your current feelings or attitudes toward people with disabilities in general?

Debriefing

Many of the attitudes that we possess today are a result of our earlier experiences related to people with disabilities. These experiences could have occurred directly or indirectly. At times, we may have directly encountered a person or people with disabilities. During these times, the way in which our parents, siblings or friends interacted with the person or people with disabilities may have strongly influenced the way we now think about people with disabilities. In addition, we are exposed to people with disabilities in indirect ways. People with disabilities are presented in books, magazines, movies, television programs, and in many other media forms. Again, the manner in which these individuals are represented often influences our perceptions of people with disabilities. Consider the following questions when reflecting on the orientation activity:

1. What are advantages in improving your attitude toward people with disabilities?
2. What barriers do you see as you consider improving your attitude toward people with disabilities?
3. Do you see your attitude toward people with disabilities improving?

Introduction

In response to the observation that attitudes of recreation professionals significantly impact the leisure opportunities and lifestyles of individuals with disabilities, strategies which would reduce or eliminate prejudice toward individuals with disabilities have been identified. Development of these strategies has been further encouraged by federal legislation mandating the integration of people with disabilities (e.g., The Americans with Disabilities Act, The Individuals with Disabilities Education Acts). The outcome of legislation mandating integration and equal opportunity will, unfortunately, be unpredictable until people develop positive attitudes toward individuals with disabilities (Donaldson, 1980). Therefore, examination of attempts directed toward positively influencing attitudes of professionals toward individuals with disabilities appears warranted.

Cultivate a Sense of Professional Competence

Rizzo and Wright (1987) reported that professionals' perceived ability to work with people with disabilities is related to attitudes. The quality rather than merely the amount of experience is important in fostering favorable attitudes

(Rizzo & Vispoel, 1991). Recreation professionals who perceive themselves as more competent tend to be more positive in their attitudes toward people with disabilities being integrated into their programs. For example, Patrick (1987) and Bedini (1992) demonstrated that attitudes toward people with disabilities could be changed in a positive direction as a result of exposure to a course on recreation for people with disabilities. Both studies indicated that students completing the course expressed more positive attitudes toward people with disabilities. Patrick reported that the results of his investigation have the potential for yielding more positive behaviors based on the development of a learned positive mind-set by the students (Yuker, 1988). Bedini concluded that an introductory course on recreation for people with disabilities utilizing a combination of techniques can become an arena for change and enlightenment.

People responsible for professional preparation can play an important role in enhancing positive attitudes toward and perceived competence in providing recreation services for all people. Rizzo and Vispoel (1991) suggested that attitudes and perceived competence are influenced either directly or indirectly by academic preparation and experience (factors at least partially under the control of those who design the curriculum), and may be important in enhancing attitudes and perceived competence. For example, previous exposure to courses about people with disabilities has been linked to the development of favorable attitudes (Rees, Spreen, & Harnadek, 1991). More favorable attitudes and greater perceived competence in turn are likely to lead to a more beneficial learning experience (Rizzo & Vispoel, 1991).

Attitudes toward people with disabilities can be improved through information, persuasion, vicarious experience, and direct contact (Shaver, Curtis, Jesunathadas, & Strong, 1987). The use of multiple methods such as presentations and discussions, simulations, and direct contact are advocated by Bedini (1992) and have been demonstrated to provide significant positive changes in attitudes toward people with disabilities (e.g., Jones, Sowell, Jones, & Butler, 1981). Rizzo and Vispoel (1992) reported that a planned, systematic intervention using all these procedures had a positive effect of attitudes toward providing services for people with disabilities. In addition, examination of one's own attitudes has also been used as an agent of attitude change.

The remaining portion of this chapter presents information on methods which can influence attitudes and cultivate a sense of professional competence as illustrated in Figure 2.1 (see page 32). The first strategy focuses on indirect exposure through presentation and discussion of information about people with disabilities and methods that help facilitate their participation in programs. This book was developed to help achieve this goal. The second technique described in this chapter is the development of an awareness of what attitudes people possess and possible ways their attitudes were formed. This

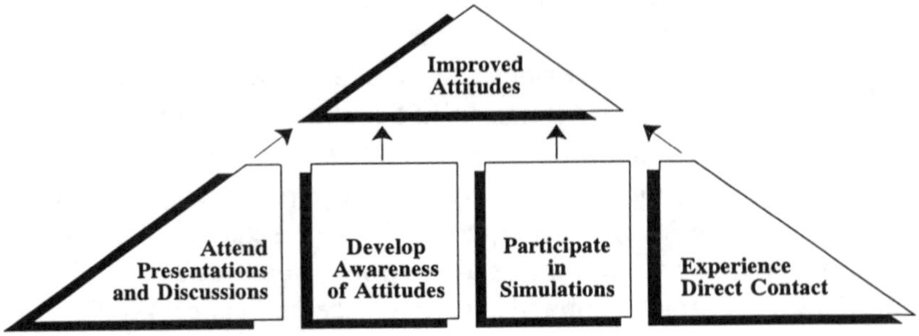

Figure 2.1 Methods influencing attitudes to cultivate a sense of competence.

technique of self-awareness is intended to help people become more responsive to information that may improve their attitudes. The third strategy, simulation of disabilities, can promote a vicarious experience of disabling conditions that may enhance the development of positive attitudes. Finally, the fourth strategy, direct contact with people with disabilities, facilitates the development of an understanding and appreciation of people's lives and, thus, tends to improve attitudes.

Attend Presentations and Discussions

As an extension of their earlier research (i.e., Stainback, Stainback, & Jaben, 1981; Stainback & Stainback, 1983), Stainback, Stainback, Strathe, and Dedrick (1983) conducted a study to determine whether professionals' attitudes or behavioral intentions toward the integration of children with disabilities could be modified by having them read and discuss materials on the integration of students with disabilities. Stainback and colleagues reported that the presentation of reading materials and subsequent small group discussions modified the attitudes and behavioral intentions of professionals toward the integration of children with disabilities. In addition, Austin, Powell, and Martin (1981) examined the use of class presentations to modify recreation and leisure studies students' attitudes. Results indicated that the presentation positively influenced participants' attitudes toward people with disabilities.

The aforementioned findings provide support for presenting information to recreation professionals on methods to facilitate successful integration of people with disabilities into community recreation programs. However, Kennedy, Austin and Smith (1987) warned that results of studies examining the influence of class presentations to modify attitudes are ambiguous; additional techniques are often helpful to influence attitude development. Therefore, Rizzo and Vispoel (1992) advocated the use of several techniques (e.g., information, direct contact, vicarious experience, and persuasive messages) to influence professionals' attitudes toward people with disabilities.

Develop an Awareness of Personal Attitudes

An important aspect of developing positive attitudes toward people with disabilities involves an examination of one's attitudes and values. Once people become aware of their values, they are more prepared to assume responsibility for making their own decisions (Tinsley & Tinsley, 1982).

Examples of Awareness Activities

An example of an awareness activity is included as the orientation activity for this chapter. Additional examples of awareness activities are presented in this section of the chapter.

ATTITUDE SURVEY ABOUT PEOPLE WITH DISABILITIES

Directions: Please respond with only one answer per statement that best describes *your* reaction to the statement. On a separate sheet of paper write the numbers 1-14 and record the response in the space to the right of the number. The possible answers are:

SA = Strongly Agree	A = Agree	MA = Mildly Agree
MD = Mildly Disagree	D = Disagree	SD = Strongly Disagree

1. People with disabilities have similar needs and desires as other people.
2. People with disabilities are entitled to the same rights as other people.
3. People with disabilities can experience pleasure as often as other people.
4. It is unlikely that a person with disabilities will lead a productive life.
5. People with disabilities do not possess the potential to acquire the skills needed to participate in meaningful leisure experiences.
6. Most people with disabilities should be admitted to a large residential institution.

7. You should not expect as much from a person with a disability as you do a person without a disability.
8. All people with disabilities require assistance to complete their daily activities.
9. Most people with disabilities prefer associating predominately with other people with disabilities.
10. People with disabilities are more aggressive than other people.
11. A person can be disabled physically, mentally, emotionally, and/or socially.
12. People with disabilities are entitled to experience meaningful leisure.
13. People with disabilities are more similar to other people than they are dissimilar from other people.
14. It is difficult to make generalizations about people with disabilities because every person is unique.

Debriefing

Statements that reaffirm similarities between people with and without disabilities (statements 1-3, and 13) are often identified as representative of a more positive attitude than those that emphasize differences (statement 7). In addition, statements that avoid making overgeneralizations about any group of individuals and recognize differences within a group (such as statements 11 and 14) often reflect more positive attitudes than statements that tend to miss individual differences (statements 4, 5, and 8-10). Finally, statements that reflect support for the inclusion of people with disabilities into the mainstream of community life (statement 12) are often more positive than those focusing on segregation (statement 6).

1. How did you feel about responding to these questions?
2. How did you differ with the responses indicated in the debriefing?
3. What are some actions you could take to improve your attitudes toward people with disabilities?

ATTITUDE SURVEY ABOUT RECREATION FOR PEOPLE WITH DISABILITIES

Directions: Please respond with only one answer per statement that best describes *your* reaction to the statement. On a separate sheet of paper write the numbers 1-37 and record the response in the space to the right of the number. The possible answers are:

SA = Strongly Agree	A = Agree	MA = Mildly Agree
MD = Mildly Disagree	D = Disagree	SD = Strongly Disagree

1. People with disabilities should be prevented from attending an activity if you feel the disability will hinder the person's performance in the activity.
2. You should change the location of a recreation activity to accommodate people with disabilities, even if the new location is inferior to the original one.
3. You should promote interaction between people with and without disabilities during recreation participation.
4. Adaptation of activities should occur if the changes will make participation opportunities more equal.
5. Someone should be available to assist you in maximizing learning opportunities for people with disabilities.
6. You should be willing to spend extra time assisting a participant with a disability in a recreation program.
7. Providing aids and services is likely to impinge on your leadership freedom.
8. You should alter your leadership style to enhance communications with participants with disabilities.
9. You should integrate people with disabilities into the recreation programs you offer.
10. Each recreation agency should conduct meetings to increase service delivery to people with disabilities.
11. An interpreter for a person with a hearing impairment is a distraction in a recreation program.
12. You should design group activities in which people with disabilities can participate with other people.
13. People with disabilities can participate in team and individual sports with people without disabilities.
14. People with disabilities are able to make decisions about their leisure participation.
15. People with disabilities have more free time than people without disabilities.
16. The main purpose of recreation programs for people with disabilities is therapy.
17. Most people with disabilities prefer individual activities to group activities.
18. You should provide similar activity opportunities to people with and without disabilities.

19. Making arrangements for people with disabilities is likely to lower program objectives.
20. Background information concerning participants' disabilities would be useful.
21. You should help people with disabilities receive assistance for maximum recreation participation.
22. It may be better to exclude people with disabilities from participation if it is difficult to evaluate them.
23. You should consult with the person with disabilities concerning conditions for optimal participation.
24. People with disabilities are more likely to be injured in activities than people without disabilities.
25. Therapeutic recreation specialists are the only personnel who should provide recreation activities for people with disabilities.
26. Most people with disabilities would rather participate with other people with disabilities.
27. People with disabilities are unable to participate with other people in competitive recreation activities.
28. Segregated recreation programs should be provided for people with disabilities.
29. People with disabilities are more easily frustrated than other people.
30. People with disabilities should be allowed to participate in all public recreation programs.
31. All recreational facilities should be made accessible to people with disabilities.
32. People with disabilities need more supervision in activities than other people.
33. People with disabilities should not become highly excited in recreation activities.
34. Attendance in recreation programs will decline if people with disabilities attend the programs.
35. It is harmful to expose people with disabilities to ridicule by encouraging them to participate in community recreation programs.
36. Parents do not want their children without disabilities playing with children with disabilities.
37. People with disabilities are able to participate in selected high risk activities.

Debriefing

Many people agree that treating people with disabilities in the same way you treat all participants is the best practice. Making accommodations without undue burden is stipulated in the Americans with Disabilities Act. Remember to think of each participant as an individual and take actions to include people in community recreation activities. Consider the following questions:

1. How did you feel about responding to these questions?
2. How did your responses differ from other people's responses?
3. What are some actions you could take to improve your attitudes toward people with disabilities participating in recreation programs?

Include Debriefings

Professionals attempting to enhance people's attitudes toward individuals with disabilities are encouraged to use awareness activities such as the two surveys presented above; however, these awareness activities should be immediately followed by debriefings.

Debriefings can consist of a series of questions that require participants to reflect on the learning activity (Dattilo & Murphy, 1991). In addition, debriefings can provide a forum for participants to report on their responses and allow them to ask questions that arose during the completion of the activity. Dattilo and Murphy (1991) stated that debriefings encourage participants to consider the relevance of the learning activity and identify accomplishments and barriers experienced in the learning activity.

McDonald and Howe (1989) reported that debriefings enabled participants to experience self-expression, enlightenment, and empathy. The debriefings described by McDonald and Howe (1989) were led by a facilitator who possessed a thorough understanding of the content. Professionals intending to use awareness activities should consider having a person who is sensitive to the issues surrounding the lives of people with disabilities conduct debriefings after the activities.

Participate in Simulations

To alter attitudes toward people with disabilities, distorted ideas that are supported by deeply felt emotions must be confronted (Tripp & Sherrill, 1991). According to Tripp and Sherrill, the first step in the reeducation process must focus on the individual at an emotional level. One strategy that affects people at an emotional level is participation in a simulation of disabling conditions, called "vicarious simulation" by Curtis and Shaver (1987). For example, after a five-hour program that included a disability simulation, children's attitudes toward other children with disabilities were more positive than their attitudes prior to the educational program (Jones et al., 1981). Both role-playing and vicarious experience of observing role plays can be effective methods of modifying at least some dimensions of attitudes toward disability. Through disability simulations, participants can develop some sensitivity to the experiences that people with disabilities encounter on a regular basis.

Simulation of disabilities can be effective in the modification of attitudes; however, the simulation should require participants to observe reactions of other people. Movement through a largely unfamiliar group of people as a single role player may further enhance realism, allowing the person to experience the possible frustrations of the condition but, perhaps more importantly, to experience other people's reactions.

Perlman (1987) suggested that if people would like to become sensitive to the indignities and frustrations experienced by people with disabilities, they should spend a day or two in a wheelchair. Perlman provided the following guidelines for people engaging in a wheelchair simulation:

> Tell yourself that you cannot get up—then try to get into a car. Try to go shopping or use the toilet in a restaurant. See what it feels like to be all dressed up and have to ride to your appointment in a freight elevator with the garbage. I can tell you how that makes me feel—furious . . . What we need is an attitude that we're all human beings, and as such, we all care about each other (p. 64).

Many individuals have participated in simulations of a disability while enrolled in introductory courses related to disability. The rationale for the assignments is often to encourage participants to become more sensitive to the requirements placed on an individual with a disability and to develop an awareness of the barriers, both physical and attitudinal, that confront a person who happens to have a disability. Simulations are learning experiences as opposed to recreation activities. The primary intent of a simulation is to develop sensitivity rather than simply provide participants with a "fun" experience. However, it is hoped that participants experience enjoyable and amusing moments during the simulation.

Conduct a Simulation with a Wheelchair

One specific example of a simulation requires participants to pretend they have paralysis of the legs and use a wheelchair to move. The duration of the simulation can vary according to the learning situation, but a simulation that is brief in duration may not have the desired effect. When providing such a simulation, extensive information and guidelines should be presented to prevent problems and increase the chance that participants will approach the task in a mature, understanding fashion (McGill, 1984). The following are some possible suggestions that can be made when involving people with a simulation requiring the use of a wheelchair.

When encountering friends and family members, participants are encouraged to explain to them that the experience is an assignment and provide them with the rationale for the simulation. In some cases, it may be advisable for participants to describe the assignment in advance to people with whom they have close relationships. The most appropriate responses to questions about participants' condition while they are conducting the simulation are those that are direct and honest.

Participants are encouraged to place themselves in challenging situations but to use sound judgment. It is recommended that participants carefully preplan all experiences before charging ahead. Providing sufficient time to arrive at planned destinations on time is a necessity. Often, participants will experience that even the "best laid plans" will lead them into the unexpected. Therefore, when possible, participants are encouraged to have a friend accompany them. The participant's friend should assist only when absolutely necessary. Typically, it is suggested that if a transportation system is in place specifically for people with disabilities, participants in the simulation should not use this transportation service because it may be reserved only for persons with disabilities. Participants are also discouraged from conducting their simulation with another person using a wheelchair.

Throughout the experience, participants should attempt to remain in the wheelchair as much as possible. If, for any reason, participants must get out of the wheelchair (e.g., the person is alone and they are stuck in the mud) they should attempt to do this discreetly while others are not watching. This may mean that participants might need to wait a few moments before breaking character. If it is unavoidable to break character in front of other people (e.g., the participant is in danger), participants should attempt to briefly explain the situation truthfully to those present. It is hoped that participants do not break character at all during the time they are using the wheelchair.

After completing the simulation experience, participants will not know what it is like to actually have the particular disability, due to many physical and psychological factors which exist in actual disabling conditions. In certain situations, participants may experience more problems than an individual who regularly uses a wheelchair due to lack of skill and problems with the wheelchair. In other situations, participants may experience less difficulty as they realize that they can literally walk away from the experience. However, their awareness of disability and attitudinal and physical barriers will be enhanced.

In any simulation, participants should be notified that if they have personal concerns, fears, or reservations about the experience, they should be discussed immediately with the person supervising the simulation. Figure 2.2 summarizes the suggestions for simulation participation.

In response to employees of a hospital in his hometown participating in a simulation requiring the use of a wheelchair, Scott Balko had a few of his own suggestions for the participants that illustrate the limitations of such an educational experience. He recommended that people conduct their simulation for one year, and, during this year, participants should get a skin ulcer that does not heal so that plastic surgery is required, experience some urinary tract

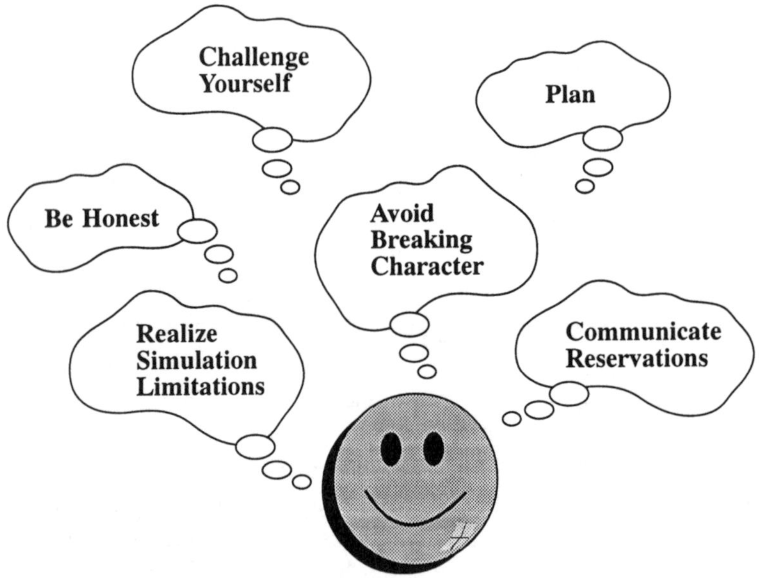

Figure 2.2 Considerations for simulations.

problems, encounter calcium deposits, have some muscle atrophy, experience respiratory problems such as pneumonia, and encounter cardiovascular problems. In conclusion, Balko warned people participating in an educational simulation that it is no game. Balko's sentiments are a reminder that although participation in educational simulations of disabling conditions can heighten awareness, once participants have completed the simulation, they will not know what it is like to be disabled for a considerable length of time.

Encourage Participants to Learn from the Simulation

To enhance the effectiveness of the simulation, participants are often encouraged to record their impressions of the experience. The topical areas presented in this section are provided to help guide participants in their organization of such a report (see Figure 2.3).

Frequently with any professional paper, it is useful to write an introduction that presents an overview of the paper and introduces the sections contained within the paper. Participants are encouraged to briefly describe the sequence of their experience during the simulation.

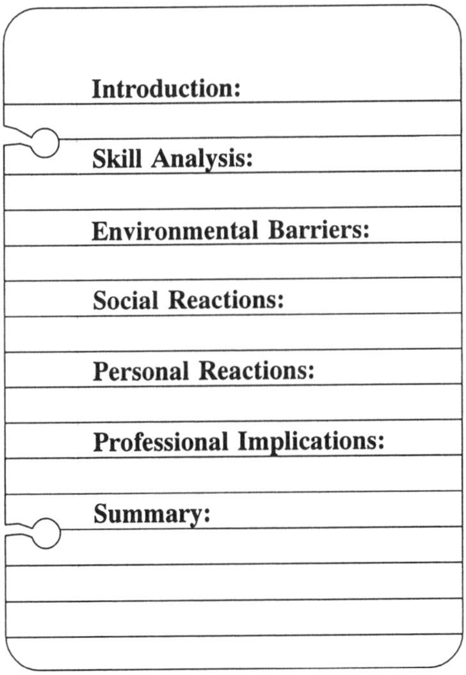

Figure 2.3 Possible components of a simulation report.

An analysis of the skills participants needed while completing the simulation can be enlightening. It is often helpful to provide specific examples of skills demonstrated while participating in the simulation and of some tasks which were no longer able to be completed independently (e.g., cooking, eating, personal hygiene, leisure skills).

Another area for consideration is the environmental barriers that participants experienced. A description of the various architectural barriers (constructed by people, such as steps), ecological barriers (found in the natural environment, such as steep hills), and transportation barriers encountered throughout the experience and participants' responses to these barriers can be informative.

The section of the report which appears to be critical in influencing the development of positive attitudes toward people with disabilities is one that describes the social reactions that participants experienced. Identification of the verbal and nonverbal responses of people who were encountered can be very revealing. Participants are encouraged to describe specific communication behaviors and avoid making assumptions about people's intentions. The identification of specific examples of different people's reactions can help participants become aware of how they would now treat people with disabilities.

When attempting to process the simulation that has influenced participants' emotions, a section of the report devoted to personal reactions can be helpful. Participants may attempt to explain their feelings before, during, and after the simulation. This comparison can develop insights that were not initially apparent to the participants. Trying to find the answers to such questions as: "What was your response to your abilities and disabilities?" and "How did you feel about other's reactions?" can help participants develop insights into the lives of people with disabilities.

Since the intent of many simulations is to enhance attitudes toward people with disabilities by professionals working with human services, a section of the report focusing participants' attention on professional implications may be valuable. Participants are encouraged to provide specific examples of how this experience will improve their ability to successfully meet the demands of their intended career responsibilities (e.g., municipal recreation professional, environmental interpreter at a state park, coordinator of recreation for a resort, a therapeutic recreation specialist at a community recreation center). The identification of specific actions that could be taken as a professional to provide accessible programs helps individuals develop action plans for inclusion of people with disabilities into leisure services.

As with other professional papers, the inclusion of a summary that reviews the highlights of the report can bring the experience into clearer focus. Participants are encouraged to draw conclusions based on their experiences and consider how participation in the simulation influenced their attitudes.

Responses to a Simulation with a Wheelchair

Yaccino, a former student in recreation and leisure studies, reported on her experience of participating in a simulation that required her to use a wheelchair for half a day. Yaccino reported that she always felt slightly uneasy when she was around people with disabilities. And she stated that:

> It was always very scary to me. I was always very intimidated. It's made me much more comfortable being around people with disabilities. It's opened my eyes to how people with disabilities are treated in our society. And how to treat people with disabilities in a way that is appropriate.

Yaccino said using the wheelchair showed her just how many barriers exist for people using wheelchairs. She explained that she still does not know what it is like to have a disability because she was able to stand up and put the chair away.

Eichmiller (1990) interviewed several college students who were using an earlier draft of this text for a course in which they participated in a simulation. The simulation required them to use a wheelchair for half a day. One student, Chrissy, said she had not thought about it before, but in the future her attitude would not be patronizing. "People think they (people with disabilities) are in need of constant assistance. Now I realize that they're not. To have people constantly offering help makes you feel childlike," she said. The class prepared students for what they might encounter, including people staring. "Definitely, yes," people stared, Chrissy said. "People were more friendly than usual, then they would stare at my legs," she added. Although she does not think that anyone without a disability could fully understand, Deborah reported that after the simulation, she could relate much more to those with disabilities.

The course syllabus stresses, "After completing your experience you will *not* 'know what it is like' to actually have the particular disability." Linda reported that "You can only understand to a point. I could build my upper body strength, but I couldn't get used to the staring." Nancy explained that "I sat in with a student who uses a motorized wheelchair. He thinks everybody should spend time in a wheelchair. He told me, 'You'll definitely learn from this.'" Dave admitted that "Normally girls will look at me, but when you're in the chair, it's like you're being looked right over. They don't see you, they see the chair." Bob reported that "I think I will, in the future, approach a person with a disability differently. I won't just look at their disabilities, but at their abilities." Nancy exclaimed that "It was definitely an eye-opening experience, definitely!" Dave added, "You don't forget an experience like that." "Even now (two weeks after the simulation), I'll go somewhere and take note if places are accessible," Deborah said. "Will this stick with me? . . . Definitely, yeah."

Lawrence Young (1990), a columnist for the Pennsylvania *Centre Daily Times,* reported in an editorial that being temporarily disabled was an "eye-opening experience" for him. His strongest realization was how inaccessible the world is for people with disabilities. He observed that although many buildings have access ramps, some were angled too steeply or were in such a state of disrepair that efforts at access were hazardous. What was most surprising and disconcerting to him was the number of public facilities that had no access ramps. At times, he felt a sense of outrage at his helplessness and dependency upon the graciousness of others that he withdrew from the public. Young expressed the feeling that seeing himself as a burden to others was quite sobering. Throughout his experience, he reported that many of his friends were generous with their time and energy. Yet, Young reflected that the many years most people spend learning to be self-sufficient are difficult to ignore, and the desire for self-sufficiency can lead one to eliminate events and activities where self-sufficiency is not possible. Young's comments teach us that although it is helpful to provide assistance when individuals require help, an even more effective action to help people with disabilities access community recreation programs is to create a supportive and accessible environment that allows people to participate as actively as possible without the need for assistance.

After reading Young's editorial, a person responded that he had a friend, Brian, who will use a wheelchair for the remaining portion of his life. The anonymous writer reported that, fortunately for those people who know Brian, he has refused to give up life in the mainstream to just stay at home where life, while perhaps easier and safer, would deprive him of leading as normal a life as possible, and from being the exceptional role model he is. The writer stated that if people would increase their awareness of people with disabilities, all would benefit. Although awareness has improved in the last few years, communities have a long way to go to provide a workable public transportation system, rest rooms that have doors that open easily for both entry and exit, properly constructed curb cuts on both ends of sidewalks, seating that does not relegate wheelchair users to out-of-the-way areas of theaters and usable ramps which do not become barriers because they have a locked door at the end of them. Finally, the writer suggested that it is not an issue of "them and us;" rather, we are all in this together. At any time, those people who today consider themselves not to be disabled may acquire a disability tomorrow.

Thompson and Vierno (1991) reported that Don Smitley likes to refer to people who do not use wheelchairs as people who are "shoe-bound." He relates using his wheelchair to other people using their shoes. "You would only think about shoes if they are uncomfortable, and I view the wheelchair the same way," Smitley said.

Become Familiar Through Direct Contact

Evans (1976) observed that a strain in social interactions representing uneasiness, inhibition, and uncertainty experienced by persons without disabilities in their interactions with people with disabilities, appeared to be a strong factor in the development and maintenance of negative attitudes. Therefore, the use of structured experiences, such as guest speakers, with people who represent nonstereotypic images of disabilities and are of equally valued status in relation to participants, appears to be effective in attitude modification.

The lack of long-term behavioral effects of in-services devoted to attitude change (e.g., Stainback & Stainback, 1983) suggests that only providing written information and discussions about individuals with disabilities may not be sufficient to change the attitudes of some people. To increase the likelihood of long-term behavioral change by recreation professionals, educational experiences that include opportunities for direct exposure to persons who present nonstereotypic images of people with disabilities are suggested (Dattilo, 1985). The direct exposure could involve the use of people with disabilities as guest lecturers, viewing people on videotapes, the pairing of a recreation professional and a person with a disability to work on a specified task, or the involvement of recreation professionals in integrated programs (Anthony, 1969). For example, Rowe and Stutts (1987) observed improved attitudes toward people with disabilities when college students participated in a practicum experience requiring them to interact with people with disabilities. Using a different approach to direct contact, Lazar, Gensley, and Orpet (1971) reported on the effectiveness of providing guest speakers with disabilities in enhancing the attitudes of those in attendance.

Conclusion

Education of recreation professionals about the capabilities of individuals with disabilities may improve their attitudes. To maximize the usefulness of such educational attempts, the following strategies can be employed:

(a) positive indirect exposure through readings, discussions, and videos;
(b) completion of self-awareness exercises and associated briefings;
(c) involvement in simulations; and
(d) positive direct contact with individuals with disabilities in a variety of contexts.

The strategies presented in this chapter are intended to help people without disabilities reduce their discomfort around people with disabilities. A reduction in discomfort around people with disabilities will increase the likelihood of positive attitudes being developed. As recreation professionals develop more positive attitudes toward people with disabilities, leisure opportunities for individuals with disabilities will increase. When opportunities to experience leisure increase, the quality of the life for individuals with disabilities often is enhanced.

Discussion Questions

1. How can you cultivate a sense of professional competence?
2. What is the value of attending presentations and engaging in discussions about people with disabilities?
3. How can you become aware of your attitudes toward people with disabilities?
4. What is the value of participating in simulations of disabling conditions?
5. What are some guidelines to follow when conducting or participating in a simulation requiring the use of a wheelchair for an extended period of time?
6. How can you encourage people to learn from a simulation?
7. What have been some responses of people who have participated in a simulation of a disabling condition?
8. What is the value of participating in situations that provide you with an opportunity to become familiar with a person with a disability?
9. What are some techniques you could use to improve other people's attitudes about people with disabilities?
10. What is the value of reducing some people's discomfort around other people who happen to have disabilities?

Chapter 3

Improve Others' Attitude

"There is something that is much more scarce,
something finer far, something rarer than ability.
It is the ability to recognize ability."
—Elbert Hubbard

Orientation Activity: Examine Societal Attitudes

Directions When Alone: Read each statement. On a separate sheet of paper, record your feelings about the person making the statement. Describe what you might say if the person directed the statement to you.

Directions With Others: Find a person, introduce yourself and find out that person's name. Discuss the implications of one statement on recreation participation. Make notes as you talk for later discussion. Once you finish discussing your responses, find another person and discuss another statement. Try to discuss all of the following statements.

1. "No, we cannot handle any cripples at this bowling lane. We had retarded kids here last year and it was a big pain."
2. "She could not belong to the ceramics class—she's got the mind of a 6-year-old, even if she is 48 years old."
3. "We're going camping this summer, and it is the first time we have had this many blind adults together in a camping trip."
4. "We want the handicapped at the recreation center, that's why we have special-needs classes."
5. "It is nice to have the youth group be so active in offering daytime dances for the elderly from the nursing home."
6. "He can play in the volleyball league; however, if his cerebral palsy becomes a problem then he must leave.
7. "Our movie theater offers discounts to handicapped persons with proper identification."
8. "I saw that a girl who attends the Thursday evening social group is missing a leg—I could not look at her all night."

9. "It is expensive to make our resource room accessible to the disabled—it is better if they order resources from home."
10. "Sure she wants to learn sports, but our clinics are not set up for retarded people."
11. "Make sure your older brother does not get wet on the bird-watching trip—you know he will not take care of himself."
12. "We like to keep people busy because the idleness is hard on them —that's why we developed our diversional program."

Debriefing

According to Patrick (1987), people often fear what they do not know, what is different, and what makes them feel vulnerable. Negative attitudes based on fears create barriers to full participation in society by individuals with disabilities. Conversely, positive attitudes create opportunities for people that enable them to pursue active participation in their communities. The development of positive attitudes can begin with exposure to individuals to allow people to develop an understanding and an appreciation for those that may differ from them in some way. Consider the following questions when reflecting on the activity you have recently completed:

1. What are the problems associated with the aforementioned statements?
2. What attitudes do you feel are being represented by these statements?
3. How would you change these statements to turn them into statements reflecting positive attitudes?

Introduction

Frequently, ignorance resulting from a lack of exposure can facilitate the development of negative attitudes. A direct result of ignorance is fear, as illustrated in the following quotation by Bart, who happens to have an observable physical disability.

> People do not know how to act towards you. They're afraid they'll say something wrong, they're afraid that they'll do something different that will make you upset, they don't know how to act with you.

Fear is the strongest feeling people with disabilities elicit from people without disabilities, and it is fear that underlies compassion for the poster child and celebration of the "supercrip" (Shapiro, 1993). According to Murphy (1990), a researcher with paraplegia, people with disabilities "serve as constant, visible reminders to the able-bodied that the society they live in is a counterfeit paradise, that they too are vulnerable. We represent a fearsome possibility."

Guskin (1981) reported that while there is a widely-held belief that many people hold negative views about individuals with disabilities, there is also the assumption that public attitudes and perceptions become increasingly positive as people become more knowledgeable about and familiar with people with disabilities. Allport (1954) observed that interaction between people with differences produces changes in attitudes.

Previous exposure to people with disabilities can result in the development of positive attitudes toward these individuals (Jansma & Shultz, 1982). For example, Stewart (1988) reported that students who participated in an integrated university weight-training course involving contact with two students with disabilities improved their attitude toward people with disabilities significantly more than participants in a university weight-training course that was not integrated. As another example, Kisabeth and Richardson (1985) documented significant positive changes in the attitudes of students toward people with disabilities as a result of a person with a disability being integrated into a university racquetball class.

Although exposure to people with disabilities is an important first step in enhancing people's attitudes, it is only a first step. Tripp and Sherrill (1991) reported that the direction of attitude change—that is, whether the change is positive or negative—depends largely on the conditions under which contact has taken place. Favorable conditions tend to produce positive attitude shifts, whereas unfavorable conditions tend to produce negative attitude shifts.

The increase in acceptance of people through previous positive exposure has been demonstrated for people who are aging. For example, Barber and Magafas (1992) reported that college students with previous positive experiences with people who are aging had a more positive attitude toward associating personally and professionally with these individuals. According to Knox, Gekoski, and Johnson (1986), quality was considered to be the more reliable indicator of preference compared to the quantity of contacts; that is, the more positive attitudes toward people who are aging were a direct result of quality contact. The challenge to recreation professionals is to determine ways to provide exposure that results in the development of positive attitudes toward all of their participants.

Adopt Inclusive Beliefs that Help Improve Attitudes

The next portion of the chapter will provide some ways to think about and treat people with disabilities. The ways of thinking presented in Figure 3.1 are intended to set the stage for beneficial contact and the development of positive attitudes.

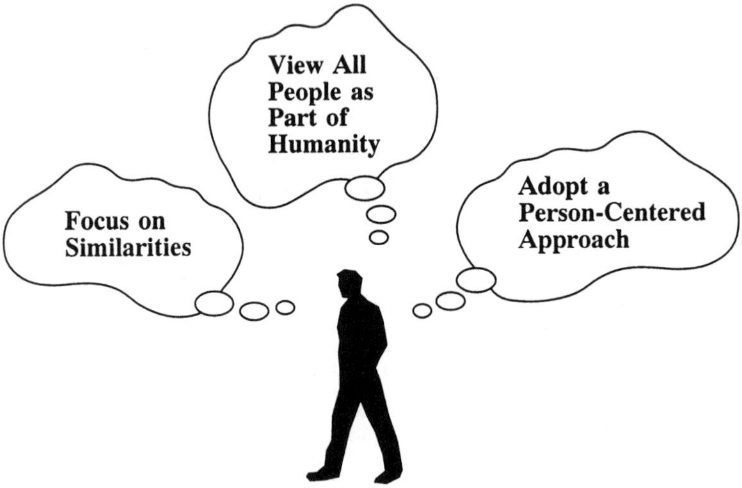

Figure 3.1 Some inclusive beliefs that help improve attitudes.

Focus on Similarities

Yuker (1988) reported that in the case of groups that are already disadvantaged, such as people with disabilities, ignoring similarities adds to their disadvantagement. If people focus only on other peoples' differences from them, they will develop a different impression of those differences than if they perceived them within a system that includes similarities as well (Yuker, 1988). Therefore, recreation professionals can encourage participants to discover leisure interests and abilities they share with other participants. Friendships help people focus on positive qualities and commonalities, rather than on differences (Hutchison & McGill, 1992).

Positive relationships are often established between people who believe they share common characteristics with other people. According to Yuker (1988), there are many factors that encourage the feeling that two people belong together in some way. Among the strongest is the factor of **similarity.** When a person identifies with someone because of similarity, there will be a tendency to like the other person.

With the development of a common bond between individuals resulting from focusing on similarities, people's ability to accept differences of others is enhanced. Differences between people can be viewed negatively by requiring conformity, or differences can be seen as exciting ways to learn new ways of looking at the world. Diversity is what allows people to grow and learn. Shapiro (1993, p. 4) emphasized this point when he stated that people with disabilities:

> . . . no longer see their physical or mental limitations as a source of shame or as something to overcome in order to inspire others. Today they proclaim that it is okay, even good, to be disabled. Cook's childhood polio forced him to wear heavy corrective shoes, and he walked with difficulty. But taking pride in his disability was for Cook a celebration of the differences among people and gave him a respectful understanding that all share the same basic desires to be full participants in society.

The orientation activity presented at the beginning of this chapter was provided to encourage readers to begin considering the implications of focusing on similarities with people and identifying differences between people. Statements by two people following their rehabilitation from spinal cord injuries emphasize this point:

> "I forget that I'm in a wheelchair sometimes, I totally forget that I'm any different than anybody else and it just doesn't bother me."

> "I'm still the same person that I used to be, just look, you know I just sit down instead of stand up all the time, um, that I can still have as much fun as I ever wanted to and ever did, that I'm still able to do things that I used to do and want to do . . ."

View All People as Part of Humanity

Bogdan and Taylor (1992) reported that when people are accepting of individuals with disabilities, they often describe their friends and family members as possessing characteristics of "humanness." Consequently, the disability is viewed as secondary to the person's humanness. The authors offer four primary dimensions of humanness illustrated in Figure 3.2:

(a) attributing thinking to the other;
(b) seeing individuality in the other;
(c) viewing the other as reciprocating; and
(d) defining social place for the other.

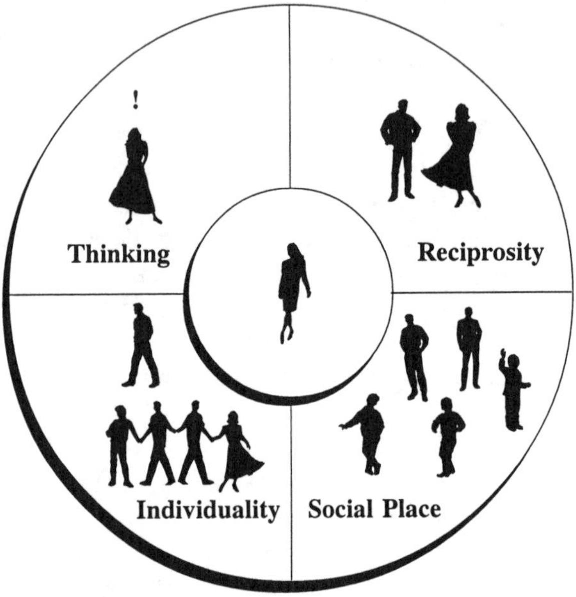

Figure 3.2 Bogdon and Taylor's (1992) four dimensions of humanness.

Belief in these dimensions enables people without disabilities to define people with disabilities as people "like us" despite their significant behavioral and/or physical differences (Bogdan & Taylor, 1992). The dimensions of assuming that a person can think, observing that each person is an individual, and believing that each person has something to contribute are fairly straight forward. However, the final dimension of defining a social place is a bit more complicated. According to Bogdan and Taylor (1992), since people are social beings they belong to groups and are part of social networks, organizations, and institutions. The authors stated that:

> Within these social groups, individuals are given a particular social place. The concept of role is often used to describe a person's social place, but social place is not merely a matter of playing a social role. It is also a matter of being defined as being an integral part of the group

> or social unit. There is a personal dimension to roles. Roles are particularized for each social unit and personalized by each occupant. Through fulfilling particular social roles, social actors are defined as being part of humanity (p. 289).

Adopt a Person-Centered Approach

Similar to Bogdan and Taylor (1992), Hutchison and McGill (1992) described what they termed as a "person-centered" approach that is based on the assumption that in an ever-changing world, one constant factor is our shared humanity. The authors described this approach by stating that:

> Our shared humanity should be what compels us to treat each other as unique human beings with unknown potential for growth and learning. A strong person-centered philosophy helps us respond to each other, first in terms of our human needs, and second in terms of our more individual requirements (p. 75).

When people adopt a person-centered approach, all people feel important, are given hope, and can begin to dream about a future of relationships and community (Hutchison & McGill, 1992). According to the authors, the cornerstone of a person-centered approach involves the belief that every person:

(a) is unique and different from all other people;
(b) is an entire person with many different qualities; and
(c) has unknown potential for growth and development.

Take Actions to Change Perceptions

In the next section of the chapter some specific strategies to help people without disabilities develop more positive attitudes about people with disabilities will be described. The strategies presented in Figure 3.3 (page 54) are intended to promote beneficial contact and the development of positive attitudes. Leisure services professionals can become actively involved in facilitating the acceptance of people with disabilities by all members of their community.

Structure Interactions

Programs that are structured to promote positive interactions among participants tend to promote the development of more positive attitudes. Following a review of the literature, Donaldson (1980) reported that structured experiences consistently resulted in positive attitude changes, but unstructured contact did not consistently demonstrate improvement in attitudes. One way to encourage the presentation of structured interactions is for recreation professionals to include the promotion of positive interactions among participants with and without disabilities as one of the goals of each program. Plans could be developed to stimulate positive interactions and methods for responding to negative interactions.

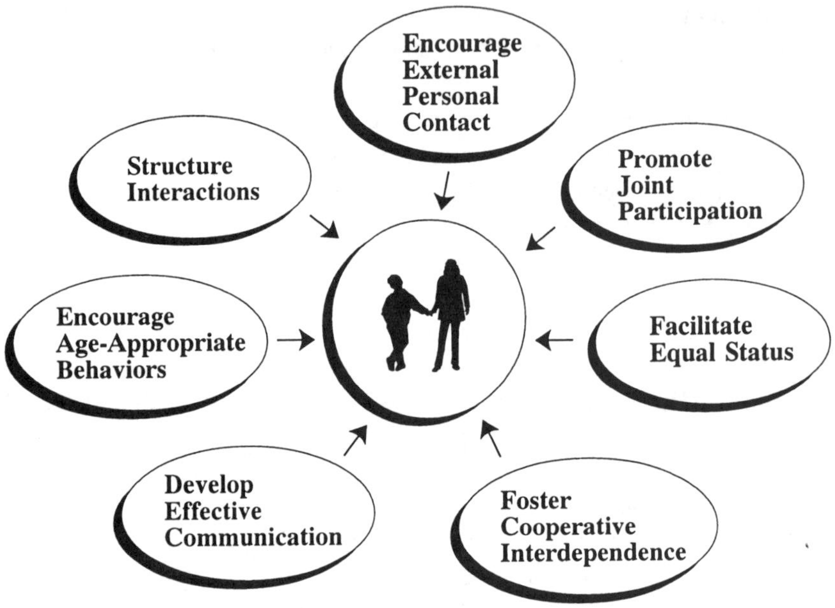

Figure 3.3 Actions promoting beneficial contact and development of positive attitudes.

Because peer tutoring is generally structured and long-term, interpersonal relationships are created that promote a balance between the experience and their sentiment (Tripp & Sherrill, 1991). **Peer tutoring** programs have been effective in improving the attitudes of children. For example, after a seven-week peer tutoring program that linked sixth graders without disabilities with children of a similar age that had disabilities, the peer tutors reported that the youths with disabilities were more capable than originally thought (Fenrick & Petersen, 1984).

Encourage Extensive Personal Contact

The extent of contact with persons with a disability is a critical factor associated with the development of favorable attitudes (Strohmer, Grand, & Purcell, 1984). This finding is consistent with previous research (e.g., Donaldson, 1980; Weinberg, 1978) that suggests a positive relationship between attitudes and contact.

The goal of providing extensive contact between people with and without disabilities is intended to increase communication and understanding (Dattilo & Weltner, 1991). For example, Hoenk and Mobily (1987) reported that children who had extensive contact with other children with disabilities in an integrated play environment demonstrated more positive attitudes toward interacting with peers with a disability than those with little contact. In addition, Rowe and Stutts (1987) demonstrated that a one-semester practicum experience which provided contact with persons with disabilities improved the attitudes of the undergraduates.

Personal contact with people with disabilities in informal settings results in the development of more accepting attitudes (Hamilton & Anderson, 1991; Patrick, 1987). Mace (1977) observed that once negative attitudes about people with disabilities have been dispelled by close personal exposure to their aspirations and abilities, cooperation seems to begin.

When practitioners employ the use of volunteers to assist people with disabilities in an integrated recreation program, they may wish to consider the implications of the volunteers' role. If volunteers are placed in situations where they have ample opportunities to interact with individuals with disabilities, it appears they may be in a better position to develop positive attitudes toward these individuals than if they were placed in situations where they encountered difficulty interacting with the participants. One-time interactions with people with disabilities that are brief in duration, such as special events, may not create an environment that fosters positive attitudes by volunteers toward participants with disabilities.

Promote Joint Participation

Recreation departments that offer inclusive recreation services will have more of an opportunity to achieve the goal of frequent contact between people with and without disabilities, as suggested by Roper (1990) and others, than those departments that do not actively promote inclusive participation. Recreation professionals should provide opportunities for people residing in the community to experience positive interaction that dispell existing stereotypes through participation in inclusive recreation activities.

People who are not disabled often positively alter their attitudes about people with disabilities as a result of joint participation in recreation activities (Evans, 1976). According to Hamilton and Anderson (1991), since recreation activity often offers a greater opportunity for close personal contact than either education or employment, participation in inclusive recreation activities can provide an effective channel for changing the attitudes of the general public toward people with disabilities. By facilitating inclusive leisure opportunities for all community members, professionals can contribute to the acceptance of people with disabilities.

Recreation programs in which people with and without disabilities jointly participate can be an effective means of changing attitudes toward people with disabilities. By encouraging joint participation of persons with and without disabilities in leisure programs, leisure services professionals can and are making a significant contribution in the acceptance of people with disabilities (Hamilton & Anderson, 1991). According to Hamilton and Anderson, if a goal of the recreation profession is to improve attitudes toward people with disabilities, the key to success is to have the public, family members, and students jointly participate in recreation activities with individuals with disabilities. Through the provision of opportunities for joint participation, recreation professionals can encourage societal acceptance of people with disabilities.

Facilitate Equal Status

The most positive attitudes result from contact between individuals with and without disabilities that are on an equal status basis (Levy, Jessop, Rimmerman, & Levy, 1992). For people to achieve the goal of equal status, members from each group must be treated as equal, and no particular group should assume superiority (Roper, 1990). Inclusive recreation activities that bring people together on an equal basis have the potential for positively influencing the public's perceptions of people with disabilities (Dattilo & Weltner, 1991).

To promote equal status of participants, recreation practitioners must clearly communicate the unique contributions that each individual makes to a given activity. Attention should be directed to the insights people gain by being exposed to diversity among participants. All participants should be encouraged to view their involvement with others as a means to facilitate leisure participation for the entire group, rather than simply helping those "less fortunate" people.

Foster Cooperative Interdependence

Johnson and Johnson (1984) reported that cooperative activities, rather than competitive ones, were effective in promoting positive interactions and good attitudes. These findings supported previous observations by Amir (1969) who reported that when the contact situation between individuals involves common goals that are higher ranking than individual goals, improved relationships and fostering of positive attitudes occur. In addition, Yuker (1988) concluded that positive attitudes result from contact between individuals with and without disabilities that are friendly, cooperative, and aimed at a common goal.

For the goal of cooperative interdependence to occur, each person must be equally dependent on the other for achieving the desired goals (Levy, Jessop, Rimmerman, & Levy, 1992). Recreation professionals can provide many different recreation activities related to areas such as team building, trust development, and adventure recreation that require cooperation and contributions by all participants (Dattilo & Weltner, 1991). The focus of the recreation activities can be on the process of collaboration to meet a challenge rather than the product of winning. Examples of cooperative activities include:

(a) gardening where everyone is assigned a particular task;
(b) making a papier-mâché project where everyone adds a layer;
(c) bowling when the highest possible team score is desired;
(d) making a quilt with a group; and
(e) cooking where everyone does at least one step of the cooking.

Develop Effective Communication

Jones and colleagues (1984) recommended that clear communication between people can reduce interaction strain. Hastorf, Wildfogel, and Cassman (1979) and Belgrave and Mills (1981) reported that simple acknowledgment of the disability by the person with the disability can reduce the other person's discomfort.

Cook and Makas (1979) noted that people with and without disabilities differed in their perceptions of what constitutes the most positive attitudes toward persons with disabilities. The authors observed that to the respondents with disabilities, "positive attitudes" meant either dispensing with the special category of disability entirely, or promoting attitudes that defend the civil and social rights of people with disabilities. For the respondents without disabilities, Cook and Makas reported that "positive attitudes" reflected a desire to be nice, helpful, and ultimately place people with disabilities in a needy situation. People without disabilities may actually be perceived by people with disabilities, therefore, as expressing negative attitudes when, in actuality, the individuals with disabilities are attempting to express what they consider to be positive attitudes (Makas, 1988).

Kleck (1968) reported that people without disabilities want to express attitudes that are acceptable to and respectful of people without disabilities with whom they come in contact. Given these good intentions, it becomes clear that people without disabilities need to be educated about areas in which their notions of positive attitudes offend people with disabilities (Makas, 1988). Makas stated that people without disabilities must be educated about disability as a civil-rights issue, and made aware that many people with disabilities reject special treatment on the basis of their disabilities and do not desire to be perceived as different, even if "different" means "better."

According to Makas (1988), in situations in which a person makes a statement or behaves in a way that demeans or insults, an individual with a disability is justified in correcting the error. However, the author warns that if the correction is accompanied by powerful negative emotions, the content of the correction is likely to be lost. Negative reactions to a person's failed attempts at positive interaction may discourage the person's good intentions and create further misunderstanding and discomfort (Makas, 1988). Communication, particularly the sharing of one another's expectations, can be valuable in reducing the barriers that contribute to this discomfort (Makas, 1988). Cook and Makas (1979) demonstrated that one way in which successful relationships between people with and without disabilities can be facilitated is through exchange of information between the two groups to clarify the situation.

Encourage Age-Appropriate Behaviors

Brown and colleagues (1979b) stated that if one goal of education is to minimize the stigmatizing discrepancies between persons with disabilities and others, it is our obligation to teach major functions characteristic of their chronological age using materials and tasks which do not highlight deficiencies. Individuals with disabilities need to develop a repertoire of leisure skills that is appropriate to their chronological age, that is based in their community, and that will facilitate successful integration into the community (Schleien, Olson, Rogers, & McLafferty, 1985).

Certo, Schleien, and Hunter (1983) suggested that leisure-skill instruction for people with disabilities be developed based on activities performed by individuals without disabilities in a wide variety of integrated community environments. Therefore, practitioners should encourage people with disabilities to acquire leisure skills that are appropriate to their age and comparable to those of their peers (Block & Krebs, 1992).

Rejection and ostracization by people without disabilities may be reduced when stigmatizing differences, such as age-inappropriate behaviors, are minimized (Rusch, Chadsey-Rusch, White, & Gifford, 1985). Calhoun and Calhoun (1993) reported that chronological age-appropriate activities may reduce the stigmatizing effects of disability on the perceptions of adults with disabilities. Participating in age-appropriate activities may lead others to view adults with disabilities—specifically, those with mental retardation, as capable of taking on more complicated and advanced tasks than would otherwise be expected.

Because some people with disabilities may have difficulty developing accurate perceptions about their capabilities (Kennedy, Austin, and Smith, 1987), practitioners should assist participants in understanding the implications of their leisure choices. Dattilo and Schleien (1994) provided the following example that, as a child, Jason loved to listen to bells ringing and children's tunes. When he got a bit older, his parents bought him a portable pinball machine. This table game was extremely reactive, as its bells rang, lights flashed, and score was kept automatically when the game was played appropriately. Jason was highly reinforced for pulling the pinball machine's plunger and pressing its flippers. Now that he is older, Jason enjoys playing with electronic pinball machines with his friends in video arcades, movie theater lobbies, and bowling alleys.

Conclusion

Although behaviors that reflect negative attitudes can limit opportunities for people with disabilities (as presented in Chapter 1), these negative attitudes, and subsequent behaviors, can be changed. The recreation professional can play an important role in moving participants' attitudes about people with disabilities from those that are negative to attitudes that reflect acceptance and understanding of diversity. Structuring interactions, encouraging extensive personal contact, promoting joint participation, facilitating equal status, fostering cooperative interdependence, focusing on similarities, and developing effective communication are some examples of ways which may be considered in developing positive attitudes toward individuals with disabilities. Perhaps, as Eisenberg (1982) suggested, with increased contact, and the maintenance of a highly visible presence, some of the prejudicial feelings toward people with disabilities shared by many people without disabilities can be eliminated.

Discussion Questions

1. What is the value of structuring interactions when people with and without disabilities are participating in recreation programs?

2. What is an example of how to structure a situation to promote positive interactions between people with and without disabilities?

3. How can you encourage extensive personal contact between participants with and without disabilities?

4. What are some methods which promote joint participation between people with and without disabilities?

5. What is the value of facilitating equal status among participants in a recreation program?

6. How might you encourage participants in your recreation programs to be of equal status?

7. How might you foster cooperative interdependence with people participating in your recreation program?

8. What are ways you can encourage people you encounter to focus on people's similarities rather than their differences?

9. What are some strategies to increase effective communication that would help improve the attitudes of people you encounter?

10. What are some specific techniques you could utilize to improve people's attitudes toward individuals with disabilities?

Chapter 4

Use Sensitive Terminology

"More people are blinded by definition than by any other cause."
—Jahoda

Orientation Activity: Change Terminology

Directions When Alone: Read the words and phrases presented. On a separate piece of paper list numbers from 1-40. Write in the space to the immediate right of your numbers the word or phrase that communicates a more positive attitude toward people with disabilities. Circle the numbers of those words or phrases that are the most difficult for you to change.

Directions With Others: After dividing into small groups, discuss the words or phrases that posed the most difficulty for each participant. Other members of the group attempt to explain the rationale for their choices for these items. After a specified time, discuss your responses with the entire group based on the information presented in this chapter.

1. a special kid
2. crippled
3. the retarded
4. autistic people
5. the blind
6. AIDS victim
7. the deaf
8. a CP
9. those MDs
10. wheelchair bound
11. dependent on crutches
12. suffers from MS
13. mental age of 3
14. confined to a wheelchair
15. stricken with epilepsy
16. borderline retarded
17. dummy
18. feeble-minded
19. a nervous breakdown
20. a spinal-injured man
21. maniac
22. crazy
23. deaf
24. dumb
25. deaf mute
26. handicapped person
27. normal
28. able-bodied
29. a paraplegic
30. afflicted with autism
31. imbecile
32. the amputee
33. the special woman
34. lunatic
35. moron
36. deformed person
37. a spina bifida child
38. the schizophrenic
39. a neurotic person
40. psycho

Debriefing

Mary Johnson, editor of *The Disability Rag,* identified language and words as probably the biggest handicap facing persons with disabilities (*Rag Time*, 1989). Although breakthroughs in technology, medical treatment, and legislation are opening doors to full and independent lives for persons with disabilities, language persists in developing barriers (National Easter Seals Society, 1981).

The use of insensitive language to describe other people often creates tension between the persons who are being referred to inaccurately and the people using the inappropriate terminology. To reduce this barrier to interaction, Jones and colleagues (1984) recommended that, during interactions, people use clear and accurate communication. In addressing the challenge to improve attitudes toward people with disabilities, Alderson (1985) suggested breaking away from words with connotations conveying fear, insensitivity, stereotyping and discrimination. The intent of this chapter is to supply information on terminology that encourages the communication of positive attitudes toward people with disabilities. As you examine the words and phrases you substituted for the previous words, consider the following questions:

1. In what situations are you not sure of how to refer to people with disabilities?
2. What general rules can you offer when attempting to describe people with disabilities?
3. Why is it important to focus on the words you use to describe people with disabilities?

Introduction

People with disabilities want access. New laws such as the Americans With Disabilities Act, approved in July 1990, bar discrimination of people with physical or mental disabilities in public accommodations, private employment and government services. By passing laws, the federal government hopes to empower people with disabilities, but the battle for access may be better fought on the communication front. Educators can help the next generation of writers and the working press learn to use language that promotes the notion that people with disabilities are entitled to access. The day the ADA bill passed, *The Atlanta Journal and Constitution* announced, "Handicapped Rights

Bill Awaits Final Approval" (1990, p. 11.). This usage may seem innocuous enough, but it is off the mark. The preferred usage is people with disabilities (Smith, 1992, p. 1).

The information presented in this chapter is based on an article by Dattilo and Smith (1990). This chapter provides information on sensitive terminology that communicates positive attitudes toward people with disabilities. Suggestions for using terminology that focuses attention on similarities shared by all people rather than differences are made. A "people first" philosophy is described with implications for terminology. Encouragement is given to emphasize individuals' abilities rather than their disabilities by using specific words and phrases. Recommendations on using language that communicates dignity and respect are also presented. An attempt is made to alleviate confusion with some words and promote the use of consistent terminology that represent people with disabilities in a positive manner. In addition, information is provided on preferred terminology to describe people without disabilities. Debate and controversy surrounding some words and phrases is also presented. Finally, encouragement is provided for professionals and students to act as agents of change to help other people use the most appropriate terminology to describe individuals with disabilities. These major sections of the chapter are illustrated in Figure 4.1 (see page 64).

Kleck (1968) determined that people typically desire to express acceptable attitudes that demonstrate respect for people with disabilities they encounter. Based on these findings, Makas (1988) recommended that people should become aware of behaviors that offend individuals with disabilities. Therefore, terminology should reflect the equality of all its citizens, as well as being sensitive to the situation (Beaver, 1993).

Obviously, the behaviors and attitudes of professionals providing leisure services that include people with disabilities can affect the quality of life, self-concept, and degree of general acceptance of those individuals by others (Stewart, 1988). One particular behavior that has been identified as frequently offending people is the use of insensitive terminology to describe people with disabilities. Since leisure services providers frequently interact with people with disabilities, it is critical to project a positive attitude through the use of sensitive terminology.

After conducting an experimental investigation, Byrd, Crews, and Ebener (1991) reported that students who were briefed on rules for appropriate use of language when referring to people with disabilities performed significantly better than students who did not. Byrd and colleagues (1991, p. 41) concluded that: "There apparently is benefit to providing this instruction to students who are in a course where disability, disease, or exceptionality is being discussed."

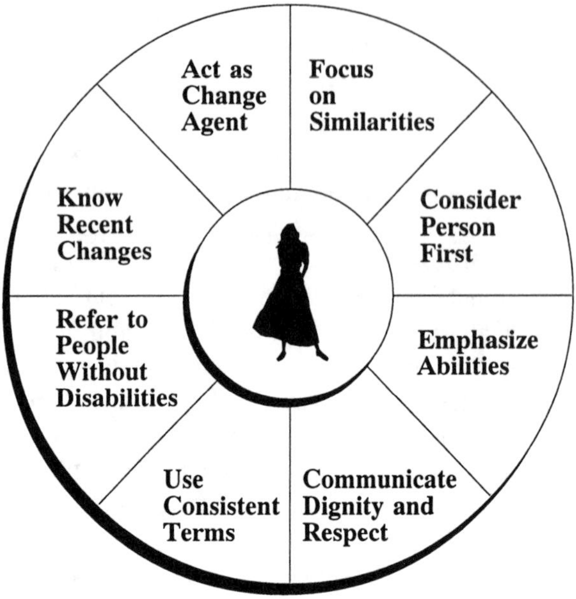

Figure 4.1 Guidelines for using sensitive terminology.

Focus on People's Similarities

Focusing on a person's uniqueness can be a positive way to view the individual. However, Howe-Murphy and Charboneau (1987) warned that an overemphasis on unique and unusual traits can become so overwhelming that the similarities shared by all people are ignored. According to the authors, failure to recognize that all individuals have the same basic needs sets people apart from one another and results in the development of barriers to interpersonal relationships. Typically, it is easier to interact with a person if we initially concentrate on similarities we share with this person as opposed to differences. People's attitudes tend to be more positive when they focus on the similarities they share with persons with disabilities as opposed to their differences (Snell, 1988).

One way that people mistakenly focus on differences rather than similarities between people is by identifying some individuals as being "special." Typically, people with disabilities express the desire to be treated with the same respect as any person. Charles Greenlaw, an official associated with the Boy Scouts, summarized the involvement of Tim Fredricks, a scout who happens to have mental retardation, in a community scouting program. "The other scouts see nothing unusual about having Tim in the group, nor do they treat him 'special.' The only way that Tim is 'special' is that he is an Eagle Scout" (Fredricks, 1987, p. 27).

When people are identified as "special," as a result of their disability, the implication may be that their disability limits all that they do. When this generalized impact of their disability is accepted, people tend to lower their expectations of individuals with disabilities. Bree Walker, a coanchor of an evening television newscast who in addition to many other characteristics has a physical disability, stated that "We have to reach a point where having a physical difference doesn't matter. When we do, I will feel that my time has come and I am no longer regarded as 'special'" (Dietl, 1988). Deborah McFadden, 1993 Commissioner of the Federal Administration on Developmental Disabilities, stated that:

> We're trying to (prevent use of) the word 'special,' because every time you have a 'special' person, you make (that person) different. We must have the dream and the hope that our future will be inclusive of everyone (McFadden & Burke, 1991, p. iii).

Leisure service providers should avoid identifying people as a member of a "special population" or a "special child." These phrases may encourage people to treat individuals with disabilities differently than people without disabilities. Treating people differently occurs when we fail to focus on similarities shared by people.

According to Wright (1988), when a person identifies with someone because of similarity, a tendency for that person to like the other person will be induced. However, the author suggested that focusing on individuals' differences can be perceived in a way that promotes prejudice. Therefore, when leisure services providers use terminology to describe people with disabilities, they should only use a label when absolutely necessary. For example, a supervisor may be educating her staff about the needs of a person being integrated into a program and may say, "Because John has mental retardation, he may have some difficulty with abstract concepts; therefore, you may want to provide some demonstrations when providing verbal directions."

The Research and Training Center on Independent Living (1984) suggested that journalists not refer to a person's disability unless it is critical to the story. According to the National Easter Seals Society (1981), emphasizing the worth of all persons, rather than differences between people, will encourage portrayal of people with disabilities in a positive fashion.

Consider the Person First

When relating to people who have been grouped together, for whatever reason, it is helpful to consider these individuals as people first and then, if relevant, consider their group affiliation. If it is relevant to use a label, place the person first to avoid the tendency to make stereotypic generalizations about people who, in addition to many of the other characteristics that affect their humanness (i.e., sense of humor, reliability, honesty), happen to have a disability. To place the person first, use the label only as a noun referring to a condition (e.g., "a person with mental retardation") rather than a noun referring to the person (e.g., "the retard") or an adjective (e.g., "the mentally retarded person").

By making reference to the person first, professionals demonstrate respect for the uniqueness and worth of the person (National Easter Seals Society, 1981). Coulter (1992) reported that the use of disability-first language (such as "the retarded" or "retarded persons") shows a lack of respect for people with disabilities. According to Coulter, in the current language of the street, those who use this language are "dissing" ("disrespecting") people with disabilities.

Another suggestion to encourage focusing on the individual is to avoid labeling persons into groups according to medical diagnoses or disabilities (e.g., "the blind," "the amputee"); rather, you are encouraged to focus on people first (e.g., "individuals with visual impairments," "persons with amputations," "people with hearing disorders"). In general, attempts should also be made to avoid using acronyms such as "CP" for cerebral palsy, "MR" for mental retardation, or "MD" for muscular dystrophy. The use of such acronyms emphasizes the condition rather than the person.

Use of acronyms may create confusion and make some people feel ignorant because they are unaware of the meaning of some acronyms. This breakdown in the communication process can only hurt your ability to present a positive image of people with disabilities. However, if it is relevant to identify the person's medical diagnosis, the name of the condition is lengthy, and there is high recognition of the acronym within a given society, the acronym may be appropriately used. For example, Acquired Immune Deficiency Syndrome is most frequently identified as AIDS. The acronym "AIDS" appears to have a higher recognition rate than "Acquired Immune Deficiency Syndrome." Therefore, in some limited situations, the use of an acronym may be accepted.

When identifying individuals, it is useful to recognize their humanness and identify them as "people" or "program participants" rather than "patients" or "cases." The use of words "patients" or "cases" implies that individuals are ill and in need of medical assistance. Many people with disabilities are not receiving medical care, are in excellent health, and therefore should not be identified as "patients." Most of us, at some time, will be receiving medical care and be identified as a "patient" in the context of the medical environment; however, this does not imply that we should then be identified in all contexts of our lives as a "patient." The condition of being a "patient" or a "case" varies according to the situation and, therefore, the use of these terms as a label for people with disabilities is often inaccurate.

The word "client" may be used to describe people receiving a variety of recreation services. If the word "client" is used consistently to describe all recreation participants, then it is more acceptable than when the word "client" is used only to describe those individuals with disabilities.

An example of the trend to use "People First" terminology occurred on May 10, 1988, when former President Reagan signed Executive Order 12640 establishing the 41-year-old President's Committee on Employment of the Handicapped as The President's Committee on Employment of People with Disabilities. The name change was enthusiastically received by consumer advocates who are working to improve the language concerning disability (*Rag Time,* 1989). Chairperson Harold Russell stated that the new name placed the President's Committee firmly into the forefront of demonstrating sensitivity to the desires of people with disabilities. In addition, other more recent legislation such as Public Law 99-457, the Individuals with Disabilities Education Act (IDEA), formerly known as the Education of the Handicapped Act, and Public Law 101-336, the Americans with Disabilities Act (ADA), clearly demonstrate a focus on "People First" terminology.

Emphasize Each Individual's Abilities

When describing people with disabilities, it is important to emphasize individuals' abilities rather than focusing on their limitations. For example, it is more accurate to say "a woman who uses a wheelchair" rather than "she is confined to a wheelchair" or "she is wheelchair-bound." The use of the phrase "he walks with crutches" is more accurate than "he is dependent on crutches." Typically, when people access forms of transportation other than walking (i.e., automobile, bicycle, skateboard) they are not described as being "confined to" or "dependent on" that particular means of transportation. Be consistent with this line of reasoning when describing people with disabilities who use alternative forms of transportation or mobility.

Many of the words used to depict individuals with disabilities reflect concepts of dependency and helplessness, which perpetuate negative attitudes and corresponding patterns of response and expectation (National Easter Seal Society, 1981). At times, fund-raising efforts have employed the use of counter-productive terminology that is intended to evoke impressions of needy, fragile persons requiring special treatment (Brolley & Anderson, 1988). Organizations using such tactics to raise funds intended to promote independence may, in fact, foster a sense of dependency through the fund-raising campaign. It is important, then, to avoid sensationalizing or exploiting a person's disability. Describe people as simply having a disability rather than using words that imply pain and suffering. Phrases such as "afflicted with . . . ," "suffers from . . . ," "a victim of . . . ," "crippled by . . . ," or "stricken with . . ." sensationalize the disability and tend to evoke sympathy toward individuals. Instead, it would be more appropriate to say "the person has . . . ," "the condition is caused by . . . ," or " "a disability resulting from . . ."

In a 1988 February issue of *Time* magazine entitled "Roaming the Cosmos," the lead sentence to the article describing the renowned physicist, Stephen Hawking, was: "Physicist Stephen Hawking is confined to a wheelchair, a virtual prisoner in his own body." This description can be contrasted with the lead sentences in the article entitled "Black Holes Figured Back in Time" reported in a June, 1988, issue of *Insight* magazine: "Through the intricate equations devised over two decades, cosmologist Stephen W. Hawking has advanced intriguing visions of the universe's origin and structure." The differences between the two representations of Stephen Hawking are striking because of the terminology used in the articles.

Frequently, sympathetic views evoked by such words as "confined" or "prisoner" restrict people's independence by limiting other people's tendency to treat individuals who have disabilities with dignity and respect. For instance, at the second AIDS forum in Denver in 1983, individuals with AIDS condemned attempts to label themselves as "AIDS victims." People attending the conference stated that the phrase "AIDS victims" implied defeat and, therefore, identified the phrase "persons with AIDS" as the most preferred terminology.

Communicate Dignity and Respect for Each Individual

The practice of classifying individuals according to mental age has been drastically reduced in recent years. Avoid using the phrase "mental age," because the label tells the practitioner nothing about the particular pattern of the person's cognitive strengths and weaknesses (Baroff, 1986). For instance, when discussing the implications of following written directions by a woman, say "a woman who is 35-years-old that currently identifies a few words" as opposed to stating "the woman who has the mind of a 3-year-old." Use of the phrase "mental age" may result in the mistaken treatment of a person with a mental impairment such as Alzheimer's Disease, mental retardation or learning disability as a child.

Practitioners must avoid using terminology that conveys adults with mental impairments as children (e.g., "he is childlike" or "our kids") and instead communicate dignity provided to other adults in our society (Wolfensberger, 1972). Using age-appropriate terminology to describe individuals will encourage the development of programs that are appropriate for the age of the participants and do not require the participants to compromise their dignity.

Use terminology that demonstrates respect by avoiding the use of any terms to describe people with disabilities that communicate racism or ethnocentrism. For instance, sometimes people with mental retardation who have Down's Syndrome are referred to as "Mongoloid." This term was used because of one of the characteristic features of persons with Down's Syndrome; that is, their eyes resembled individuals of Oriental descent. Therefore, if it is relevant to describe the specific form of mental retardation caused by an extra number 21 chromosome, professionals are encouraged to use the phrase "Down's Syndrome" rather than the term "Mongoloid."

Many words that have been used in the past to describe people with disabilities have communicated ideas of deviancy, helplessness, dependency and a variety of negative traits. Words such as "imbecile," "lunatic," "moron," "borderline," "dummy," "feeble-minded," "maniac," "crazy," "deaf and dumb," or "deaf-mute" are no longer acceptable words because of their strong negative overtones. Instead, use phrases such as "people with developmental disabilities," "individuals with mental retardation," "persons with psychological disorders," "individuals with communication disorders," or "persons with speech and hearing disorders." Through the use of these words and phrases, you will be able to better communicate a positive attitude about people with disabilities.

Use Consistent Terminology to Enhance Understanding

The words "impairment," "disability," and "handicap" are three distinct words that are defined in different ways. Unfortunately, many people use the words interchangeably and often, inaccurately. It is the intent of the author to clarify confusion surrounding the use of these words in this section of the chapter.

The word **"impairment"** means to diminish in strength (Alderson, 1985). According to Gunn (1975), "impairment" refers to identifiable organic or functional conditions that may be permanent (e.g., amputation) or temporary (e.g., sprain). When an individual possesses an impairment, the focus is on the problem (e.g., disease, injury) with a specific portion of the body. For instance, a visual impairment involves a deficit with the eye such as that caused by clouding of lenses resulting in cataracts. When cataracts are mentioned, the problem with the eye is emphasized. Another example may be that a person has a neurological impairment, such as cerebral palsy, that prevents independent leg movement. In this situation, when the phrase "neurological impairment" is used, attention is directed toward the central nervous system that was damaged. The focus of the discussion related to impairment is not on the person; rather, the discussion is directed to the actual condition.

According to Webster's New Collegiate Dictionary (1977) "able" is defined as having sufficient power, skill or resources to accomplish a task. When the word "able" is combined with the prefix "dis," which refers to being deprived of, the definition of the word **"disability"** becomes apparent. The word "disability" describes the reduction or deprivation of a skill or power. This reduced ability is a result of an impairment. For instance, a person with cataracts has a visual impairment that may result in a reading disability even when corrective lenses are used. When the word "disability" is used, attention is given to the interaction of the visual impairment with the functioning ability of the individual. The person who has a neurological impairment, such as cerebral palsy, may possess a mobility or ambulation disability. When discussing a person's disability, it is necessary to examine the individual and the effect that the impairment has on that person.

The word **"handicap"** was originally used to denote a disadvantage in sport and is a concept that is open to change (Hale, 1979). According to the Merriam-Webster Dictionary, "handicap" is a game in which forfeits were held in a cap (hand in cap), a content in which artificial advantage is given, or disadvantage imposed on a contest to equalize chances of winning; a disadvantage that makes achievement difficult. Howe-Murphy and Charboneau (1987) identified the word "handicap" as being linked with the practice of beggars who held "cap-in-hand" to solicit charity. These definitions demonstrate that the labeling of people as "handicapped" represents an impression of society that these individuals are dependent on others.

The important aspect of the word "handicap" is that a handicap varies from one situation to another. In effect, a handicap is an interaction between environmental conditions and the individual, rather than simply inherent in the person. For instance, a person with a visual impairment may be handicapped when going to the theater to watch a movie but may not be handicapped when listening to music on the radio. A person with a neurological impairment who uses a wheelchair may be handicapped when playing soccer but may be extremely skilled at billiards. Because a person may be handicapped in one situation and not handicapped in another, it is inaccurate to label the person as "handicapped." The word "handicap" implies that the person is handicapped in every situation. This generalization of a condition to all life situations imposes unnecessary restrictions on the individual.

Based on Lord's (1981) observation that being "handicapped" is a social phenomenon influenced by our society, Kennedy, Austin and Smith (1987) reported that people with disabilities can handicap themselves by believing that they cannot do something and society can handicap people with disabilities by refusing them opportunities to participate.

The National Easter Seals Society (1981) recommended that "disability" be used rather than "handicap" because a disabling condition may or may not be handicapping. Many people with disabilities have communicated a desire to be identified with a disability rather than a handicap. For instance, Karol Davenport, a therapeutic recreation supervisor for a rehabilitation hospital who also happens to use a wheelchair, explained to reporters that she preferred to be referred to as a "person with a disability" rather than "handicapped" (Jesiolowski, 1988). Ms. Davenport's preference was supported by a survey conducted by *The Disability Rag* (The results are in!, 1986) that reported the preferences of 25 percent of the magazine's readership. Nearly three-fourths of the sample who possessed disabilities stated that they would prefer the phrase "a person with a disability" in referring to themselves, while only three percent preferred "handicapped person." Shapiro (1993) stated that the term "disabled" has replaced "handicapped" in recent years and is becoming the first word to emerge by consensus from people with disabilities.

Refer to People without Disabilities

The word "normal" is acceptable when people are referring to statistical norms and averages; however, this term is demeaning to people with disabilities when used in reference to persons with no disability (National Easter Seals Society, 1981). The use of the word "normal" to describe people who do not possess an apparent disability implies that a disability is the one distinguishing factor that separates people into two primary categories, "normal" and "disabled." Not only is the word "normal" demeaning to persons with disabilities, but many people without disabilities resent being labeled as "normal." "Normal" implies that people act similar to many other people in almost all aspects of their lives. This view stresses conformity and ignores individuality, creativity and diversity.

When describing people without disabilities, apply the same principles described earlier in this chapter. If not having a disability is not relevant to a particular situation, then avoid labeling the individual. However, if it is important to identify the person as not having a disability, the National Easter Seals Society (1981) recommended using the phrase "persons without disabilities" to refer to people who do not possess an apparent disability. Some people use the phrase "able-bodied" to describe individuals without disabilities.

This phrase can cause confusion, because individuals with disabilities may also possess bodies that are very able (e.g., people with mental retardation, autism, and learning disabilities).

Recent Controversy About Most Preferred Terminology

Currently there are some words and phrases that are being considered by persons with disabilities and their advocates as demonstrating a positive view toward people with disabilities. For instance, Ted Kennedy, Jr. (1986) dislikes the terms "handicapped" and "disabled," because they imply inability and are negative descriptions that promote undesirable stereotypes. Instead, Kennedy prefers "physically and mentally challenged" or "persons with a disability," to stress human beings first and limitations second. Kennedy's desire to emphasize the person first is in keeping with most people's preferred terminology. However, some people view the phrase "physically challenged" as vague and ambiguous.

Some newer terminology describing people with visual impairments, such as "partially sighted," has met controversy. Some individuals feel the phrase "partially sighted" implies an avoidance of the acceptance of having a disability, while others feel it accentuates positive aspects (sight). Rana Arnold, co-founder and president of the Sight-Loss Support Group of Central Pennsylvania, reported that when polling members of the Sight-Loss Support Group, views regarding the phrase "partially sighted" varied from person to person.

Another controversy relates to ways to describe people who are deaf. Some people who are deaf reject "people first" terminology and prefer being described as "Deaf people." According to Dolnick (1993, p. 38), "the uppercase D is significant. It serves as a succinct proclamation that the deaf share a culture rather than merely a medical condition." The argument of deafness as culture relates to the belief that over a half a million Americans who are deaf share a common language (American Sign Language) and, as a result, share a common identity. However, according to Dolnick (1993), the view that deafness is akin to ethnicity is far from unanimously held.

One problem that arises when using phrases that have yet to receive general support from people associated with a particular group is the difficulty in receiving services such as financial aid, specialized education and recreation. Although phrases such as "partially sighted" and "physically challenged" seem to accentuate the positive for some people, these same phrases may create problems in acquiring services and seem to offend other individuals. *The Disability Rag* (The results are in!, 1986) reported that only a few of their subscribers indicated a preference for the phrases "physically challenged" or "inconvenienced." In describing the perceptions of the hundreds of people with disabilities whom he interviewed, Shapiro (1993, p. 33) writes:

> Concoctions like "the vertically challenged" are silly and scoffed at. The "differently abled," the "handi-capable," or the "physically and mentally challenged" are almost universally dismissed as too gimmicky and too inclusive. "Physically challenged doesn't distinguish me from a woman climbing Mt. Everest, something certainly I'll never do," says Nancy Mairs, an essayist and poet with multiple sclerosis. "It blurs the distinction between our lives." Only by using direct terminology, she argues, will people think about what it means to be disabled and the accommodations she needs, such as wheelchair accessible buildings or grab bars in bathrooms. Dianne Piastro, who writes the syndicated column "Living with a Disability," complains that such terms suggest that disability is somehow shameful and needs to be concealed in a vague generality. "It's denying our reality instead of saying that our reality, of being disabled, is okay," says Piastro.

Therefore, at this time, it is difficult to recommend the consistent use of such phrases. It is important, however, to realize that identification of the most preferred terminology to describe persons with disabilities is a continuously evolving process. If you are unsure of which words to use when in contact with people, ask the person with a disability what terminology he or she prefers.

Words that are currently creating controversy, and have yet to receive a general consensus, may be the words of choice in the future. In all situations, listen to your constituents to determine the terms and phrases they most prefer and attempt to understand their reasons for these choices. This sentiment is reflected by Coulter (1992, p. 2):

> I believe that people have a right to call themselves whatever they want, and that others should respect their choice. We should not be surprised when these choices change over time. We have seen several such changes recently: people preferring to be called gay or lesbian instead of homosexual, or people preferring to be called African-American instead of colored or black, for example. If this choice reflects a reasonable consensus of those who may be so described, then I believe we should respect it. People with disabilities have made it perfectly clear that they want us to use people-first language, and so we should.

Act as a Change Agent

Based on the premise that changing social attitudes through language has been a powerful tool for the civil rights movements, Medgyesi (1988) encouraged advocates for people with disabilities to insist upon terminology that is empowering rather than demeaning. According to Medgyesi, the use of empowering terminology establishes people with disabilities as a social and economic force to be considered and respected. The Research and Training Center on Independent Living (1984) reported that the words and images used to portray persons with disabilities can create an insensitive, negative portrayal or a clear, positive view.

The use of insensitive terminology may occur because well-intentioned people are not aware of the most accurate words or phrases to describe people. Therefore, if a person makes a statement or behaves in a way that demeans or insults, Makas (1988) suggested that people are justified in correcting the error. She warned, however, that if the correction is accompanied by powerful negative emotions, the content of the corrections is likely to be lost. Therefore, after reading this chapter and gaining knowledge of the most appropriate terminology, consider the perspective of the people using the inappropriate terminology when educating them about the most desired behaviors to exhibit as they interact with or represent individuals with disabilities.

Conclusion

This chapter contains information on the most appropriate terminology to be used when describing people with disabilities. You are now encouraged to become change agents within society. Considering Yuker's (1977) definition of an attitude as a positive or negative reaction to a person, accompanied by specific beliefs that tend to impel the individual in a particular way toward that person, you are encouraged to communicate and engender positive attitudes toward persons with disabilities. Although the intent of this chapter was to describe what many people with disabilities and professionals are espousing as the most preferred terminology, it is important to consider that the use of acceptable terminology is an evolving process. Therefore, you are encouraged to continuously respond to the most recent information presented, demonstrate a willingness to listen to and consider other people's perspectives (Beaver, 1993), and be eager to revise your terminology to best represent people with disabilities.

Finally, in reporting on the life of Judy Clouston, a recognized poet, Crabtree (1994) presented a quote by Clouston that demonstrated how she felt about sensitive terminology:

> . . . when the clerk shouts, "Hey, Joe, there's a crippled lady up here who needs some sour cream," I wince. When a stranger says, "My aunt is an invalid . . ." I can't hear the rest of the sentence. When I hear the phrase "confined to a wheelchair" I want to jump out of mine. They're words, but they make a difference.

Discussion Questions

1. What is the "People First" philosophy?
2. What are the six general suggestions provided in this chapter for using sensitive terminology?
3. Why is it important to focus on individuals' similarities?
4. Why is it best to avoid the use of the term "special?"
5. Why should acronyms be avoided? When is it appropriate to use acronyms?
6. What is the difference between the terms "patient," "client," and "participant?" Which term is preferred and why?
7. What are two ways the federal government acknowledged the importance of People First terminology?
8. Why should you avoid using terminology that sensationalizes or exploits people with disabilities?
9. What is meant by the terms "impairment," "disability," and "handicapped?"
10. What is the best way to refer to people who do not have disabilities?

Chapter 5

Support Families

"It's a tough balancing act."
—Jan Walters

Orientation Activity: The Family Balancing Act

Directions When Alone: Collect 10 large empty cardboard boxes. Set them on the floor in front of you. Begin to read the following list of possible problems a family might experience. All families may experience these situations; however, families that have a member who has a disability often are likely to experience these situations. As you read each situation, pick up one of the boxes. Continue reading and adding boxes until you drop a box.

Directions With Others: Divide into small groups and discuss how you felt when you were attempting to carry as many boxes as possible. Describe how you felt when a box or more than one box fell. Discuss your perception of the requirements of family members of individuals with disabilities. Generate some ideas on how leisure service providers may be able to alleviate the stress experienced by these families.

1. Since there is no afternoon recreation program for your child to attend, you hire someone to be with your child.
2. The person you have scheduled to watch your child is sick and you are required to take a day off of work.
3. Since there is no summer recreation facility open to your sister, you must watch her instead of working and earning money.
4. Because of the unwillingness of preschool to accommodate your child, you must stop working and stay home with your child.
5. One of the members of your household becomes ill and you must take care of them.
6. Your child is injured while playing out in the street.
7. A person working at the bowling alley tells you that you should not bring your brother there in the future.
8. You decline an invitation to a party because the last time you were there people did not make your family feel welcome.

9. You are unable to afford to go on a family vacation this year because of the medical expenses you incurred.
10. Your friends make fun of you because a member of your family has a disability.

Debriefing

Families must respond to a variety of circumstances that influence their lives. Each circumstance requires the family to make an adjustment. In the orientation activity, the family circumstances were represented by you taking on a cardboard box to carry. As families acquire "boxes," they must readjust their strategy of working together to keep the "boxes" from falling and to maintain an intact family. Through a life cycle, the family accumulates numerous "boxes," which they attempt to share and carry as a group. Eventually, this simulation required the addition of so many adjustments that you could no longer carry all the boxes. You are then identified as being in crisis and could not remain stable without outside community support and intervention. Consider the following questions when thinking about the orientation activity:

1. How did you feel while participating in the activity?
2. What did you learn from this learning activity?
3. How can leisure services providers support families who have a member who has a disability?

Introduction

Mary Ulrich is a woman who has been an active advocate for people with disabilities. She is a contributing member of her community and is a leader in several national organizations. In addition, Mary is a wife and a parent. One of her children happens to have a severe disability. Based on her personal experiences, Mary made a significant contribution to this chapter.

Behind every person with a disability is a family. Each family tries to manage the needs of each member of the family, as well as their collective needs. Some families meet their needs, others do not. At times, families are placed in a position of having to choose which needs in the family will be met and which ones will not. "Because we could not find after-school care and daily respite care, we had to place our son in a group home. We want him home now, and I cannot bring him home because there is no place for after-school care, vacation, etc." (Fink, 1988).

Braddock, Hemp, and Fujiura (1987) reported that the trend within the last couple decades of moving people out of large residential institutions (deinstitutionalization) has resulted in an increase in the number of people with disabilities residing in their communities (see Figure 5.1). Therefore, families have become a major source of caregiving for these individuals (Singer & Irvin, 1989). Attempts to provide this care creates major challenges for the family unit (Krauss, 1986).

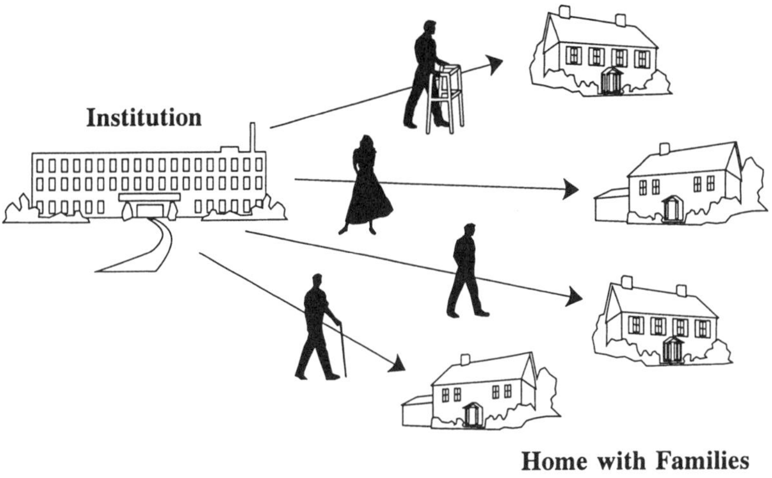

Figure 5.1 Movement of people with disabilities from institutions to community life with their families.

Examples of Community Support

Community Support for Beverly

Many local communities have responded to the needs of typical families. For example, Beverly's parents accessed the services of daycare for Bev when she was younger. Currently, they piece together public and private community programs to help support their family. During the summer when school is not in session, Bev, who is now 13 years old, rides her bike to the Recreation Community Center at 8 a.m. as her mother and father go to work. She begins diving lessons at 8:30 a.m., swim team practice at 9:30 a.m., and free swim with her friends until noon. She then rides her bike to a nearby park for tennis lessons from 1-3 p.m. After a short bike ride home, Bev calls her mother or father at work to provide them with an update on her status and then starts a few chores for dinner.

If you conduct a life-space analysis (Brown, Shiraga, York, Zanella, & Rogan, 1984) of Bev's life during the school year and in the summer, the time blocks would be similar: classes, free time, classes, home, and chores. During the summer, Bev's family is able to adjust their routines to accommodate their needs. As a result of a little creative planning, the availability of financial and community resources and Bev's growing skills and independence, Bev's family is able to maintain a balance between their needs and community support.

Community Support for Karen

Now, let us examine the balance of family needs and community supports for the family of a person with severe intellectual challenges. Many unprepared families have been thrust into becoming advocates for family members with disabilities (Shapiro, 1994). For example, Karen (age 13) lives in the same neighborhood as Beverly. She goes to the same school, and her mother works with Bev's mother in the same business. Karen, however, cannot go alone to the neighborhood community recreation center. The swimming program for children with disabilities is only on Thursdays from 3-4 p.m. Karen is currently not able to ride her bike to the park independently and is not eligible for tennis lessons because of her disabilities. The sports leagues, Bible schools, Scout camps, community camps, and recreation centers in Karen's community either have no programs for children with disabilities, or they have programs at specific times which are suitable for personnel working with these programs and are inconvenient for Karen's family (Gallagher, Beckman & Cross, 1983). Daycare centers will not accept Karen either (Fink, 1988). Although Karen's family contacted the school and many social-service agencies, they were unable to locate any ongoing programs that would meet Karen's needs (Ulrich, 1991). Further, though many professionals were sympathetic to the family's problem, it was clearly the family's problem. The inability to provide community leisure services added more stress to the family (Turnbull & Summers, 1985).

Karen's family must become active problem-solvers by searching the community for options. They were devastated that the school professionals determined Karen had met all her IEP objectives and would not "qualify" for an extended school year. Therefore, next year, they will attempt to encourage the development of broad individualized educational plan objectives that leave more room for interpretation (Martin, 1986a, 1986b). The family regretted not having a knowledgeable attorney or the energy for a due process hearing.

The family is worried about Karen's future. They know she is going to learn proportionately fewer skills than most, if not all, of her peers (Brown, et al., 1984). Karen is going to need an increased number of teaching trials to learn those few skills. She frequently will forget skills she does not practice, and then it takes Karen longer to relearn these skills. Karen has problems with transfer and generalization of skills from one place to another. Karen's family must help develop and choose her goals and objectives carefully because they are waging an important battle against time. The family is also aware that Karen enjoys a variety of recreation activities and wants to be with other people. Unfortunately, instead of engaging in opportunities for growth and enjoyment (Barton, Johnson, & Brulle, 1984), frequently Karen finds herself alone and wasting time.

Karen's mother and father, reluctantly, have taken their vacation days on consecutive Mondays during the summer when Karen was not in camp and procured the services of different babysitters for the remainder of the week. They resented that they could not plan an extended, relaxing, and fun vacation. The additional emotional stress certainly affected their jobs and other relationships (Strully & Strully, 1985). Karen's mother also resented that the caregiving responsibility for Karen was almost totally hers.

Karen has very little to do during her free time. A life space analysis of Karen conducted during her school year yields dramatically different results than an analysis completed during the summer. She has no friends and spends a great deal of time engaging in self-stimulatory and destructive behaviors (Ulrich, 1991). Her behaviors reflect an attempt by Karen to communicate her desire to actively participate in enjoyable and satisfying activities (Donnellan, Mirenda, Mesaros, & Fassbender, 1984) through behaviors identified by others as being inappropriate. Because Karen's schedule during the summer was not physically demanding, Karen did not sleep through the night. By the end of the summer, 12 babysitters had resigned their services for Karen. During the summer, Karen had not received opportunities for practice and growth of many of the skills she had mastered during the school year. Karen also had no one in her life—except a very exhausted family—who saw her strengths, gifts, and talents (Mount & O'Brien, 1988). It appeared there was no one who wanted to be around Karen in the beginning of the summer, and now that Karen's skills had regressed throughout most of the summer and her maladaptive behaviors increased, the likelihood of finding someone who would care about Karen seemed remote. Although Karen's family tried desperately to listen to her and made many attempts to meet her needs, in the end they realized they had failed the young woman for whom they cared so deeply.

Karen's family was under tremendous stress and felt extremely frustrated with their lack of options, community support, and their inability to support their daughter (Schwier, 1988). They began to see themselves not as a "family with one member who happens to be severely disabled," but rather as a "Handicapped Family" (Ulrich, 1987). Karen's family began to question their parenting skills and their ability to meet Karen's needs. They sadly joked that in their county, the only way to receive after-school, school holiday, or summer vacation programming was to place Karen in an institution (Friedrich, Wilturner, & Cohen, 1985).

Unfortunately, if Karen's family does become dysfunctional through divorce, abuse, or other tragedies, some people in the community will conclude they failed because a member of the family had a disability—rather than attributing the failure to a lack of community resources and supports. Wolfensberger (1989) wrote:

> Valued people in our society rarely die from broken arms, broken teeth, or hangnails—but as we see over and over all the time, societally devalued people do. For instance, in Bill's case, it seemed that for want of a tooth, the whole denture was lost; for want of the denture, appetite was lost; for want of appetite, nourishment was lost; for want of nourishment, bodily weight and strength were lost; for want of strength, three falls occurred . . . So it might have been that for want of a tooth . . . his life itself was lost.

Community Support for Aaron

Public schools are designed to support families in educating their children. Unfortunately, many people perceive the support of public schools as all that is necessary for families with children with disabilities. However, it is important for us to keep the amount of support received from the public schools in perspective. For example, Aaron (age 15) has a life expectancy of 74 years. His school has a responsibility for his education for approximately 22 years. In a 365-day calendar year, the school year is usually about 180 days, and the school day is approximately 8 a.m.-4 p.m. (including transportation), which totals eight hours or one-third of a 24-hour day. Therefore, the school has responsibility for one-third of the 180 days of the 22 years, a total of 1,300 hours. Aaron's family's responsibility totals 25,700 hours, or approximately 20 times the amount of time their child is under the supervision of the public schools.

During the eight hours of the school day, Aaron has a large support staff (e.g., teacher, aides, therapists, administrators, maintenance and transportation staff, cafeteria workers, clerical personnel), but the other 16 hours he has only the support of his family. The school also places further demands on the parents by expecting them to follow the usual supportive roles of other Parent Teacher Association parents of children without disabilities (Salisbury & Evans, 1988). Although there have been exciting reports of integration facilitators, community developers, leisure and recreation support staff (e.g.,

Ray, Abery, DePaepe, Cameron, & Green, 1989), the only way that Aaron can be in any extracurricular activity such as the school cross country team) is for one of his parents to attend and assist him (Ulrich, 1989). The literature also contains exciting trends for better quality lives and the process for connecting people to their communities (e.g., Vandercook, York, & Forest, 1989). However, in Aaron's last evaluation, his circle of friends was desperately small (O'Brien, 1988). There are some wonderful resource materials to help families learn to choose their priorities, address stress, and manage their problems (Goldfard et al., 1987). Yet, many family members pray that their child dies before they do, because even with their strongest advocacy efforts, they cannot meet their child's needs, especially if they choose the value system which embraces integration.

Whose Responsibility Is It Anyway?

A research team from the University of Minnesota—Minneapolis asked professionals from community education agencies: "Who should be responsible for the educational and recreational programs of their students on weekends, holidays, and in the summer?" They asked the same question of professionals in parks and recreation. The investigators reported that 93 percent of community education agencies named the parks and recreation staff, and 78 percent of the parks and recreation staff chose the community education agencies (Schleien & Werder, 1985). This inability of professionals to assume responsibilities for meeting the leisure needs of students with disabilities is extremely disconcerting for families. Families are often forced to compromise needs of family members with disabilities in order to access leisure programs and services (Shapiro, 1994).

To illustrate the many frustrations parents feel toward the absence of adequate community leisure support, Mary Ulrich continues to have a dream that haunts her. The dream begins in a community recreation center during a "handicapped family swim night." Her family (husband Tom, sons Tommy and Aaron, and Mary) and friends from a parent coalition are all splashing and playing in the water. The pool is an excellent facility which has very new equipment and has been carefully painted with black racing lines across the bottom. On "handicapped swim night" professionals with an "LG" (Life Guard) on their T-shirts are stationed between each black line. The LG has been assigned the responsibility of saving the lives of people drowning in his or her area. Their areas are divided by the large black lines at the bottom of the pool. Each LG has had specialized training in specific aspects of lifesaving and possesses the necessary education and credentials to make it obvious he or she is an expert.

As the families are swimming, they notice that the pool water starts to change. Instead of calm water, now there are swift currents. The water keeps rising and whirlpools are pulling them under. Tom and Mary attempt to keep Aaron and Tommy above water. The rest of the families are also struggling. The participants paddle and try to go to the side of the pool, but they continue to be thrown back into deeper water. They cry to the LGs on the side of the pool, but the LGs do not seem to hear them. Every time a family member sinks to the bottom of the pool, it seems they land on a black line. Finally, the families all gather in the middle of the pool and shout in one loud voice, "Help, please help, we cannot do it ourselves." The families' shouting causes the LGs to look at the family members. However, the LGs appear confused because the family members continue to land on the black lines, and the LGs cannot decide whose territory the family members are in. Each LG has specific rules and guidelines regarding who they can save. The situation gets grave. One or two of the LGs throw life preservers into the pool or shout encouragement (e.g., "Swim faster," "Remember the strokes I taught you," "We are doing all we can," "You parents just need an organized effort," and "It is up to you, parents, you can do it!"). In time, the water begins moving more swiftly, and the families become weaker. As the situation gets desperate, the first LG turns to the second LG and says, "What do you think?" The second turns to the third LG and says, "What do you think?" This line of questioning continues from one LG to another until finally, all eyes are on the Head LG (who is sitting high in a chair in the middle of the facility). As the families sink into unconsciousness, the Main LG begins shaking his head as he frantically pages through a rule book (Ulrich, 1986).

Coping with Stress Through Family Support

According to Brazelton (1983), children produce an element of stress for parents, and children with disabilities are no exception (Rousey, Best, & Blacher, 1992). Although children with disabilities can contribute in positive ways to their families (Turnbull & Behr, 1986), they have daily care needs and associated problems that exacerbate difficulties for parents (Rousey, Best, & Blacher, 1992). In addition, the transition periods are almost always a time of great stress for families (Olson et al., 1983). However, the family who has a child with a disability may encounter greater stress during transition, especially if the transition period is delayed or does not occur (Wikler, Wasow, & Hatfield, 1983).

Rowitz (1992) reported that many families who have a member who has a disability perceive they do not have control over what happens to them. In addition, they often do not know how to access resources and feel intimidated by the system. Saetermoe, Widaman, and Borthwick-Duffy (1991), described the situation where many parents who have a child with a disability are working and report that they have no free time and are barely able to take care of their own responsibilities. These families often must struggle with the rising costs of many services such as respite care, transportation, and medical support (Stark, 1992). Stark and Goldsburg (1990) reported that family members become frustrated because they feel there are very few resources provided to them to continue their efforts in taking care of their son or daughter.

For some people, having a relative with a disability alters family roles (Gill, 1994). According to Gill (1994), children often feel a deep sense of anger and loss when a parent no longer functions in an accustomed manner as a result of a disability or caring for a family member with a disability. Struggles faced by families of people with disabilities include financial and time constraints, searching for and accessing resources, experiencing fatigue, and social isolation (Gill, 1994). Family duties and responsibilities may change from member to member as the realities of living with a person with a disability become apparent.

Cobb (1976) stated that "social support" emphasizes personal interactions that lead a person to feel cared for, valued, and included in mutually dependent relationships. Social support influences families' ability to cope and adjust (Flynt, Wood, & Scott, 1992; Gill, 1994). Family support programs should be designed to prevent or delay out-of-home placement of a family member with disabilities and improve the caregiving capacity of the family (Krauss, 1986). Agosta, Jennings, and Bradley (1985) reported that family support programs have accelerated dramatically in the past decade.

Since resources remain a significant factor in closing the gaps in family support programs, Herman and Hazel (1991) called for public policy to place greater emphasis and reliance on family-based care for people with disabilities. Herman and Hazel noted that responsible public agencies (such as leisure services providers) need to emphasize family-centered approaches to services as indicated in Figure 5.2 (see page 86). Family-centered approaches to leisure services delivery will require support by each professional to help families overcome barriers to leisure participation.

In a review of family leisure and leisure services, Shaw (1992, p. 13) reported that "family leisure is an important aspect of leisure and an important part of life for many people in our society." Shaw also noted that family-oriented activities within and outside the home are the most common forms of leisure activity. Research has consistently demonstrated that family time and family leisure are highly valued (Shaw, 1992). Based on her thorough review of families and leisure, Shaw suggested that recreation programming for

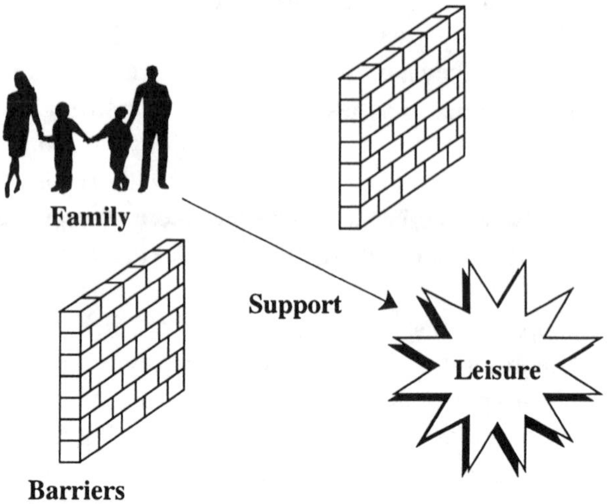

Figure 5.2 Family support by leisure services providers that reduces barriers.

families represents a challenge because of the mix of ages and both sexes, and because of the variety of interests, skills and needs that individual family members bring with them. This challenge is often increased when a member of the family possesses a disabling condition.

Conclusion

Leisure is not an "extra" or luxury; it is a right of all human beings. As a result, a recommendation to service providers for individuals with severe disabilities is in order. If we truly embrace the concepts of integration and normalization, and if we really want families to resist institutional care in favor of the community, then stronger support systems must be developed to facilitate community-based leisure participation for persons with severe disabilities and their families. Therefore, in addition to the areas of "family support," "supported education," "supported work," and "supported living," another area should be developed and encouraged entitled "supported leisure." Supported leisure would require professionals to examine the individual desires and needs of people with severe disabilities and concentrate on coordination of resources and development of community support systems. As exemplified in the simulation described at the beginning of this chapter, through a cooperative approach to meeting individual leisure needs, professionals will be in a position to assist families by helping them carry some of their boxes.

To illustrate the value of participating in community recreation with one's family, the following statement by Wanda is provided. Wanda made this response when discussing how she felt when going to an amusement park with her family. The trip to the amusement park occurred soon after Wanda returned to her community following completion of a treatment program conducted at a rehabilitation center.

> I just had so much fun, I loved it and I was out with my family and I had like aunts and uncles and cousins were there with my parents and brothers and sister and it was really fun. It was . . . and you know we just had a great time and didn't care about anything and it was just terrific.

Discussion Questions

1. What are five suggestions for community support that could help Karen, the adolescent described in this chapter, and her family?

2. What is social support?

3. Why is it helpful for families with members with disabilities to receive social support?

4. Why is it important for community education agencies and parks and recreation staff to work together to meet the leisure needs of individuals with disabilities and their families?

5. How does support help families to alleviate their stress?

6. What is supported leisure?

Chapter 6

Be Aware of Barriers to Leisure

"I have learned that success is to be measured not so much by the position that one has reached in life, as by the obstacles which one has overcome by trying to succeed."
—Booker T. Washington

Orientation Activity: Whose Problem is it?

Directions When Alone: Read the following scenario. On a separate piece of paper, write a brief paragraph describing what you feel the relevance of the scenario is to understanding people with disabilities.

Directions With Others: After dividing into small groups, have each person describe their interpretation to the group. Everyone record the most important points. When everyone has presented their ideas, determine how many different interpretations there were of the scenario. After a specified time, discuss your response with the entire group.

> I thought my wife was losing her hearing, so one day I decided to test it. I quietly walked in the front door and stood 30 feet behind her. "Suzanne," I said, "can you hear me?" There was no response so I moved 20 feet behind her. "Suzanne," I repeated, "can you hear me?" Still no reply. I advanced to 10 feet and asked, "Now can you hear me?" "Yes dear," Suzanne answered, "for the *third* time, yes!"

Debriefing

Many recreation professionals have observed that people with disabilities have problems. Some people with disabilities may rarely initiate contact with others, at times individuals may not follow rules and "misbehave," some people may completely withdraw from participation, and others may even indicate a lack of interest in available recreation programs. If recreation professionals view these problems as originating from the person as a result of their disability, little can be done to facilitate inclusive leisure services. The man in the above scenario had determined that the problem was his wife's, not his.

If the problems experienced by people with disabilities are viewed from the perspective that professionals, family members and community members contribute to these problems, then we are in a position to assist individuals with disabilities in many ways. For example, some people may rarely attempt to communicate, because many of us may control communication exchanges by not waiting long enough to allow an individual who may take a bit longer to communicate to actually do so. In addition, at times, we may allow people with disabilities very few opportunities to make choices; these people may misbehave because they feel that their few freedoms are threatened. Other people may withdraw from participation as a result of repeated failures within a program. In these situations, without intervention, people may begin to feel helpless. As a final example, some people with disabilities may not appear interested in participating because of an overemphasis on external rewards such as prizes and trophies.

In situations where people with disabilities encounter problems, examination of what we do may be helpful in determining the best way to overcome these barriers to participation. This chapter will highlight some of the barriers encountered by people with disabilities and the role we may play in these problems. Ways to overcome some of these barriers have been discussed in previous chapters and will be addressed in subsequent chapters. As you consider the orientation activity ask yourself the following questions:

1. What are some other problems people with disabilities may encounter when attempting to participate in community recreation programs?
2. How might recreation professionals be contributing to these problems?
3. What can be done to overcome these problems?

Introduction

When asked to describe the leading barrier they experience, people with disabilities consistently report that negative attitudes is the most devastating barrier. These negative attitudes, described in Chapter 1, do not occur in isolation. People with disabilities perceive these negative attitudes and respond accordingly.

There are some explanations of human behavior which provide insight into the problems people with disabilities experience relative to their leisure participation. Therefore, at the beginning of this chapter, information describing "reactance" is provided to help identify one reason why some people may disregard a professional's directions. In addition, a description of one reason why some people seem to give up and stop attending recreation services is presented. The perception of "helplessness" some potential leisure participants possess and the negative impact this perception can have on participation is also provided. Other information presented in this chapter includes a description of the impact that environments which are controlling or unresponsive have on people's motivation to participate. Warnings against an overemphasis on direct competition and problems associated with discrepancies between challenges and skills conclude the chapter.

Psychological Reactance

Brehm (1977) stated that the experience of freedom involves a set of behaviors which requires physical and psychological skills. In addition, individuals must have the knowledge and understanding that they are able to make a choice in order to experience freedom. Behaviors that are free include only those acts that are realistically possible for the individual. According to Brehm, given a set of free behaviors, "reactance" will occur when any of these behaviors is eliminated or threatened. The relationship between freedom and reactance is illustrated in Figure 6.1.

People demonstrate reactance when they try to regain free behaviors that are eliminated or threatened. The occurrence of reactance increases the desirability of the eliminated or threatened behavior; that is, the behavior

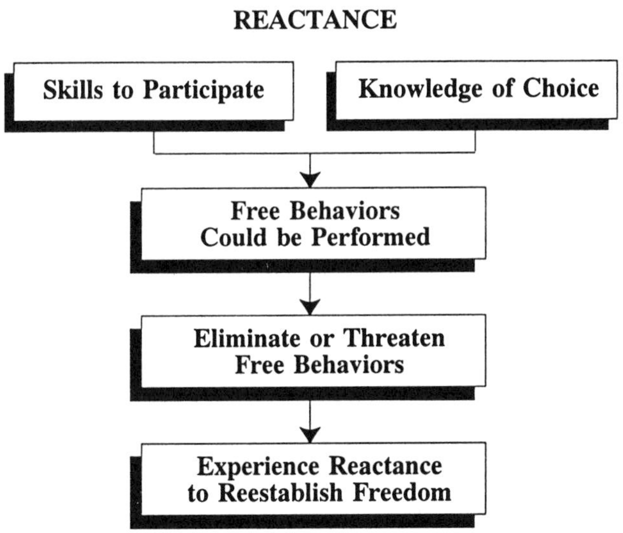

Figure 6.1 Relationship between freedom and reactance.

becomes more attractive to the individual. For instance, as depicted in Figure 6.2, when a child is about to select one recreation activity from among several alternatives that are all attractive (e.g., hiking, dancing, reading), elimination of one alternative by an adult (e.g., hiking) will result in that activity becoming more attractive and desirable.

A person who experiences reactance will be motivated to remove the threat to the free behavior or regain the lost free behavior. When reactance occurs, the person tends to engage in the threatened free behavior, engage in behaviors that imply continued engagement in free behaviors, and encourage

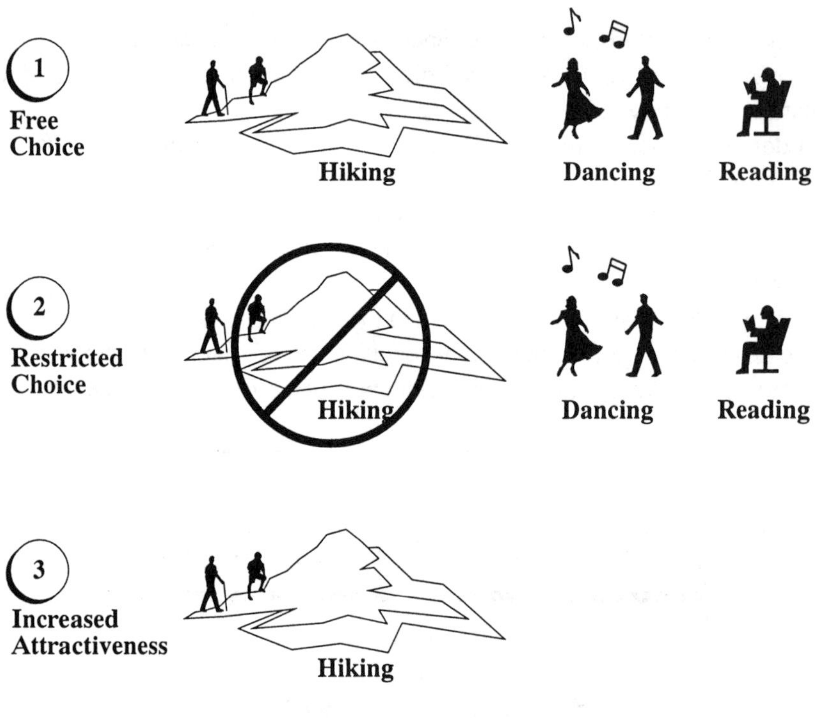

Figure 6.2 With reactance comes an increased attractiveness of unavailable alternatives.

other people of similar abilities and status to engage in threatened or eliminated behaviors. For example, a person playing a basketball game is told by a recreation professional to stop yelling obscenities. The individual may continue or even accelerate the use of obscenities, may reduce the use of obscenities but increase physical aggression, or may encourage other players to use obscenities.

Relinquishing Freedom

When people expect to influence a certain outcome, but find their control and freedom jeopardized, initially they exert more effort to establish control (reactance). However, Wortman and Brehm (1975) reported that the perception of helplessness will occur if people become convinced that further attempts will not produce an outcome. Leary and Miller (1986) explained that people find it difficult to assess their ability to control a situation when they first encounter events that are troublesome for them to control. Often, people initially assume that the cause of difficulty is unstable and specific to the situation. Therefore, they increase their attempts to exert control. That is, they feel that their failure may be related to factors that could change the next time they try (e.g., the difficulty of the recreation activity, people associated with the activity, their luck, the amount of effort and concentration they expend). However, if they are still unable to gain control after repeated attempts to do so, they may begin to assume the outcome is uncontrollable and will experience helplessness.

A person will eventually give up the desire for freedom when reestablishment of freedom proves impossible. The length of time required for individuals to stop believing that they have freedom to engage in the eliminated or threatened free behavior depends, in part, on the certainty of elimination. The more apparent the inability to experience the free behavior becomes, the more quickly the person will give up that freedom. Given the obvious elimination of an important freedom, an initial demonstration of a sharp increase in the desire to engage in the eliminated behavior will occur (Wortman & Brehm, 1975). Eventual surrendering of freedom will follow. The surrendering is equivalent to the condition referred to as "learned helplessness."

Learned Helplessness

Seligman and colleagues first used the phrase "learned helplessness" to describe responses of animals to uncontrollable shock (Overmier & Seligman, 1967; Seligman & Maier, 1967). Following investigations with animals to test the theory, Seligman (1975) described helplessness as a psychological state that frequently results when events are uncontrollable. Events are uncontrollable when they are independent of a person's voluntary responses. Voluntary responses can be modified by reinforcement or punishment. That is, certain consequences of voluntary behavior will increase the likelihood of the occurrence of the behavior (reward) or decrease the likelihood of the behavior (punishment). Those behaviors that are not voluntary are reflexes or instincts.

As individuals are exposed to uncontrollable events, they begin to learn that responding is futile. That is, they feel that it just does not matter what they do because they will fail. This learning of helplessness reduces the incentive to respond, which decreases motivation. Learned helplessness undermines a person's motivation to respond, reduces the ability to learn that responding works, and results in emotional disturbance (e.g., depression, anxiety). The occurrence of learned helplessness is presented in Figure 6.3.

Human Helplessness

Experiments conducted in the 1970s substantiated the presence of learned helplessness in humans (e.g., Abramson, Seligman, & Teasdale, 1978). Garber and Seligman (1980) recognized that once people perceive the absence of a relationship between their actions and the desired consequence, they attribute their helplessness to a cause. In other words, the person believes that no matter what he does, he will be unable to achieve his goal. Two types of learned helplessness will now be described and are presented in Figure 6.4.

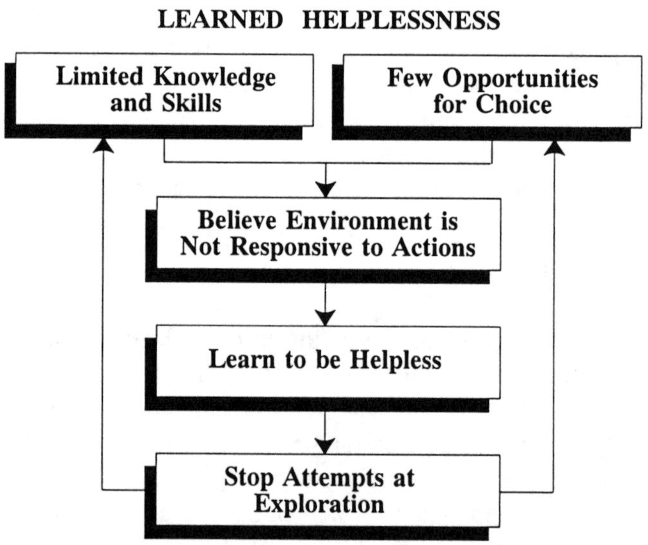

Figure 6.3 Conditions encouraging learned helplessness with subsequent results.

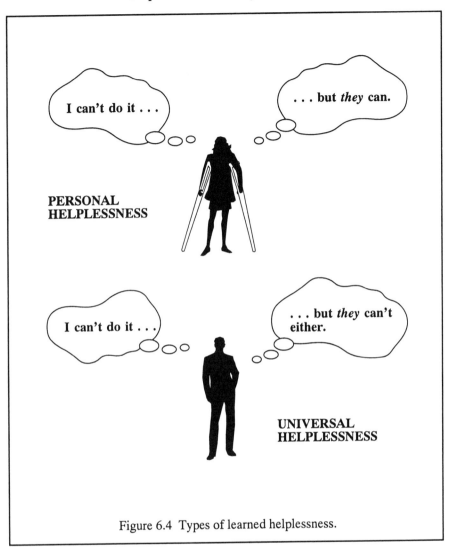

Figure 6.4 Types of learned helplessness.

Personal Helplessness

Human helplessness is perceived at a level related to oneself and related to other people. When people expect outcomes not to be contingent on their own responses yet expect the outcome to be contingent on others' actions, personal helplessness is experienced. This personal helplessness results from failures that erode self-determination. For example, Laura may see other people receiving instruction in snow skiing and think that it is fine for those people to learn to ski, but she could never learn to do it.

Universal Helplessness

Some people also may expect outcomes not to be contingent on their own responses; however, they may expect that outcomes are not contingent on other people's actions, either. This form of helplessness is identified as universal helplessness, and produces feelings of hopelessness. For example, Matthew may decide not to attend a program on volunteerism, thinking that nobody really wants anyone else's help and, even if other people try to help, it would not do any good.

In each of the aforementioned situations, the outcome expectancies are not absolute; rather, they are on a continuum ranging from the expectation that outcomes are totally noncontingent on one's responses to expectations of limited controllability. That is, helplessness comes in degrees. People do not necessarily adopt the perception of helplessness or mastery in every situation. The challenge for leisure services professionals is to attempt to move participants in their programs away from perceptions of helplessness toward a more mastery-oriented orientation.

Consequences of Helplessness

Learned helplessness may be revealed in a person's cognition, emotional level, and motivation. These three consequences of helplessness are important considerations for professionals attempting to facilitate leisure participation.

Cognition

In reference to cognition, people who learn to be helpless will experience difficulty understanding that their responses produce outcomes. Consequently, they will have problems learning to take control of their lives. For example, Thomas, who is attending a dance class, may feel that no matter how hard he tries, he will never learn to dance. As a result of this belief, he finds it difficult to concentrate and learn what is being presented.

Emotions

Learned helplessness also can be manifested at an emotional level. People who expect that outcomes are independent of their responses will tend to have a depressed affect. Depression is likely when people perceive that they cannot control an outcome that is possible. As individuals attribute their negative outcomes to internal, stable, and global factors, and their positive outcomes to external, unstable, specific behaviors, they experience a reduction in self-esteem. For example, if each time Samuel experiences failure in outdoor adventure recreation activities he attributes his failures to his abilities (which are internal, stable, and global), and attributes his successes to luck (which is external, stable, and specific), he may experience a reduction in self-esteem and be unhappy.

Motivation

Individuals' levels of motivation can be directly influenced by a perception of helplessness. As individuals expect that their responding is futile, they will experience a reduction in their initiation of voluntary responses. If Cleo feels that no matter how hard she tries to learn judo she will never learn it, she will not be motivated to go to judo class.

Typically, people with disabilities have less knowledge and fewer skills than their same-age peers. Consequently, they are afforded fewer opportunities to make choices and demonstrate self-initiated leisure participation (Dattilo, 1991). At times, the environment does not respond to their attempts to initiate leisure participation. Repeated futile experiences result in the perception that one is helpless. With the perception of helplessness comes an elimination of attempts to explore the environment. As exploration decreases, opportunities to experience enjoyment also decline.

Interaction of Failure and Helplessness

People respond to failure in different ways at different times. The manner in which people react to failure is dependent on their perspective. Two different orientations (mastery and helplessness) are presented.

Mastery Orientation

For some people (on some occasions), failure can result in escalated effort, intensified concentration, increased persistence, heightened sophistication of problem-solving strategies, and enhanced performance. When people respond in this way, they are identified as having a mastery orientation (see Figure 6.5, page 98). If they assume a mastery orientation, they may:

(a) perceive their mistakes are rectifiable;
(b) view their failure as a result of a lack of effort;
(c) look forward to the future;
(d) emphasize the positive aspects of their failures; and/or
(e) engage in active problem solving (Dweck & Light, 1980).

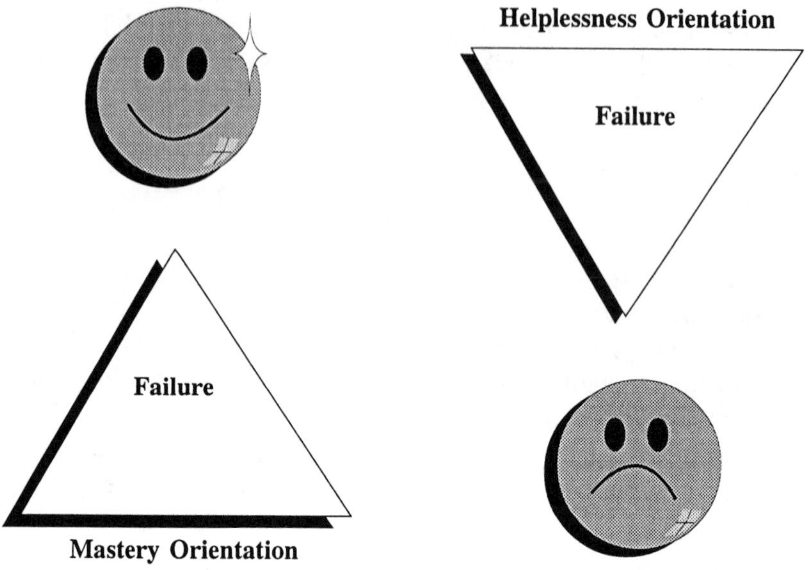

Figure 6.5 Different perspectives on failure from a mastery versus a helplessness orientation.

Helplessness Orientation

Other people (on other occasions) may respond to failure with curtailed effort, reduced concentration, decreased persistence, a deterioration of problem-solving strategies, and a disruption in performance. These responses are indications that a person has learned to be helpless. Dweck and Light (1980) stated that if people come to expect that they cannot control outcomes, they may:

(a) perceive that their mistakes are inevitable;
(b) view their failure as a result of a lack of ability;
(c) dwell on the present and focus on negative aspects of a situation; and
(d) stop attempts at solving the problem associated with failure.

As previously stated, individuals with disabilities have an increased chance of experiencing reactance and, with repeated failure to produce an effect, perceptions of helplessness. The presence of these conditions decreases the ability of the individual to experience the self-determination necessary for enjoyment. Therefore, services provided by recreation professionals that try to enhance self-determination are needed.

A Controlling Environment

A controlling environment does not respond to people's initiatives; however, it does demand behaviors from individuals. When an environment directs and controls people, they often experience extrinsic motivation. The presence of rewards and deadlines that pressure people toward specific outcomes tends to undermine intrinsic motivation, promote extrinsic compliance or defiance, and inhibit enjoyment. Deci and Ryan (1985, p. 57) noted that:

> research has substantiated that extrinsic rewards and controls can affect people's experience of self-determination. In such cases, the events will induce a shift in the perceived locus of causality from internal to external, a decrement in intrinsic motivation for the target behavior, less persistence at the activity in the absence of external contingencies, and less interest in and enjoyment of the activity.

Studies by Lepper and Greene (1978), among others, have demonstrated such effects. Typically, children are "playing" at some activity (e.g., drawing) and then experimenters offer to pay the children for the products they produce (e.g., drawings). "Productivity" increases while rewards are offered (the children draw more). However, when rewards are withdrawn, children show less interest in the activity than they did before rewards were offered and less than children who were not offered rewards. Referred to as the **"over-justification effect,"** such studies show that intrinsic motivation can be undermined by extrinsic rewards. The relationship between motivation and overjustification is illustrated in Figure 6.6 (see page 100).

As an example, Deci (1971) had two groups of students work on a set of puzzles. Half the students were rewarded with a dollar for each puzzle they solved, and the others received no reward. All students were then observed in a subsequent free-choice period, and results indicated that the students receiving rewards spent significantly less free-choice time with the puzzles than did the students who were not rewarded. Deci and Olsen (1989) reported that numerous other studies have shown that across ages, sexes and tasks, extrinsic rewards such as money (Deci, 1972), prizes (Harackiewicz, 1979), food (Ross, 1975), and good-player awards (Lepper, Greene, & Nisbett, 1973) all tend to decrease intrinsic motivation.

MOTIVATION AND OVERJUSTIFICATION

Figure 6.6 The relationship between motivation and overjustification.

In another example related to sport, Orlick and Mosher (1978) initially provided children with a free-choice pretest period. Next the children played in either a reward condition where they received a task-contingent trophy or a no-reward condition. Four days later, they returned for a post-test free-choice period. The children who had participated to obtain the trophy displayed a decrease in free-choice time spent on the task, as compared to the students who did not receive any rewards. Results of the Orlick and Mosher study and similar studies (e.g., Halliwell, 1978) suggest that extrinsic incentives can undermine intrinsic motivation for interesting recreation activities (Deci & Olsen, 1989). For example, when a coach overemphasizes the need to win the championship trophy, the enjoyment associated with participation in a baseball league may be reduced for many of the participants.

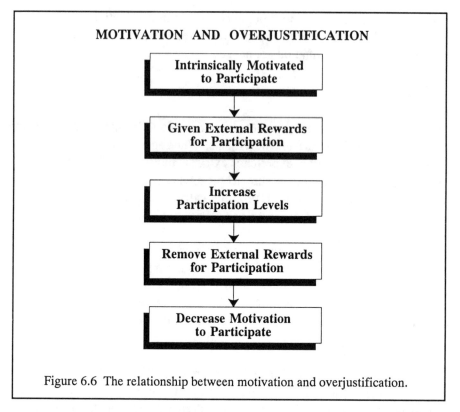

Unresponsive Environments

Some individuals experience environments which do not respond to their initiatives. As a result, outcomes are perceived to be unrelated to their behaviors. In this type of an environment, contingencies (the relationship between an action and associated consequences) are not clear and cannot be mastered by the individual. According to Deci (1980), capricious environments that contain negative feedback and noncontingencies tend to erode all forms of motivation, result in impersonal causality, and stifle instrumental behavior. When professionals provide general (i.e., nonspecific) praise or criticism to people with disabilities as they attempt to learn a new leisure skill without regard to the effectiveness of their responses, professionals will inhibit, rather than stimulate, learning and a desire to master the skill. Participants will have difficulty determining the efficacy of their actions when professionals fail to provide them with informational feedback.

Overemphasis on Competition

Competition can make many recreation activities fun and exciting. Deci and Olsen (1989) stated that in such activities—swimming laps, for example, or shooting baskets—people can compete against themselves (i.e., against some internal standard that a person has set). This **indirect competition** (Ross & Van den Haag, 1957) provides purpose and direction and is the basis for satisfaction when the standards are met. **Direct competition**, which involves pitting oneself against another, can add even more fun, excitement, and challenge, and as such can encourage intrinsic motivation (Deci & Olsen, 1989). Doing well at a competition (direct as well as indirect) provides clear competence feedback and could enhance a person's intrinsic motivation.

Deci and Ryan (1985) have warned us that a focus on winning, rather than on doing well at an activity, can be problematic. The focus on winning makes the activity into an instrument for winning rather than something that is enjoyed for its intrinsic properties (Deci & Olsen, 1989). Direct competition can cause mutual distrust and deceit (Kelley & Thibaut, 1969), as well as impaired performance and aggression (Berkowitz, 1962; Deutsch, 1969). For example, when participants in a painting program are only told that they need to use more highlights and avoid overshadowing even after they have made considerable progress, they may become frustrated. At the same time, if a person completes a project and the instructor never seems to have time to provide useful feedback, the participants may lose their desire for the activity.

As an example, Deci, Betley, Kahle, Abrams, and Porac (1981) had two groups of students work on puzzles, with each student working in the presence of another person. Students in one group were instructed to solve each puzzle faster than the other person, while students in the other group were told to solve the puzzles as quickly as they could. When given a chance for free choice afterwards, the direct, face-to-face competition led to a decrease in intrinsic motivation. In a similar example, Vallerand, Gauvin, and Halliwell (1986) reported that competition undermined the intrinsic motivation of 10- to 12-year-old children. The children worked with a motor task, and those who competed at it spent less subsequent free-choice time working with the activity than those who had not competed.

People tend to experience competition as controlling and, in all likelihood, they become ego-involved in winning; they feel like they have to win (Deci & Olsen, 1989). Deci and Olsen explained that even when they do win, although they feel satisfied, participants are less intrinsically motivated for the activity itself and will be motivated to continue competing and will still want to win; however, the activity itself will no longer be inherently rewarding. Weinberg and Ragan (1979) demonstrated that participants who had won a competition were more eager to compete again than those who had not, but considering the aforementioned examples, they are less eager to engage in the activity in the absence of the competition.

Boredom and Anxiety

Although recreation activities can offer people opportunities that allow them to control their lives, increase their personal development, experiment with roles, and take part in self-appraisal (Kleiber & Rickards, 1986), leisure and free time themselves are not necessarily positive, nor do they necessarily produce positive results (Caldwell, Smith, & Weissinger, 1992). Negative leisure behavior often is motivated by a lack of optimal arousal or a need for challenge (Iso-Ahola & Crowley, 1991).

Boredom and anxiety may occur because of an incompatible match between skill level and challenge. For example, as seen in Figure 6.7, too little challenge coupled with a high skill level is likely to produce boredom and, conversely, too much challenge and too little skill may produce anxiety (Caldwell, Smith, & Weissinger, 1992). People tend to be motivated to participate in activities that require performance at their maximal level or require them to "stretch" and expand their skills to some degree.

At times, **boredom** may occur as the result of activities being perceived as worthless, meaningless, frustrating or monotonous (Hamilton, 1983). Iso-Ahola and Weissinger (1990) suggested that frustration is a result of perceived or actual constraints that limit the availability of satisfying experiences. For example, Nathan attended a promotion for a cruise and immediately had difficulty understanding the terms used by the cruise leader. Nathan may become frustrated and bored with the presentation and elect not to go on the cruise because of the boring presentation.

On the other hand, Martens, Vealey, & Burton (1990) referred to **anxiety** as negative expectations about personal success in an activity. For example,

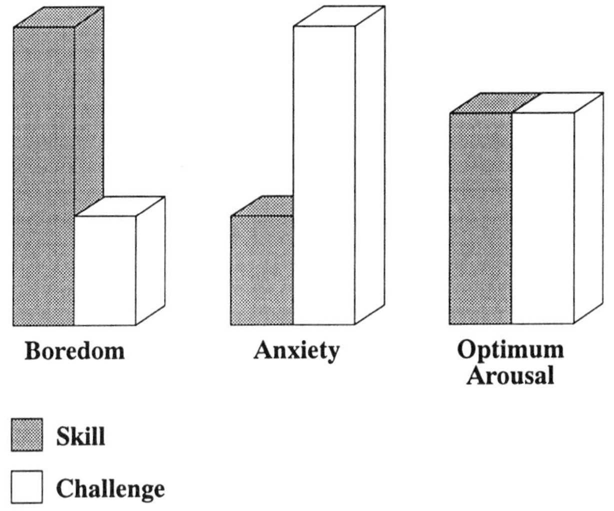

Figure 6.7 Impact of levels of skill and challenge on motivation.

many people with disabilities experience repeated failure when engaged in various activities. As repeated failure is experienced by some people, their fears may increase and result in anxiety.

People tend to gravitate to recreation activities providing them with challenges that require some effort and concentration while permitting some degree of success. For example, a group of people were given the choice to play ring toss. They were first instructed to throw several rings to a post at their feet (where they consistently achieved ringers), one a few feet away (which they had about a 50-percent success rate), and one several yards away (where they rarely, if ever, achieved a ringer). After being given the opportunity to try each post, participants were asked to throw rings toward the post of their choosing. The majority of the participants chose the post a few feet away because it required them to concentrate and afforded them the opportunity for success. They reported that throwing rings at the post at their feet was boring and throwing at the post far away was frustrating.

Conclusion

Theories such as reactance and learned helplessness help clarify difficulties experienced by some individuals in becoming self-determined. These difficulties often result in the failure to experience enjoyment. Sensitivity to barriers experienced by people with disabilities such as reactance, learned helplessness, overjustification, boredom, and anxiety, should help professionals design recreation programs that help alleviate these barriers rather than contribute to their development.

Discussion Questions

1. What is the leading barrier to participation as reported by people with disabilities?
2. How can reactance influence leisure behavior?
3. What causes people to perceive helplessness?
4. What is learned helplessness?
5. What are two types of learned helplessness?
6. What are the three consequences of helplessness?
7. What are the two different reactions people experience to the interaction of failure and helplessness?
8. How does the overjustification effect undermine intrinsic motivation?
9. What are two types of competition?
10. How do the two types of competition influence motivation?
11. What is the relationship between skill, challenge, boredom and anxiety?

Section B

Facilitate Participation

Chapter 7

Respond to the Americans with Disabilities Act

"Ignorance of the law excuses no man."
—John Selden

Orientation Activity: Describe ADA

Directions When Alone: On a separate sheet of paper, write a brief paragraph describing the Americans With Disabilities Act (ADA). Write it as if you were explaining the ADA to someone who was not aware of this piece of legislation.

Directions With Others: With your description of ADA, move about the room, find a person, introduce yourself and find out the person's name. After introductions, read the paragraph to the person. Have that person tell you what he or she learned from your description. Record the key points that the person reports back to you. Listen to that person's description. Tell the person what you learned from the description. Make notes on important ideas you learned from this person. Move about the room and repeat this exercise with other people until you are given a signal to stop. Come together as an entire group and discuss what you have learned.

Debriefing

Essentially civil-rights legislation for persons with disabilities, the ADA guarantees the rights of full inclusion into the mainstream of American life. While there have been some improvements toward integration during the last decade, segregation and discrimination of individuals with disabilities continues to be a pervasive social problem. The opportunities created by ADA should transform the quality of life for all persons in society (Wehman, 1993, p. xxi).

Reflecting on the orientation activity consider the following questions:

1. What are some of the implications of the ADA?
2. Why was it necessary to have the ADA?
3. Who is influenced by ADA?

Introduction

John McGovern is considered by many to possess extensive understanding of Public Law 101-336, The Americans with Disabilities Act (ADA), which was signed into law on July 26, 1990. Attorney McGovern's work experience in the field of recreation and leisure provides him with a unique opportunity to help professionals understand the impact of ADA on public and private community recreation agencies. Many of his writings and notes from his presentations (e.g., McGovern, 1990; 1991a; 1991b; 1992) were consulted during the development of sections of this chapter. In addition, the text entitled "ADA Mandate for Social Change" by Paul Wehman (1993) also was found to be helpful in the preparation of this chapter.

ADA is a civil-rights law that is intended to eliminate discrimination against people with disabilities by the guarantee of equal opportunities, full community participation, enhanced independent living, heightened self-sufficiency, and access to every critical area of American life. Other disability rights laws preceded the ADA. The Architectural Barriers Act, enacted in 1968, requires that all facilities built in part or in whole with federal funds be accessible to individuals with disabilities. The Rehabilitation Act of 1973 requires agencies that receive federal funding to make their programs, services and activities accessible. Compared to the ADA, these earlier laws are limited in both scope and impact. Under the ADA, protections found in the public sector are now extended to the private sector as well.

Public facilities, such as quasi-public recreation agencies, restaurants, hotels, theaters, retail stores, museums, libraries, and parks, cannot discriminate on the basis of disability. Only private clubs and religious organizations are exempt. Reasonable changes in policies, practices, and procedures must be made to avoid discrimination. According to Parent (1993), prior to the ADA people with disabilities were segregated in employment, housing and recreation. It is hoped that this landmark legislation will encourage and empower people with disabilities to explore preferences and pursue choices, including recreation and leisure experiences (Breslin, 1994).

Consider the Major Sections of ADA

The ADA contains five major Titles illustrated in Figure 7.1. The five sections are described briefly below.

Title I prohibits employers from discriminating against "otherwise qualified individuals with a disability" in any employment action.

Title II, Subtitle A, prohibits the more than 85,000 state and local government agencies from discriminating against people with disabilities in the provision of services and opportunities. Title II, Subtitle B, prohibits providers of public transportation from discriminating against people with disabilities.

Title III prohibits private entities that offer public accommodations, goods, facilities and services, such as restaurants, theaters, hotels, zoos, and museums that provide public accommodations, from discriminating against people with disabilities.

Title IV requires the availability of communication systems for individuals with hearing impairments.

Title V covers a variety of miscellaneous issues, including regulation and enforcement.

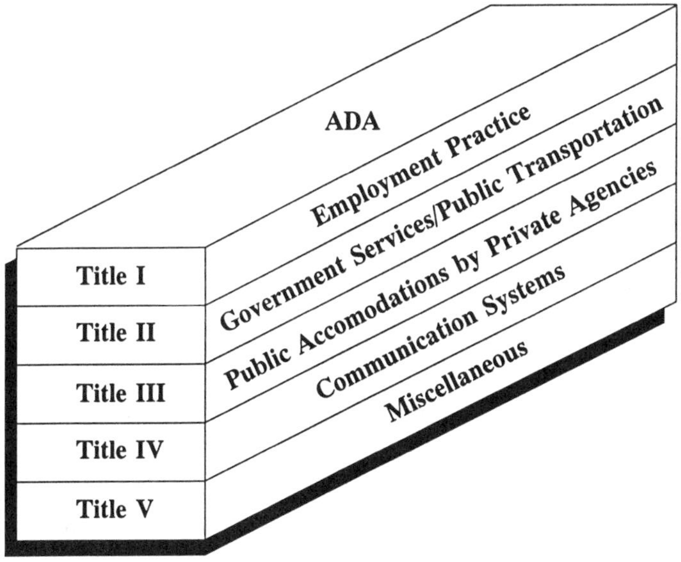

Figure 7.1 The five major titles of the Americans with Disabilities Act.

The ADA addresses many issues that facilitate realization of the rights of each person. The major areas ADA addresses relate to:

(a) employment;
(b) transportation;
(c) private agencies;
(d) government agencies; and
(e) telecommunications.

Know Who Must Comply

Employment

Employers may not discriminate against an individual with a disability in hiring, promotion, or other employment activity, if the person is otherwise qualified for the job. Employers can ask about one's ability to perform a job, but cannot inquire if someone has a disability or subject a person to tests that tend to screen out people with disabilities. Employers will need to provide "reasonable accommodation" to individuals with disabilities. This includes steps such as job restructuring and modification of equipment. Employers do not need to provide accommodations that impose an "undue hardship" on business operations. Employers of fewer than 15 people are exempt from Title I, unless the employer is a state or local government.

Transportation

Public transit buses that have been ordered after Aug. 26, 1990, must be accessible to individuals with disabilities. Transit authorities must provide comparable transportation services to people with disabilities who cannot use fixed-route bus services, unless an undue burden would result.

Private Agencies

Private entities that offer goods, services and facilities to the public may not discriminate against people with disabilities. Auxiliary aids and services must be provided to individuals with disabilities, unless an undue burden would result. Physical barriers in existing facilities must be removed, if removal is readily achievable, inexpensive and easy to do. If not, alternative methods of providing the services must be offered, if they are readily achievable. All new construction and alterations of facilities must be accessible.

Government Agencies

State and local governments may not discriminate against qualified individuals with disabilities. All government facilities, services, and communications must be accessible.

Telecommunication Systems

Companies offering telephone service to the general public must offer telephone relay services to individuals who use text telephones (TTs) or similar devices.

Take Necessary Actions

Although ADA requirements vary according to the type (e.g., state, private) and size of the agency, many procedures outlined by ADA would be beneficial for any recreation agency to follow. The guidelines presented in Figure 7.2 (page 112) are procedures that have been gleaned from ADA and would assist agencies in providing inclusive community based programs. Not all of the following suggestions are required of all agencies by ADA; however, they are being made in an attempt to assist recreation professionals in meeting the spirit of ADA.

Plan for Inclusion

Provide notice of compliance. The intent of the agency to comply with the ADA and how this intent will be achieved should be provided. For example, some agencies may report that compliance to ADA will occur by:

(a) making reasonable accommodations such as changing rules, policies, and procedures;
(b) removing barriers of architecture, transportation, and communication, and
(c) providing auxiliary aids and services to enable people with a disability to enjoy the benefits of participation.

This information should be reported in all agency materials. Business cards and letterhead should also include the agency TT phone number.

Conduct a self-analysis. To determine deficits in delivery systems and barriers to participation which result in discrimination against people with

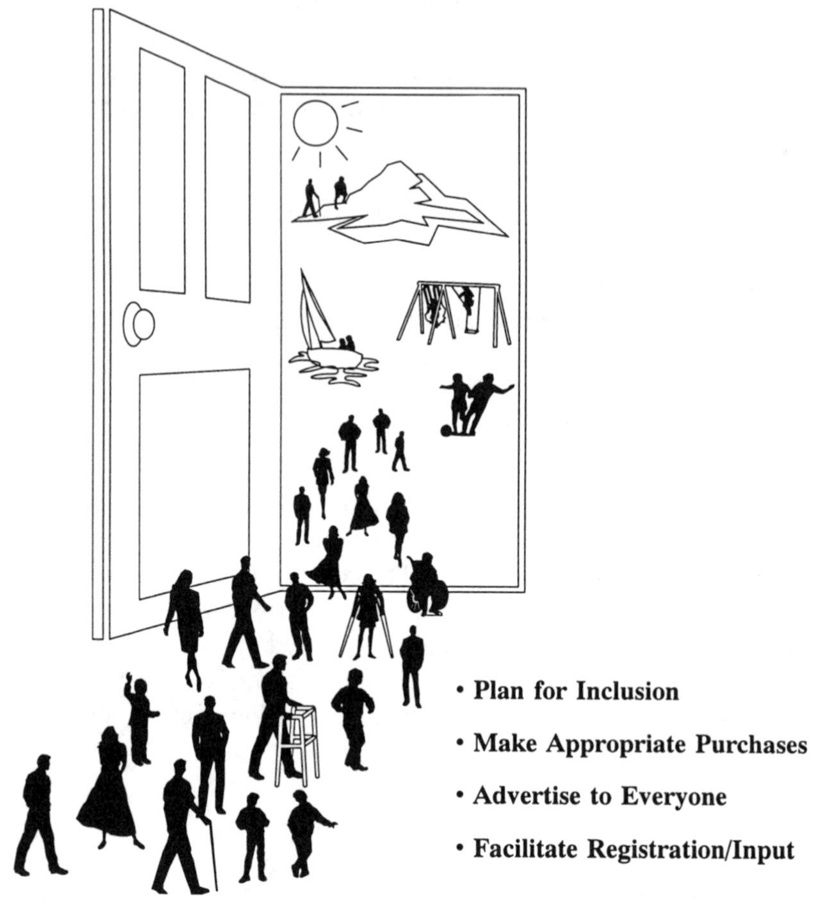
• Plan for Inclusion
• Make Appropriate Purchases
• Advertise to Everyone
• Facilitate Registration/Input

Figure 7.2 Actions to take to respond to the Americans with Disabilities Act.

disabilities, the initiation of a self-analysis is suggested. Professionals must examine all recreation programs to determine how to accommodate a person with a disability who meets essential eligibility requirements for participation. It is important to identify any architectural, transportation, communication, or service barriers, and identify programs where such barriers may exist. Recreation services providers must invite comment from interested people with disabilities or advocacy organizations. The ongoing self-analysis should be available for public review, contain a list of the interested persons consulted, and provide descriptions of areas examined, problems identified, and modifications made since the self-analysis.

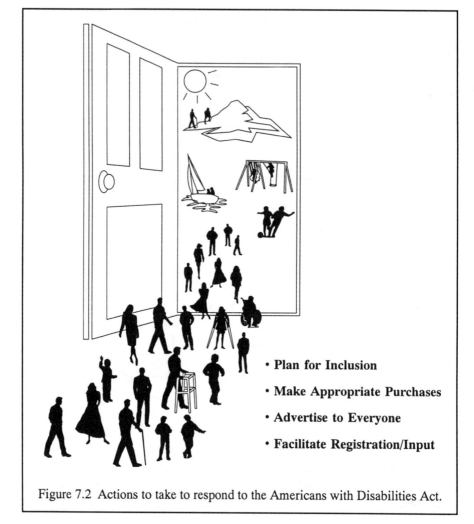

Determine essential eligibility. According to McGovern, essential eligibility is the set of factors examined by a leisure services provider to determine who participates in which service. These factors often include whether the person registers before the capacity is exhausted, whether required fees are paid, and whether the individual agrees and adheres to reasonable rules of conduct, with a reasonable accommodation made by the agency.

Complete a transition plan. A transition plan for the removal of barriers which will require structural modifications should be developed. The transition plan must describe alterations required to achieve accessibility, identify the cost of alterations, and indicate when alterations will be completed.

Ensure coordination. Designate at least one employee to coordinate agency efforts to comply with the ADA. This employee must have authority to make decisions regarding compliance, ensure cooperation of staff, and be responsible for investigating alleged complaints against the agency. The name, office address, and office telephone number of this employee must be made available to the public.

Adopt a procedure for handling complaints. It is necessary to develop a procedure for responding to complaints of noncompliance against the agency. This procedure could be similar to procedures for employee grievances, and must allow for prompt attention to allegations of noncompliance.

Consider employment concerns. Consider supplemental unpaid leave for qualified people with disabilities who, because of their disability, may require additional time from work. Individuals associated with a person with a disability, such as a family member, may also require additional unpaid leave.

Make Appropriate Purchases

Vehicles. Ensure that requests for bids to buy or lease vehicles for transporting participants in programs or activities specify that the vehicles are readily accessible to, and usable by, people with disabilities. This requirement should be followed regardless of whether any individual with a disability is known to require the use of such a vehicle. In addition, all donated or leased vehicles used for the transportation of participants need to be readily accessible to, and usable by, individuals with disabilities.

Furniture and equipment. Leisure professionals must purchase furniture and recreation equipment so that at least a portion of the product being purchased (perhaps at least 30 percent) is accessible. In the absence of guidelines from the federal government, perhaps when purchasing products such as playground equipment, at least three of every 10 distinct play areas could be accessible to wheelchairs.

Capital purchases. It is necessary to include consideration of accessibility and use by individuals with disabilities for all capital purchases. According to McGovern, if a capital purchase request form is used, and if this form asks the purpose of the purchase, a check-off box or additional question could be included on the form. The question or check-off could read as follows: "Could this product be purchased with modifications which would make it usable by individuals with disabilities?" Capital improvement plans must include removal of architectural and communication barriers.

Advertise to Everyone

Include compliance statement. Agencies should include a statement in all brochures and publications regarding ADA compliance plans. Example are:

(a) the agency does not discriminate on the basis of an individual's disability, and
(b) the agency does make reasonable accommodations (e.g., changing rules, removing barriers, and providing auxiliary aids and services) to enable a person with a physical or mental disability to participate.

It is also helpful to include a statement inviting communication of needs. For example, include a statement saying, "To assist staff in planning programs, please call in advance of programs if you or your child requires an accommodation."

Provide alternative formats. Leisure services professionals should develop brochures in alternative formats such as large print, Braille, and cassette tape for use by individuals with sight or cognitive impairments. It is helpful to examine copier technology for the creation of large-print materials. Professionals are encouraged to identify organizations that work with people who are blind and seek assistance in creating Braille materials when required. The creation of a brochure on cassette as part of the program planning and brochure planning processes is easy, and may have other uses, too.

Make advertisements accessible. It is imperative that leisure services providers ensure that brochure display areas are accessible to and usable by individuals with disabilities. Features of such displays include a shelf of the correct height for an individual using a wheelchair, or making staff available to hand out brochures that may be out of reach of an individual in a wheelchair. A Braille message regarding the type of brochures available and how these may be obtained should be made available.

Facilitate Registration and Input

Modify registration. Professionals must be prepared to change registration procedures to accommodate an individual with a disability who, because of that disability, cannot perform registration in the manner required by procedures. Alternative registration procedures may include, but are not limited to, mail-in registration, phone registration, or personal registration by appointment. As a precaution, McGovern suggests that personnel may request that a person provide proof of disability in exchange for the opportunity to register in an alternative manner. However, personnel shall permit the individual accommodation in the registration process, pending submission of proof. If satisfactory proof is not provided within a reasonable time, or if proof is insufficient, the registration may be canceled. To register a person who uses a TT, receptionists and other personnel answering the telephone must identify a TT call. In addition, they should be familiar with and be able to use the relay services available through the phone company.

Make meetings accessible. It is necessary to ensure that any public committee or advisory group meetings are conducted in an accessible fashion. McGovern suggests that notices for such meetings include the following language:

> If you plan to attend the meeting and will require an accommodation because of a disability, contact our office at least one full working day in advance of the scheduled meeting.

Agencies must be prepared to provide an accommodation, such as an interpreter, when a person with a hearing impairment calls ahead and indicates plans to attend a meeting. It is important to be ready on short notice to seek an interpreter or provide other accommodations necessary for participation by an individual with a mobility, sight or hearing impairment, even if the notice requirement is not met. Leisure services providers should plan all meetings for rooms without architectural barriers.

Obtain input. It is critical to ensure that nominees for advisory boards, citizen panels, or other groups of citizens involved in advising or guiding the agency include people with disabilities. Invitations to participate should be posted in large print or Braille, or available in alternative formats.

Determine Essential Eligibility Requirements

The ADA requires that people who meet essential eligibility requirements, or could meet them with reasonable accommodations, be given the opportunity to participate in recreation programs regardless of age, sex, presence of a mental or physical disability, race, or religious beliefs. McGovern suggests that an individual meets essential eligibility requirements for participation in most recreation programs if the following conditions are present:

(a) capacity;
(b) fee;
(c) rules of conduct;
(d) safety;
(e) skill;
(f) age; and
(g) residence.

Capacity. The person must register for the recreation program before other registrants have filled the program to capacity. For example, if a program has a capacity of 50, and a person is the 51st individual desiring registration, the person may be denied the opportunity to register. This may occur whether or not the individual has a disability.

Fee. The person must pay (or have paid) the appropriate registration fee for the recreation program. For example, if a fee of $20 is required for a one-hour golf lesson, the individual registered for the lesson must pay the fee or have the fee paid by another, such as a parent, sibling, guardian or sponsor. Individuals may not be charged a higher fee to offset the costs of accommodations.

Rules of Conduct. The person must agree to abide by any reasonable rules of conduct for participation in that recreation program. For example, in a swimming lesson, the individual must not dive from the deck into the shallow end of the pool. In a sports program, the individual must not strike other participants. In a public outing to a theater, the individual must not speak so loudly during a performance or presentation as to disturb the enjoyment or listening of others in the audience. These examples are applicable to all participants, whether a disability is present or not. If an individual violates reasonable rules of conduct, the agency may suspend or modify that individual's involvement after reasonable accommodation has been made.

Safety. Safety concerns may be a factor when a direct threat of imminent physical harm exists. This threat must be real, and not perceived. Particularly, employees must be cautioned against allowing their perceptions of an individual's disability to result in an inaccurate belief that the threat of harm is imminent. For example, where a registrant is an individual who has harmed other participants and could not be reasonably accommodated, employees may elect to refuse that individual admission to a general swimming program. However, the opportunity to swim must still be considered through such methods as individual lessons. Employees may not assume that all people with mental health disorders pose a direct threat of imminent physical harm. This is a belief based on a misconception and results in discriminatory treatment of people with mental health disorders who are not aggressive.

Relative skill. Relative skill may be a factor in a few programs, such as highly competitive sports programs. An individual could not register to participate in an annual musical performance for the public without basic competencies. This is applicable whether or not the person has a disability. Therefore, staff could refuse to permit a person with a disability to perform in a concert, but should consider providing other music options, such as joining a choir or enrolling in music lessons.

Age. The age of participants may also be a factor in an analysis of essential eligibility. It is inappropriate for a 15-year-old to be registered in a program for children ages 3 to 5. Regardless of whether the 15-year-old has a cognitive impairment, it will likely be inappropriate to place the older child with the younger children.

Residence. If agencies exclude nonresidents from certain programs for legitimate reasons (e.g., limited capacity), then nonresidents with disabilities may be excluded. Where fees charged for nonresidents are higher than those for residents, that standard may be applied to people with disabilities. However, whenever possible, services should be available to residents as well as nonresidents. No person living outside the geographic boundaries may be excluded solely because of disability.

In summary, eligibility requirements are associated with capacity of the program, the ability to pay, the need to follow rules and maintain safety, the skill and age of participants and their residence (see Figure 7.3) These criteria must be applied equally to all participants, including people with disabilities.

Make Reasonable Accommodations

The ADA includes reference to a number of specific accommodations or methods of accommodations to enable people to participate. These are articulated below, and must be considered for each program. Application will vary, depending upon the type of activity (sports, crafts, social, educational, etc.), the location of the program, whether it is an individual or group activity, whether it is competitive or recreational or instructional, the age of the participants, and other similar factors. Generally, accommodations are not expensive. Some methods for making accommodations are:

(a) modify services;
(b) remove architectural barriers;
(c) remove transportation barriers;
(d) remove communication barriers;
(e) provide aids;
(f) supply personnel;
(g) reassign programs;
(h) adapt equipment; and
(i) conduct in-service training.

Modify services. Modify rules, policies, or practices that result in the exclusion of or discrimination against an individual with a disability to enable a person with a disability to meet essential eligibility requirements to participate in the program. For example, a rule prohibiting the use of personal flotation devices in swimming pools may exclude an individual with a physical impairment who requires additional support and flotation. The rule could be modified to permit certain types of flotation devices (shape, color, size, or filling) to accommodate an individual with a physical disability. In another example, a policy requiring a driver's license, instead of an identification card, to fish would be discriminatory to individuals who are 16 years old or older but do not currently have a driver's license due to impairments. As a final example, an agency which forbids all animals from entering particular areas of their facility (e.g., dressing rooms, swimming pool areas) is enforcing a discriminatory policy. This rule must be revised to accommodate animals which provide mobility assistance to people with various visual and motor impairments.

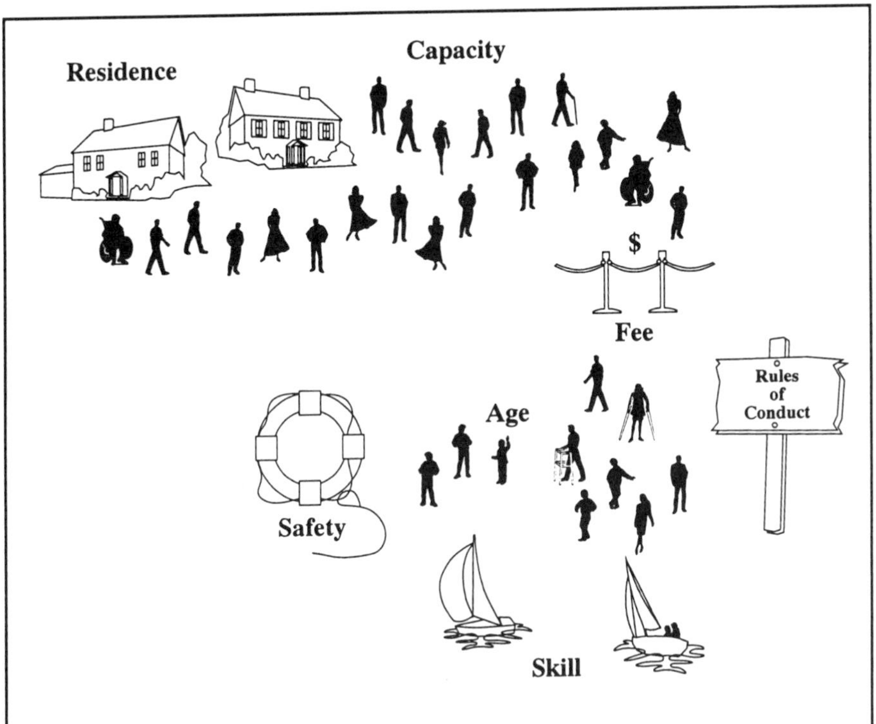

Figure 7.3 Essential eligibility requirements associated with ADA.

Remove architectural barriers. Remove architectural barriers that exclude people with physical impairments from entering a facility (e.g., the swimming pool water from the pool deck) and participating in a recreation program conducted in that facility. Such a barrier results in unlawful discrimination. If a business provides services on several floors, accommodations must be made to allow people with mobility impairments to access services on the upper floors. An immediate solution facilitating access would be to install an elevator. Although this is an excellent solution, other alternatives are possible, such as moving services to an accessible portion of the building.

Many recreation service providers own and operate historical facilities. Removing architectural barriers from a historical structure could compromise the integrity of the building. To not damage the historical significance of a facility and still accommodate people with disabilities curators could:

(a) develop a model to scale of the upper floors and display this model on the ground level;
(b) develop a videotape presentation of the upper floors;

(c) develop photographic and other displays of the upper floors; and
(d) provide a cassette tape or narrator to describe the upper floors.

All of these options could have positive program implications for people without disabilities.

Remove transportation barriers. Remove transportation barriers when transportation is provided as a part of a program and the absence of the ability to participate in the program results in the exclusion of a person with a disability. In addition, when a program is made available to the public, and a person with a disability cannot attend the program because of a disability, a transportation barrier may exist.

Remove communication barriers. Where program participation requires communication, and the medium used for communication is not one which a person with a disability may understand because of a hearing, sight, or cognitive impairment, the communication poses a barrier to participation. For example, to register for a recreation program, an individual must complete the registration form. This requires sight and the ability to see and understand the words on the registration form. For an individual with a cognitive impairment, the written form is a communication barrier which can be removed by providing an employee to read the form to the individual. This accommodation could also help a person with a visual impairment. Other actions that could be taken for people with visual impairments are to provide cassette tapes that explain registration procedures, or registration forms with Braille instructions (if the person reads Braille). As another example, when providing food services involving consumers' use of menus, servers can prepare themselves for people with visual and cognitive impairments by being ready to read the menu to customers and develop alternative forms of menus (e.g., Braille, larger type).

Provide aids. Provide auxiliary aids and devices which will enhance participation and communication. Where the methods of leadership or instruction in a recreation program require communication between employees and participants or among participants, and a person with a hearing or sight impairment has registered, some aid must be provided to enable the person with a sensory impairment to have an equal opportunity to enjoy the program. For example, in a youth sport skills program, oral instructions and demonstrations will be used to instruct participants in skill acquisition. If a registrant has a hearing impairment, the oral instructions will be difficult to interpret, even if the participant has some lip-reading ability. An appropriate accommodation may be the provision of an interpreter for the participant during the recreation program. Another accommodation may be the instruction of an employee in elementary sign language, with an emphasis on terms used in the sport, and the eventual assignment of that employee to the sport skills program in which the individual with a hearing impairment has registered. However, care must be taken to ensure that the interpreting skill of the employee is adequate to the task.

Supply personnel. Provide additional staff as needed. This may be appropriate where a participant has a lower cognitive ability than other registrants and requires more staff time to make the opportunity for recreation program participation equivalent to that enjoyed by individuals without disabilities. Trained staff and volunteers can be used effectively to assist people in various recreation programs. For example, at a section of an amusement park that is designated for children with assistance from their parents, staff or volunteers could be available to assist children with disabilities to participate or to help children without disabilities whose parents may encounter difficulty due to restricted mobility.

Reassign programs. Reassign programs from an inaccessible site to a site which is free of architectural barriers. Make home visits where a person with a disability cannot attend a program and the inability to attend is clearly a result of the disability and not a choice made by the registrant. Consider bringing the recreation program to the participant at his or her home. In certain instances, home visits may be a less costly accommodation than transportation to and from a site where a transportation barrier exists.

Adapt equipment. Where equipment is an integral part of the recreation program, such as camping equipment or sports equipment, adaptive devices may be used to help a person with a disability use the equipment. Such devices may alter the degree of strength or dexterity required to manipulate the equipment (such as a bowling ramp) or assist an individual in holding equipment (such as a brace or Velcro™ straps) which is necessary for participation.

Conduct in-service training. Conduct in-service training for agency personnel and volunteers. Training may include program planning strategies, adaptive techniques, principles of the ADA, use of sensitive language, or awareness of attitudinal barriers. For example, an appropriate training for personnel and volunteers of a nature center would be to receive information on assisting people with disabilities with participation on interpretive tours. It is recommended that agency personnel and volunteers using adaptive equipment receive appropriate training prior to use.

In summary, people with disabilities who, with or without reasonable accommodation, meet the essential eligibility requirements have the right to participate in a purely integrated setting. Reasonable accommodations which make participation as effective as that enjoyed by people without disabilities shall be provided. People who could not meet essential eligibility requirements with a reasonable accommodation may be denied the opportunity to participate in a program and directed to begin participation in a more controlled environment.

Consider the Existence of an Undue Burden

Economic burden. The Justice Department has not upheld the denial of an accommodation solely because of an economic burden. Because of the wide range of size of entities and the tremendous range in cost of accommodations, the agency must determine the cost of the accommodation in comparison to the operating budget, availability of tax funds for this accommodation, the number of employees affected, the potential number of beneficiaries, the nature of the program and the location of the program, and other similar factors, including the availability of funds from other sources in the agency.

Administrative burden. The second portion of this test is an undue administrative burden. An example of where an undue burden may exist is if there is a severe shortage of qualified personnel needed for a specific accommodation. For example, if there are no certified interpreters in the area and if the nature of the service to be provided is most effectively met by a certified sign-language interpreter, the agency would be permitted to employ a noncertified interpreter who lived in the area.

Programmatic burden. The third portion of this test includes an accommodation which results in a fundamental alteration of the nature of the program. For example, a home visit where an employee brings the activity to the participant in his or her home could result in a fundamental alteration. If the program for which the individual registered is a team sports program, it would not be reasonable to bring the entire team and the opposing team to an individual's home. However, with a crafts program, instructional music program, or art program, which tend to be very individualized, a home visit would be an effective accommodation. Conducting arts programs or music lessons in the individual's home may be appropriate. This accommodation opposes the concept of "most integrated setting," but if because of disability the individual cannot leave the home, home visits may be appropriate.

Understand Who Enforces ADA

The Equal Employment Opportunity Commission enforces regulations covering employment. The Architectural and Transportation Barriers Compliance Board (Access Board) has issued minimum guidelines to ensure that buildings, facilities, rail passenger cars and vehicles are accessible to and usable by people with disabilities. In addition, the Access Board is developing design guidelines for recreation facilities and outdoor developed areas.

The Department of Transportation enforces regulations governing transit. The Federal Communications Commission enforces regulations covering telecommunications. The Department of Justice enforces regulations governing public accommodations and state and local public services.

Meet the Spirit of the Law

Recreation professionals must embrace the spirit of the ADA and develop inclusive leisure services. Such programs benefit the entire community.

The next section of this text contains five chapters which were developed to help professionals achieve the goal of inclusion as stipulated in the ADA. Information about self-determination and ways to encourage leisure participants to take responsibility for their leisure involvement is presented in Chapter 8. Leisure education, described in Chapter 9, can be a vehicle for increasing participants' awareness, knowledge and skills. Chapter 10 contains information designed to facilitate access to all services by all citizens. Information about integration and strategies designed to include people with disabilities in all leisure services is provided in Chapter 11. Chapter 12 expands on the information presented in this chapter about making reasonable accommodations. Finally, in Chapter 13, the responsibility of acting as an advocate for people with disabilities is emphasized. These chapters are provided to encourage leisure services professionals to embrace the spirit of ADA as well as comply with the law. This sentiment was expressed by Beland (1993, p. 62), who stated:

> Not only must professional recreators pay attention to recent federal legislation like the Americans with Disabilities Act, but more important, they must pay attention to the millions of Americans with handicapping conditions who are demanding recreation . . .

Conclusion

The ADA is intended to improve the quality of life for people with disabilities by involving them in all aspects of life, including recreation services provided by their communities. According to McGovern (1992a), recreation professionals deal with quality-of-life issues on a daily basis and have the unique opportunity to make compliance with the ADA a visible and positive statement for the entire leisure industry and, most importantly, for people with disabilities.

Discussion Questions

1. What type of leisure services agencies are covered by ADA?
2. What are the different Titles associated with ADA and what major topics do each of the Titles address?
3. What can you do to respond to ADA that helps you plan for inclusion?
4. What should you consider when making purchases that are consistent with the intent of ADA?
5. How can you effectively advertise for your programs while responding to ADA?
6. How can you facilitate the ability of people with disabilities to register for the services you provide?
7. What are essential eligibility requirements for the provision of leisure services?
8. What are typical reasonable accommodations for people with disabilities in recreation programs?
9. What is meant by the existence of undue burden?

Chapter 8

Facilitate Self-Determination

"Few human concerns are more universally central than that of self-determination."
—Edward Deci

Orientation Activity: The Choice is Theirs

Directions When Alone: Choose any recreation program that you might offer as a leisure services professional. Record the program at the top of a blank sheet of paper. Read each of the following questions. While thinking of the recreation activity you listed at the top of your paper, record answers for each of the questions. Be sure to include specific examples.

Directions With Others: One person will be assigned as recorder and will write the responses on a chalkboard or easel so that all participants can see what is being recorded. Address each question and report the different methods identified. Attempt to produce as comprehensive a list as possible.

1. How might you encourage participants to choose activities within a given recreation program?
2. How might you determine what a participant has chosen if he or she does not speak?
3. How might you encourage participants to make choices once you begin conducting a recreation activity?
4. If participants do not have the skills to respond to a survey or interview questions concerning their enjoyment associated with a program, how might you determine if they are enjoying an activity?

Debriefing

Self-determination is a highly valued personal characteristic in our society (Abery, 1994). If we identify self-determination and choice as important elements of leisure and enjoyment, then it appears logical to encourage participants in leisure programs to make as many choices as possible and take responsibility for their participation. Providing opportunities for individuals with disabilities to cultivate self-determination can be challenging and often requires systematic planning (Wehmeyer, 1994). The goal of enhancing self-determination has merit, since it appears that people's perceptions of freedom and their ability to determine their own participation patterns is more important than the specific recreation activity which they choose. The aforementioned questions are designed to encourage you to consider providing opportunities for choice at every possible opportunity within the programs you provide.

The fact that some participants may appear to have fewer skills than most participants, respond in different ways than most participants, or exhibit behaviors not demonstrated by most participants does not preclude them from valuing their freedom and from experiencing enjoyment based on their ability to respond to a challenge. Recreation professionals are in an excellent position to facilitate self-determination for individuals that possess such characteristics by supporting them. This support will help individuals experience leisure as much as possible. Attempt to answer the following questions related to the orientation activity:

1. What is the value of encouraging participants to make choices and increase their sense of self-determination?
2. What is the primary responsibility of leisure services providers to people with disabilities?
3. Why is it important to provide opportunities for people with disabilities to empower themselves?

Introduction

The intention of this chapter is to encourage leisure services providers to consider the impact of the way in which they deliver their services to people with disabilities. Leisure services are primarily designed to set the stage for people to enjoy themselves. At times, we become so concerned with "keeping people busy" that we lose sight of the more important goal of our services: facilitating enjoyment. It is valuable to consider that self-determination is necessary for the optimal experience of enjoyment. Self-determination makes effort and the investment of attention worthwhile for a person, and these are the factors that bring about enjoyable involvement. This experience serves to develop competence, thereby reinforcing self-determination. To better understand the impact of self-determination on leisure participation, the psychology of enjoyment will be explored. The following section of this chapter contains information adapted from a chapter previously developed by Dattilo and Kleiber (1993).

Examine the Psychology of Enjoyment

A purpose of leisure services is to bring about the experience of **enjoyment**. For whatever additional benefits enjoyment may bring, it is, in and of itself, the reason for the provision of services designed to include people with disabilities. Leisure professionals seek to identify the factors that interfere with and prohibit enjoyment, those that facilitate enjoyment, and other benefits that come to people who enjoy themselves. However, the nature of enjoyment itself has not always been made clear. Enjoyment is associated in the literature with recreation (e.g., Shivers, 1981), and with leisure (e.g., Mobily, 1989), but its inherent characteristics are rarely articulated.

The work by Csikszentmihalyi (1975, 1982, 1985a, 1985b, 1990) and his associates (Csikszentmihalyi & Csikszentmihalyi, 1988) on *optimal experience* offers a useful starting point for this examination. These investigators have studied, with various methods including interviews and surveys, the qualities of subjective experience that people have when they are doing what they want to do most and loving it. By examining the experiences of dancers, rock climbers, writers, and basketball players, as well as artists, surgeons and others who love their work, these investigations have isolated characteristics of enjoyment, or what is referred to more technically as "optimal experience."

The studies show that the experience of enjoyment is distinguishable from pleasure, the latter being the result of satisfying basic biological drives such as hunger, thirst, sex, and sufficient stimulation. Enjoyment is the experience derived from investing one's attention in action patterns that are intrinsically motivating. The activity is often so compelling in and of itself that one becomes deeply absorbed in it and loses consciousness of self and awareness of time.

The word used to describe the subjective quality of this optimal experience—often by actors themselves—is "flow." The sense of *movement* that this word implies is created by the merging of action and awareness around the challenges provided by an activity and the feedback that defines a person's capability to meet those challenges. While many activities can create this optimal experience, any given activity must become more challenging, in keeping with expanding skills, to maintain the experience. So unlike pleasure, enjoyment is consistent with concentration, effort, and a sense of control and competence. Enjoyment is often used colloquially as the equivalent of "fun," or simple positive affect, but it is being used here, as Csikszentmihalyi and others have, to reflect a considerable degree of psychological involvement as well.

An activity is assumed to be enjoyable, then, when one continues with it for no apparent reason beyond the activity itself. We say that such an activity is "intrinsically motivated." However, it is in the subjective experience of the activity that the factors producing this sustained interest are revealed. From the research of Csikszentmihalyi and others it is clear that concentration, effort, and a sense of control and competence are all critical aspects of the experience of enjoyment, and thus, it is these factors that must be understood and managed by leisure professionals if enjoyment is to be facilitated. See Figure 8.1 for a depiction of the conditions of enjoyment.

There are some indications that individuals are inherently, even genetically, different in their ability to generate optimal experience, or flow-type enjoyment, for themselves (see Kleiber & Dirkin, 1985). Csikszentmihalyi (1975) described an "autotelic personality," wherein the appropriation of self-generated, enjoyable action patterns seems to be most common. However, he adds that such patterns can be taught and environments arranged to make such experiences more common.

While there are other agendas for leisure professionals, teaching people to generate optimal experiences and establishing environments conducive to flow is especially important (e.g., Voelkl & Birkel, 1988). Creating conditions that help concentration, effort, and a sense of control and competence, while promoting freedom of choice and the expression of preference is the "engineering of enjoyment." However, to do that, it is necessary to understand the psychology of self-determination and the factors that interfere with it. The theories associated with self-determination and the factors interfering with it provide us with valuable information for developing strategies that enhance concentration, effort, and a sense of control and competence and, thus, foster enjoyment. Murray (1988, p. 156) supported this approach when he asked and answered the following question:

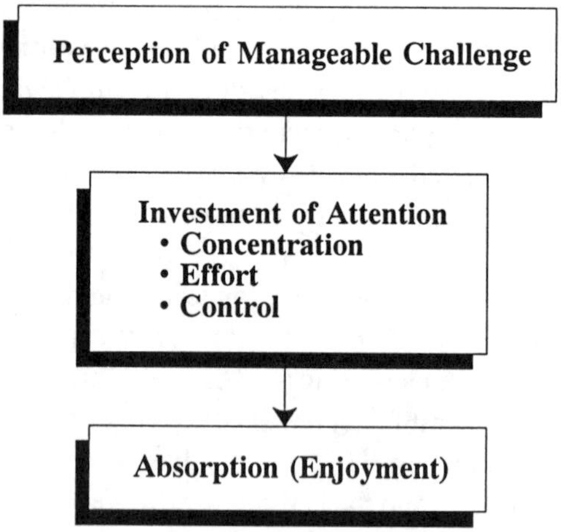

Figure 8.1 Conditions of enjoyment.

> How can social policy facilitate human enjoyment if that enjoyment is intimately linked to the exercise of competence in the face of challenge? The immediately obvious and the unthreatening answer is that social policy must facilitate the acquisition of competence by all its citizens—an answer that, among other things, can be translated into a call for better educational programs so that people will become more competent.

Also worth noting by way of introduction is that while enjoyment stands well as the culmination of intervention and as an indicator of the acquisition of self-determination, it is also a *precipitating experience* as it is described here. Thus, the creation of enjoyment serves as a reinforcing experience, leading a person on to greater challenges and to higher levels of self-determination. As enjoyment comes under one's own power, it offers an orientation for making the most of one's circumstances and enhancing the quality of one's life.

Understand Self-Determination

In the early 20th century, most psychologists believed that all motivation occurred in response to physiological needs (Deci & Ryan, 1985). However, by the 1950s psychologists came to recognize various psychological factors as very influential in human motivation. One particular psychological factor, perceived control, has received increasing attention from the 1960s to the present. This trend is based on the assumption that a sense of psychological well-being is augmented by a belief that one has some degree of control over personal events (Leary & Miller, 1986). For people with disabilities receiving leisure services, a sense of control is particularly important in establishing self-determination.

Ward (1988) referred to "self-determination" as the attitudes and abilities that lead individuals to define goals for themselves, and their ability to take the initiative to achieve their goals. The traits underlying self-determination include self-actualization, assertiveness, creativity, pride, and self-advocacy (Funk, 1987; McGill, 1987; Ward, 1988). After reviewing the literature, Ellis, Maughan-Pritchett, and Ruddell (1993) reported that, generally, people who perceive themselves as capable and self-determining are able to effectively deal with the challenges of day-to-day life and may avoid such undesirable outcomes as depression, distress, substance abuse, and physical illness (Langer, 1983; Shary & Iso-Ahola, 1989; Wassman & Iso-Ahola, 1985; Yessick, 1991).

Deci (1980) asserted that self-determination involves the flexibility and ability to choose options and to adjust to situations when only one option is available. Cognition, affect, and motivation mediate self-determination.

Limitations placed on an individual's self-determination result from environmental and unconscious forces. Self-determination reflects the interaction between freedom and constraint. When self-determination is achieved, increases in learning and perceptions of competence occur. Conversely, the experience of a lack of self-determination occurs when an individual fails to consider various options, or does not adjust to the situation when only one option is available.

Realize the Power of Intrinsic Motivation

Deci and Ryan (1985) concluded that self-determination is associated with intrinsic motivation. Motivation that is intrinsic energizes behavior and results in feelings of autonomy. Performance of the behavior does not require external rewards or control. The experiences of interest, enjoyment, and excitement provide reinforcement for such behaviors. These are the experiences most often associated with leisure and recreation.

People who are intrinsically motivated will seek challenges that are commensurate with their competencies; they will avoid those situations that are too easy or too difficult. The balancing act between competencies and challenges associated with intrinsic motivation is depicted in Figure 8.2. Intrinsic motivation is reflected in the process of seeking optimal incongruities within the environment and then reducing these incongruities. Individuals who are intrinsically motivated in certain situations are more likely to learn, adapt, and grow in competencies that characterize development. However, intrinsic motivation is vulnerable to influences from environmental forces.

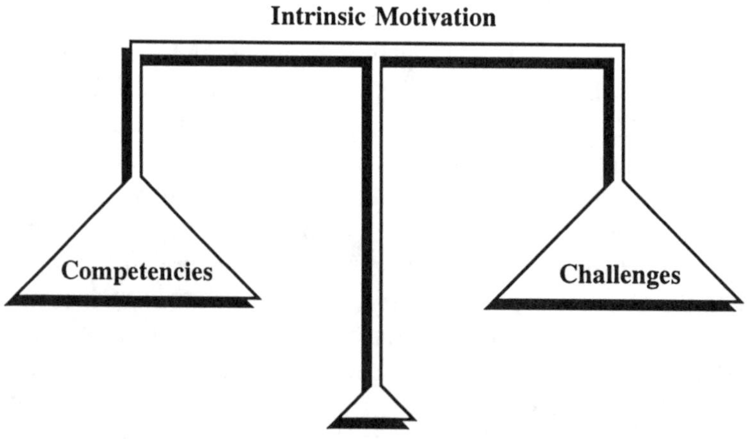

Figure 8.2 The intrinsic motivation "balancing act."

Consider the Environment

There is a continuous interaction between people's evaluation of the environment and their motivation. The environment can encourage self-determination, by being responsive and informational, or it can discourage self-determination through controlling and capricious responses to behaviors. An environment is responsive and informational if it reacts to a person's initiatives, provides data about the person's competence, and encourages further action. A responsive and informational environment fosters intrinsic motivation and internal causality. The result of this is self-determined behavior. Similarly, events involving choice and positive feedback provide information to the person thereby enhancing self-determination. For example, Maughan and Ellis (1991) demonstrated that the administration of praise and persuasion for performance accomplishments associated with a video game enhanced the efficacy judgments of adolescents.

Now that the concepts of enjoyment and self-determination have been described, strategies to facilitate self-determination are presented. Figure 8.3 previews the six strategies identified in this chapter.

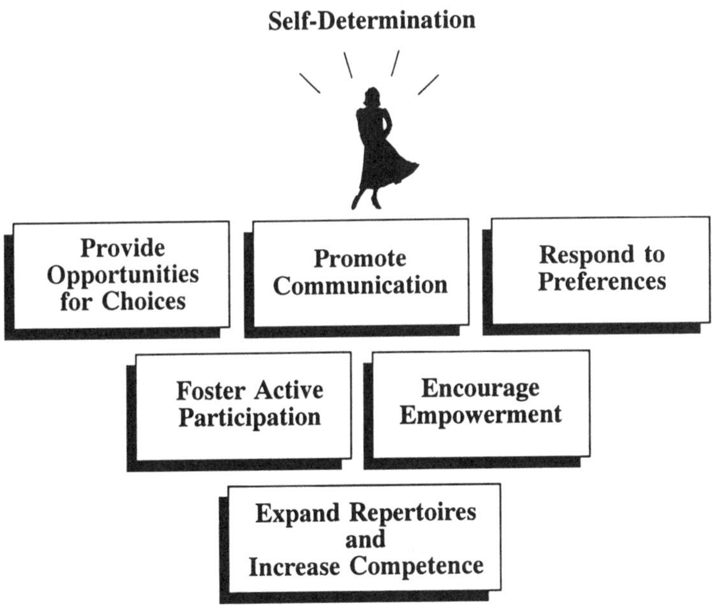

Figure 8.3 Strategies to facilitate self-determination.

Provide Opportunities for Choices

The opportunities for choice often associated with leisure participation must be systemically provided and taught to individuals with disabilities (Dattilo & Rusch, 1985). Wehman and Schleien (1981) identified the ultimate goal of any leisure program as the facilitation of self-initiated, independent use of free time with chronologically age-appropriate recreation activities. Some families and professionals make choices for people with disabilities rather than allowing participants to decide for themselves. Individuals' opportunities to express personal interests and preferences have been prevented by people who incorrectly assume that people with disabilities are incapable of making informed choices (Kishi, Teelucksingh, Zollers, Park-Lee, & Meyer, 1988).

Freedom of choice is vital to the pursuit of enjoyable, satisfying, and meaningful experience and, according to Hawkins (1993), personal autonomy for people with disabilities has become recognized as an essential aspect of independent functioning and self-reliance. Heyne, Schleien, and McAvoy (1993, p. 46) emphasize this point when they stated:

> When people with disabilities are allowed to choose activities, they are more eager to learn the skills necessary to participate, they more readily generalize those skills to other settings, and they are more likely to continue to participate in those activities.

When recreation professionals provide opportunities for individuals with disabilities to make self-determined and responsible choices that reflect their needs to grow, explore, and realize their potential, their ability to experience leisure will be enhanced. Dattilo and Schleien (1994) provided the following example to illustrate this point. Anne's favorite recreation activity is doing art work. When she attends her art class she is encouraged to select the paper she will use; she chooses between different colors, sizes, and textures. In addition, she decides to use watercolors today rather than chalk or markers. After she has her materials, Anne is invited to position her easel where she prefers and begins her chosen project while carefully selecting her color scheme.

Dattilo and Schleien (1994) reported that practitioners must maintain a delicate balance between facilitating self-determined leisure participation and encouraging development of culturally normative age-appropriate leisure behaviors for people with disabilities. Sometimes people choose to exhibit behaviors that society has identified as being offensive or detrimental. At this time, these people are often redirected to participate in socially acceptable activities of their choosing that do not bring psychological or physical discomfort to themselves or other people. Leisure instruction related to helping individuals determine the appropriateness of behaviors is often useful.

The appropriateness of behaviors may vary according to location (bedroom vs. public swimming pool), frequency (asking once vs. asking several times in a brief duration), timing (when someone is laughing vs. when someone is crying), and relationship of people present (brother vs. teacher). All people must learn that humans are rarely completely free to do anything they wish. To experience leisure on a ongoing basis, people must learn to assert their rights as well as respect other people they encounter.

Empowering individuals with disabilities to make choices and take charge of their lives is an important aspect of leisure services delivery. The earlier opportunities for choices are presented to people, the more likely it is that they will acquire behaviors associated with self-determination. One area in which children with disabilities can begin to make choices is in their play activities and partners (Jolly, Test, & Spooner, 1993). Hawkins (1993) reported that, in general, although choice by people with disabilities has received inadequate attention, especially in regard to leisure participation, leisure skills development, and overall quality of life (Bambara & Ager, 1992; Mahon & Bullock, 1992), experts suggest that, when combined with other social factors (e.g., friendship, residential placement, and opportunities for community inclusion), leisure activity choices contribute to life satisfaction and well-being (Schalock, Keith, Hoffman, & Karan, 1989).

Promote Communication

When providing leisure services to people with disabilities it may be helpful in certain situations to take a nondirective approach that strongly considers the individual's preferences and choices (Dattilo, 1993). Nondirective instructional strategies help professionals avoid instilling a sense of dependency within their students (Dattilo & Mirenda, 1987). Since a perception of freedom to choose to participate in meaningful, enjoyable, and satisfying experiences is fundamental to the leisure experience (Dattilo & Murphy, 1991), independent leisure participation is achieved more readily when reliance on directive approaches is avoided.

For a variety of reasons, some people with disabilities may take considerable time to formulate a communication turn. However, at times, professionals responding to these individuals do not provide them with adequate time to formulate a communication turn. This unwillingness to wait for people to take their turn results in the professional taking control of the conversation and, often, the entire situation.

Matson, Sevin, Box, Francis, and Sevin (1993) stated that since much of daily communication is not verbally prompted, encouraging people with disabilities to initiate communication is an important goal. As people engage in reciprocal exchanges stimulated by their ability to initiate interaction, their ability to communicate preferences, make meaningful choices, and subsequently, experience leisure is enhanced.

Dattilo and colleagues (Dattilo & Camarata, 1991; Dattilo & O'Keefe, 1992) demonstrated that simply providing people with limited communication skills with an alternative form of communication was not sufficient to shift them away from the conversational role of respondent; rather, specific attention to responding to conversational attempts was needed. Results of these studies indicated that recreation professionals should be as responsive as possible to the communicative attempts made by people that have limited communication skills.

Professionals have learned to encourage individuals with disabilities to communicate their preferences. For example, Kohl and Beckman (1990) concluded that instruction given to teachers designed to promote reciprocal interactions increased the initiations and responses of their students with disabilities. In addition, Dattilo and Light (1993) taught professionals to decrease their conversational control and provide more opportunities for people with limited communication skills to communicate. Following instruction, the professionals reduced their domination of conversations and the people with limited communication skills increased the frequency of their initiations, suggesting that the instruction of the professionals was effective in increasing communication opportunities for people with disabilities.

Since the ability to choose to initiate involvement is critical to the leisure experience, people with disabilities should be encouraged to initiate interactions and share conversations. Dattilo (1993) reported that construction of a supportive environment that is responsive to the communicative attempts of these people is important. Based on the findings of Dattilo and Light described above, a supportive environment is created when professionals:

(a) approach the person;
(b) attend to the person; and
(c) wait at least 10 seconds for that person to initiate interaction.

If the person does make a communicative initiative, speaking partners can reinforce these attempts (e.g., provide people with objects they have requested, return greetings to people, extend and expand their comments). However, if the person does not initiate interaction, professionals are encouraged to ask open-ended questions beginning with "what" and "how" as opposed to those questions that force people into a yes/no response. In conclusion, Wilcox (1993) reported on the importance of consistently recognizing a person's communicative attempts and responding in a contingent, appropriate and consistent manner.

Respond to Preferences

de Villiers, (1987) explained that **preference** refers to a desire for an option following a comparison of that option against a continuum of other options. A **choice** refers to the act of selecting one option, ideally a preferred one, from among others that are simultaneously available (Newton, Horner, & Lund, 1991). Newton and colleagues stated that although the distinction between choice and preference is subtle, it is important. For example, arbitrarily dispensing an option known to be preferred by someone robs that person of the right and pleasure of making the choice (Newton et al., 1991). Likewise, the authors reported that helping someone to choose among options that are much less preferred than others that might have been made available is only a substitute for the kind of choice-making most people value.

When attempting to provide opportunities for the expression of preferences and the making of choices, Newton and colleagues (1991) suggested that professionals determine the person's preferences, and create supporting opportunities for the person to choose among preferred options. Given the importance of choice and preference, more attention must be devoted to developing simple, valid strategies for assessing the preferences of people with severe disabilities (Newton et al., 1991). Newton and colleagues stated that whether such assessment is accomplished via participants' self-reports or via the outcomes of multiple choice-making opportunities, we should attempt to develop ways to validly and reliably assess preferences of the participants.

Each day presents many opportunities for participants to express preferences and make choices about their activities, such as activity "instances" (e.g., playing the "Space Invaders" video game vs. the "Super Mario Brothers" game), community locations where activities are to be performed, activity companions, and times when the activities are to be performed (Newton et al., 1991). To respond to the needs of people with disabilities, Newton and colleagues (1991) suggested that professionals assess participants' preferences, develop strategies for determining the *most* preferred activities, and assess the relationship between preferences honored in planning and preferences honored in daily life.

Foster Active Participation

Individuals with disabilities are often excluded from a wide range of recreation activities due to their assumed inability to perform complete skill sequences independently and in the correct order (Ford et al., 1984). However, an individual who is deemed unable to engage in an activity independently should not be denied the opportunity for partial participation (Brown et al., 1979a;

1979b). These individuals should be provided the opportunity to participate in environments in which their skills will be used rather than in artificial settings (Krebs & Block, 1992). **Partial participation** involves the use of adaptations and provides assistance needed to facilitate leisure participation, thereby affirming the right of persons with disabilities to participate in environments and activities without regard to degree of assistance required (Baumgart et al., 1982).

Adaptations to enhance participation or to make partial participation possible include: providing personal assistance; adapting activities by changing materials, modifying skill sequences, altering rules, and using adaptive devices and alternative communications systems; and changing physical and social environments to promote friendships. Through partial participation, individuals with disabilities may experience the exhilaration and satisfaction associated with the challenge inherent in a particular recreation activity (Dattilo & Murphy, 1987a).

As an example of partial participation, Jerry and his colleagues at work decided to enter a softball league sponsored by the community recreation and parks department. At the beginning of the season, a few rules were adjusted to facilitate his participation in league play. Instead of the ball being pitched to him, he was permitted to hit the ball off a tee and, following contact, a teammate ran the bases. When his teammate scored a run, the team gave "high-fives" to both Jerry and the teammate who ran the bases.

The principle of partial participation was proposed to ensure that even those people with disabilities who might never be able to acquire a large enough complement of skills to *completely* participate in recreation activities would still be able to learn enough to *partially* participate. Ferguson and Baumgart (1991) identified three problems that have arisen when professionals have attempted to promote partial participation. Some suggestions for remediation of these problems are provided below.

Some professionals have narrowly defined participation as simply presence. It is when passive participation is the dominant form of participation that the practice becomes problematic. Recreation professionals should attempt to encourage active participation by all participants, including people with disabilities.

Sometimes, professionals have failed to consider the person's preferences, long-term learning needs, family priorities, reactions of peers, and other socially validated, community-referenced guidelines when involving them in programs. It is important to gain this information from the participants and their families.

At times, professionals may interpret "doing things independently" as doing them alone, which can result in too narrow a prescription for performance. The supportive presence of another person offers recreation professionals and participants the opportunity to enhance an individual's participation by having the other person perform those parts of the activity that are burdensome, time consuming, or image-damaging for the person.

Encourage Empowerment

> Every person, regardless of the severity of his or her disabilities, has the right and ability to communicate with others, express everyday preferences, and exercise at least some control over his or her daily life. Each individual, therefore, should be given the choice, training, technology, respect, and encouragement to do so (Williams, 1991, p. 543).

West and Parent (1992) stated that for many individuals with disabilities, the opportunities for learning and practicing decision-making and self-direction are limited or circumvented. The reasons that these individuals experience such powerlessness and lack of self-direction have less to do with their limitations and impairments than with attitudes and practices of caregivers, service providers, funding agencies, and social institutions (West & Parent, 1992). Service providers do not always allow people with disabilities and their families the right to make their own major life decisions (Rowitz & Stoneman, 1990). West and Parent (1992) added that cognitive, physical, communicative, or sensory impairments may make it difficult for an individual to express his or her preferences and be accurately understood by another person.

Empowerment may be defined broadly as the transfer of power and control over the values, decisions, choices, and directions of human services from external entities (e.g., government funding agencies, service providers, social forces) to the consumers of services, resulting in increased motivation to participate and succeed, and a greater degree of dignity for the consumer (West & Parent, 1992). As previously described in this chapter, choice, a fundamental aspect of empowerment, involves a person selecting a preferred alternative from among several familiar options. This implies that choice-making requires the individual to both identify preferences and express those preferences.

Leisure service providers need to be concerned about creating environments in which people with disabilities and their family members are given the information to make rational choices as well as the opportunities to exercise their choices (Ficker-Terrill & Rowitz, 1991). West and Parent (1992) reported that learning to make good choices requires experience with the process of decision-making, with viable alternatives, and with the consequences of decisions. In areas in which independent choice-making is not feasible or safe, choice-making can be adapted or supported, and individuals may partially participate in decision-making processes (Sharpton & West, 1992). Hanline and Fox (1993) observed that most professionals agree that the development of autonomy, the importance of choice-making, opportunities for self-initiation, and environmental manipulation are all procedures that facilitate learning, enjoyment and empowerment.

Expand Leisure Repertoires and Increase Competence

Mobily, Lemke and Gisin (1991) reported that the development of a leisure repertoire is a collection of activities capable of producing perceptions of competence and psychological comfort. What people do often for their leisure they will do well, and what people do well in their leisure they will do often (Mobily et al., 1993).

Perceived competence (external competence) depends on a person's evaluation of competence compared to others of the same age and gender (Mobily et al., 1993). Perceived competence is an important feature of leisure (Smith, Kielhofer, & Watts, 1986) because it can result in feelings of personal control (Iso-Ahola, 1980). According to Mobily et al. (1993), psychological comfort (internal competence) is perceived when people compare performance to standards adopted internally and conclude that they are satisfied with their performance. Internal competence is important because its inclusion in the definition of leisure repertoire allows for the possibility that people may use a criterion other than social comparison to judge their competence (Mobily et al., 1993).

People with disabilities who have more activities to choose from when they have free time are in a better situation to experience leisure than those who do not. Participation in activities in which people perceive themselves as competent throughout their lives is important for leisure services professionals to consider when planning their services. Recreation programs designed to continuously expand the leisure repertoires and competence of people with disabilities is encouraged.

A note of caution when expanding people's leisure repertoires has been identified by West and Parent (1992, p. 75). The authors stated that:

> More activity does not necessarily mean a better quality of life. Some individuals may actually choose to engage in a few repetitive, but highly enjoyable, activities per week. The issue is ensuring that meaningful opportunities for choice are actually provided.

Conclusion

In summary, self-determination is necessary for the optimal experience of enjoyment. It makes effort and the investment of attention worthwhile for a person, and these are the factors that bring about enjoyable involvement. As seen in Figure 8.4, this experience of enjoyment serves in turn to develop competence, thereby reinforcing self-determination. According to Royal (1992), all people with disabilities need to have opportunities to take charge of their own lives. Their experiences should be organized by principles which promote self-determination (Deci & Chandler, 1986).

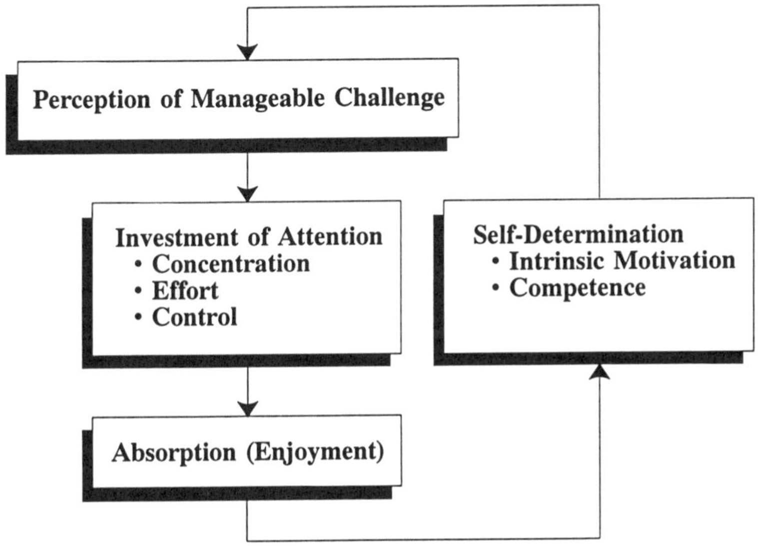

Figure 8.4 Relationship of self-determination and enjoyment.

Discussion Questions

1. What is self-determination?

2. Why is self-determination important?

3. What is pleasure?

4. What is enjoyment?
5. What is an optimal experience?
6. What is necessary to maintain the flow experience?
7. How can leisure services professionals create conditions to promote flow experiences?
8. How can the environment encourage self-determination?
9. Why is choice important?
10. What is the difference between a preference and a choice?
11. What are the six suggestions discussed in this chapter for facilitating partial participation?
12. How can leisure services providers empower participants?
13. What is perceived competence?
14. Why is perceived competence an important feature of leisure?

Chapter 9

Develop Comprehensive Leisure Education

"Education is what survives when what has been learnt has been forgotten."
—B. F. Skinner

Orientation Activity: Go Beyond Recreation Activity Skills

Directions When Alone: Select a recreation activity and write the name of the activity at the top of a blank sheet of paper. Answer the following questions to assist you in beginning to develop a comprehensive leisure education program related to this recreation activity.

Directions With Others: Record your activity on a card. Attempt to find other people who choose the same recreation activity as you. If there are more than four people that have chosen the same recreation activities, divide into smaller groups not less than two and not to exceed four. If no one else identified your activity, find another person who has identified an activity that is similar to yours. Once groups have been formed, share your ideas about leisure education with the other people or person in your discussion group. After a specified time, discuss the highlights of what you have learned with the entire group.

1. How can you encourage participants' awareness of their preferences relative to the recreation activity?
2. How can you help instill their sense of appreciation of the value of the recreation activity?
3. How might you encourage them to develop self-determination relative to this recreation activity?
4. How could you stimulate their ability to make decisions within the context of this recreation activity?
5. How might you teach them about resources associated with this recreation activity?
6. What social skills could you encourage them to demonstrate so that they may be successful when engaging in this recreation activity?

Debriefing

Limited leisure awareness, knowledge and skills of people with disabilities become major barriers for many individuals in making successful transitions into active community living. To overcome this barrier, participants in community recreation programs should be provided systematic and comprehensive leisure education. Leisure instruction that teaches and instills the following levels of awareness, knowledge and skills will assist people in their ability to experience leisure within their communities:

(a) self-awareness;
(b) leisure appreciation;
(c) self-determination;
(d) decision-making;
(e) knowledge and utilization of leisure resources;
(f) social interaction skills; and
(g) specific recreation activity skills.

Attempt to answer the following questions related to the orientation activity:

1. What is the value in addressing the six questions listed in the orientation activity?
2. What implications would offering a leisure education program have on a leisure services agency?
3. How might you incorporate leisure education into your current or future position as a leisure services professional?

Introduction

As discussed in the previous chapter, leisure is a term that describes a person's perception that he or she is free to choose to participate in meaningful, enjoyable, and satisfying experiences. As individuals get in touch with the positive feelings—control, competence, relaxation, excitement—associated with the leisure experience, they will be intrinsically motivated to participate. That is, they will participate in leisure simply to be involved in the experience, not for some tangible outcome or external reward.

Leisure education programs that are designed with the goal of facilitating the leisure experience are needed. Therefore, a rationale for leisure education for all people, including those with disabilities, is provided in this chapter. The structure and content of a leisure education model are presented to assist professionals in providing comprehensive leisure instruction. The model for leisure education presented in this chapter focuses on facilitating integrated community leisure experiences for people with disabilities, and was originally reported by Dattilo and Murphy (1991) and Dattilo and St. Peter (1991).

Understand the Rationale for Leisure Education

Voeltz, Wuerch, and Wilcox (1982) stated that a rationale for leisure education is that it is a component of appropriate preparation for life. According to Voeltz and colleagues, it is important to involve parents or family members and the person with a disability when developing a leisure education plan. In addition, specific skills and activities chosen for each leisure education program should be relevant to the participants' home and community (Nietupski, Hamre-Nietupski, & Ayres, 1984), age-appropriate, active, and fun (Wuerch & Voeltz, 1982).

Wade and Hoover (1985) identified a lack of education and training for people with disabilities as a major constraint to developing a sense of control during leisure participation. To overcome the lack of knowledge many people with disabilities possess relative to leisure, leisure education programs have been designed to encourage individuals to:

(a) raise esteem, increase satisfaction, and promote actualization (Tinsley & Tinsley, 1982);
(b) make effective leisure choices (Ross, 1983);
(c) develop leisure behaviors, skills, and the realization that behaviors can influence the environment (Peterson & Gunn, 1984);
(d) increase leisure understanding, awareness and control (Bregha, 1985);
(e) foster selection of meaningful leisure experiences, facilitating positive psychological growth by clarifying attitudes and values related to self and leisure (Munson, Baker, & Lundegren, 1985);
(f) decrease feelings of boredom by developing knowledge of leisure attitudes, awareness of psychological benefits of leisure, enhanced motivation to participate in leisure, and a diverse leisure repertoire (Iso-Ahola & Weissinger, 1987);
(g) enhance leisure involvement and knowledge retention (Lanagan & Dattilo, 1989);
(h) increase leisure wellness and thus contribute to successful transition from school to adult life (Bedini, Bullock, & Driscoll, 1993); and
(i) increase recreation participation, satisfaction and mastery (Luken, 1993).

Based on the knowledge that specific factors such as self-concept (Van Andel & Austin, 1984), social skills (Novak & Heal, 1980) and facilitation of integration into mainstream community life (Collard, 1981) can be enhanced through recreation participation and awareness, Bedini, Bullock, and Driscoll (1993) reported that the application of a leisure education program teaching these skills has the potential to prepare individuals with disabilities for transition into their respective communities. Considering the recommendations of the aforementioned authors and others, leisure services professionals should consider inclusion of leisure education programs as a component of comprehensive leisure services.

Include a Comprehensive Leisure Education Program

According to Chinn and Joswiak (1981) the term "leisure education" is applied to the use of comprehensive models focusing on the educational process to enhance a person's leisure lifestyle. Leisure education provides a vehicle for developing an awareness of recreation activities and resources and for acquiring skills needed for participation throughout the life span (Howe-Murphy & Charboneau, 1987). The need for incorporating leisure education into leisure services for persons with disabilities is strong.

This chapter provides a description of the structure and content of a leisure education curriculum for persons with disabilities who are attempting to successfully transition into adulthood. In addition, the chapter contains leisure participation evaluative procedures that can be used as indicators of successful community adjustment. The model emerged in response to the clear need for leisure education for people with disabilities and is based on previous suggestions identified in articles and texts reported throughout this chapter (e.g., Mundy & Odum, 1979; Peterson & Gunn, 1984; Witt, Ellis, & Niles, 1984; Wuerch & Voeltz, 1982).

Design a Leisure Education Program

As indicated in Figure 9.1, leisure education can contain four components that are designed to facilitate independent leisure participation for people with disabilities. One component involves development and implementation of a leisure education course. This component of the model is supplemented with community support through leisure coaching and family and friend support for leisure participation. Systematic follow-up on community leisure participation facilitates generalization and maintenance of leisure skills and knowledge.

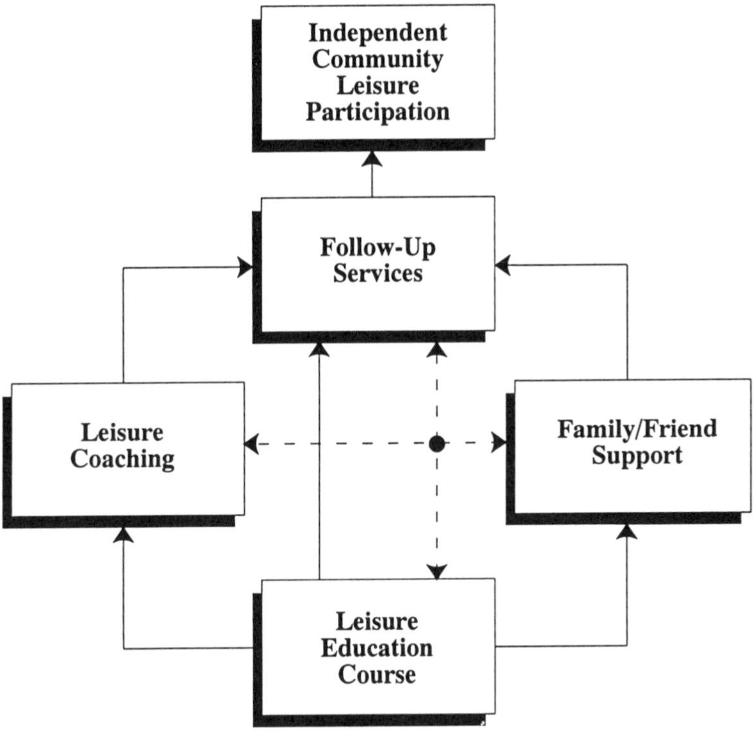

Figure 9.1 Four possible components of a comprehensive leisure education program.

Leisure education course. The leisure education model includes a structured leisure education course within the local school and/or public community recreation facility. Ideally, leisure education should begin as soon as individuals begin receiving support services. The leisure education content should help facilitate transition of an individual into active community participation.

Professionals are encouraged to develop leisure education programs that contain elements identified in this paragraph. A detailed curriculum for leisure education following the proposed format is identified in the text *Leisure Education Program Planning: A Systematic Approach* (Dattilo & Murphy, 1991). Course development is guided by goals written as general participant outcome statements. The course goals are divided into a number of behavioral objectives with corresponding performance measures. "The performance measure is a statement of the exact behavior that will be taken as evidence that the intent of the enabling objective has been achieved" (Peterson & Gunn, 1984, p. 101). The majority of information contained in the course describes content and process required to conduct the program. Each program's content specifies "what is to be done in the program to achieve the intent of the enabling objectives" (Peterson & Gunn, 1984, p. 113). On the other hand, the "process refers to the way the content is presented to the clients" (Peterson & Gunn, 1984, p. 118). The final section of each program plan contains a sequence plan with a session-by-session description of program implementation.

The course should be designed and taught through a collaborative, consultation approach. A team could be composed of community recreation professionals, classroom teachers, and therapeutic recreation specialists to help design the most effective leisure education course. The therapeutic recreation specialist can contribute specialized skills in leisure programming for individuals with disabilities while the teacher and community recreation professional can provide information regarding individual and group needs of the people with disabilities, as well as school or community resources. Participation by the classroom teacher can encourage development of a team composed of speech, physical and occupational therapists, while involvement of a community recreation professional can facilitate the participation of a variety of professional leisure services providers.

Community support through leisure coaching. The leisure education course is supplemented with systematic community-based leisure instruction and support by a leisure coach. A leisure coach can be hired by any agency that is interested in helping people with disabilities to be included in community recreation programs. The leisure coach does not conduct any activities, but rather helps participants with disabilities to participate in existing community recreation programs.

Initially, leisure coaches can meet with professionals delivering existing recreation programs providing collaborative, consultation and support for integration of people with disabilities. As indicated in Figure 9.2, leisure coaches are available to respond to questions and concerns of the community recreation professional and act as advocates for both recreation professionals and the people with disabilities.

Leisure coaches provide assistance to participants as needed while they participate in integrated community recreation activities (see Figure 9.3, page 148). A leisure coach can help identify existing community recreation activities that are compatible with interests and skills of the individual with disabilities. In addition, a leisure coach can determine the requirements of an activity, assess the skills of the participant, and identify if specific accommodations are required. A person's participation is then facilitated by systematic instruction and assistance with each activity.

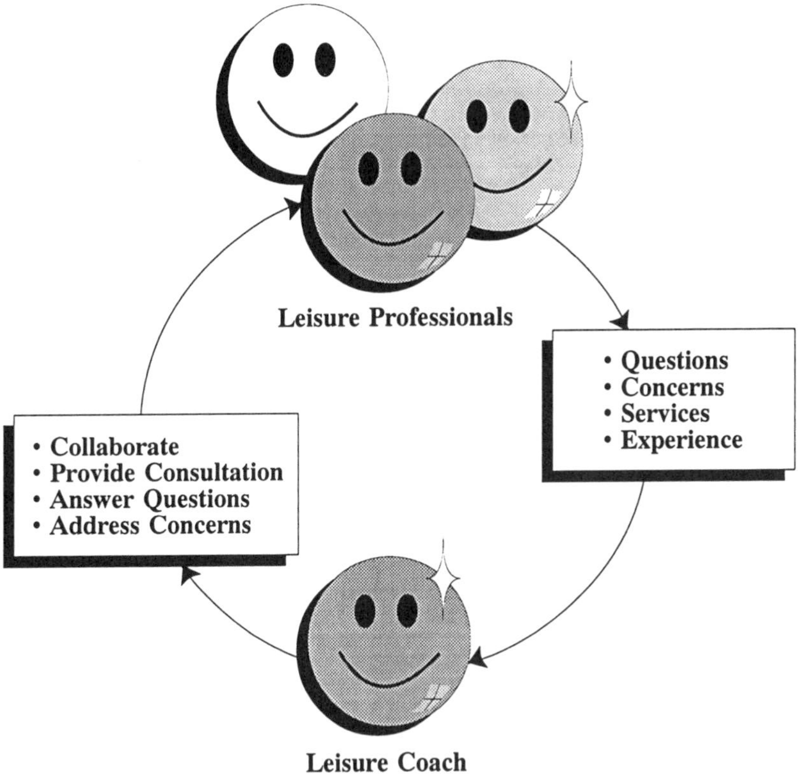

Figure 9.2 The role of the leisure coach with leisure professionals.

Leisure coaching could occur in conjunction with a formal leisure education course permitting skill enhancement and alleviation of identified barriers to leisure participation. To facilitate participant independence and autonomy, as well as create a more cost-effective system, the presence of the leisure coach is phased out systematically as the person with a disability gains skills and confidence.

In summary, the leisure coach acts as a support person. The leisure coach gives support to recreation professionals conducting programs that include people with disabilities while providing support directly to participants to help them participate in community recreation programs of their choosing.

Family and friend support for leisure participation. Parent, guardian, sibling and friend participation in the process of leisure education is stimulated through the provision of leisure transition workshops designed to increase the ability of significant others to promote rather than discourage independent

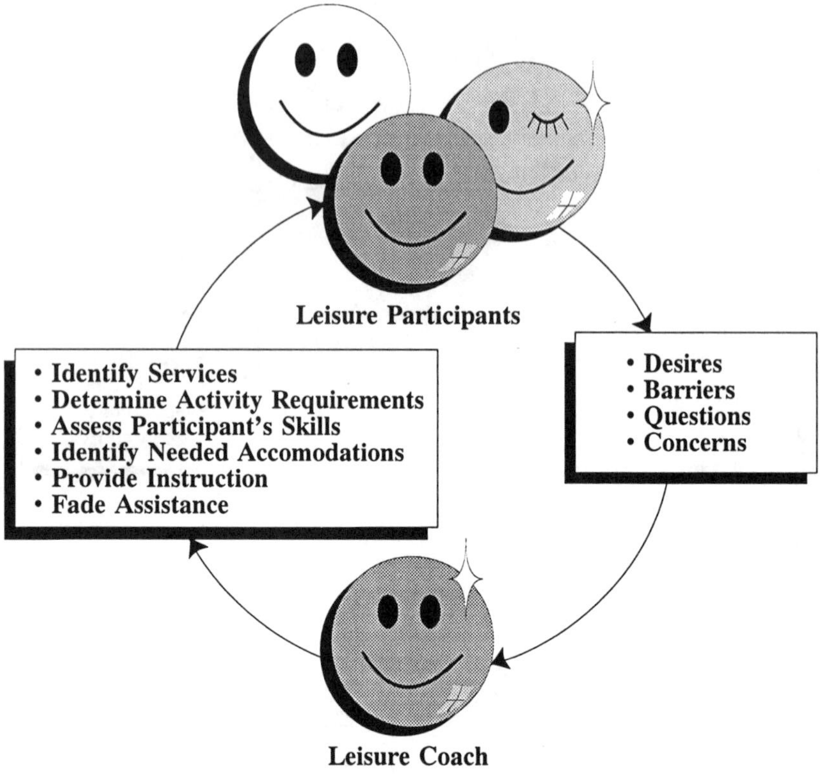

Figure 9.3 The role of the leisure coach with leisure participants with disabilities.

leisure functioning for the person with disabilities. The workshops highlight information communicated in the leisure education course, focusing primarily on identification of leisure resources available in the community.

Family and friend participation is encouraged by the leisure coach, who schedules regular meetings with families and friends to provide direct instruction about how to facilitate leisure participation for their child, sibling or friend. The leisure coach also informs family and friends of accomplishments and problems experienced by the person at community recreation agencies. Strategies encouraging continuation of the participants' successful efforts and methods for reducing barriers to community leisure involvement are addressed.

Follow-up on community leisure participation. In response to the frequent observation that many persons with disabilities fail to maintain leisure skills (e.g., Anderson & Allen, 1985), a generalization and maintenance (i.e., meaningful mastery) component is included in the leisure education model. This component requires the use of observational probes by leisure coaches to determine the degree of success experienced by people with disabilities participating in community recreation activities. The ability of individuals to maintain participation levels and generalize skills are examined. Identification of skill generalization and maintenance directly influences further instructional strategies. Therefore, the leisure coach develops generalization and maintenance reports that are shared with all human service professionals and the individual's family and friends.

Include Relevant Content in Leisure Education

Leisure education provides individuals with disabilities the opportunity to enhance the quality of their lives in leisure; understand opportunities, potentials, and challenges in leisure; understand the impact of leisure on the quality of their lives; and gain knowledge, skills and appreciations enabling broad leisure skills (Mundy & Odum, 1979). Therefore, as illustrated in Figure 9.4 (page 150), an effective leisure education program for persons with disabilities should include, but not be limited to, the three major domains of:

(a) awareness;
(b) knowledge; and
(c) application.

The awareness domain is intended to enhance individuals' sensitivity to their self-perception and leisure appreciation. The other two domains associated with the content of the leisure education model, knowledge and application, each contain the five components of self-determination in leisure, decision-making, leisure resources, social interaction, and recreation activity. The knowledge domain requires an individual to understand the concepts associated with the five components while the application domain requires people to actually demonstrate the specific leisure skills and strategies. The knowledge and application domains have been combined in the next section of the chapter in an attempt to facilitate a more rapid understanding of the components.

Awareness of self in leisure. To facilitate recreation participation, it is vital that people possess knowledge of their preferences (Montagnes, 1976). For example, small groups could go for a brief walk outside and be instructed to identify objects or activities they enjoy. Objects could be collected by participants or the leader could record the communicated preferences. Upon

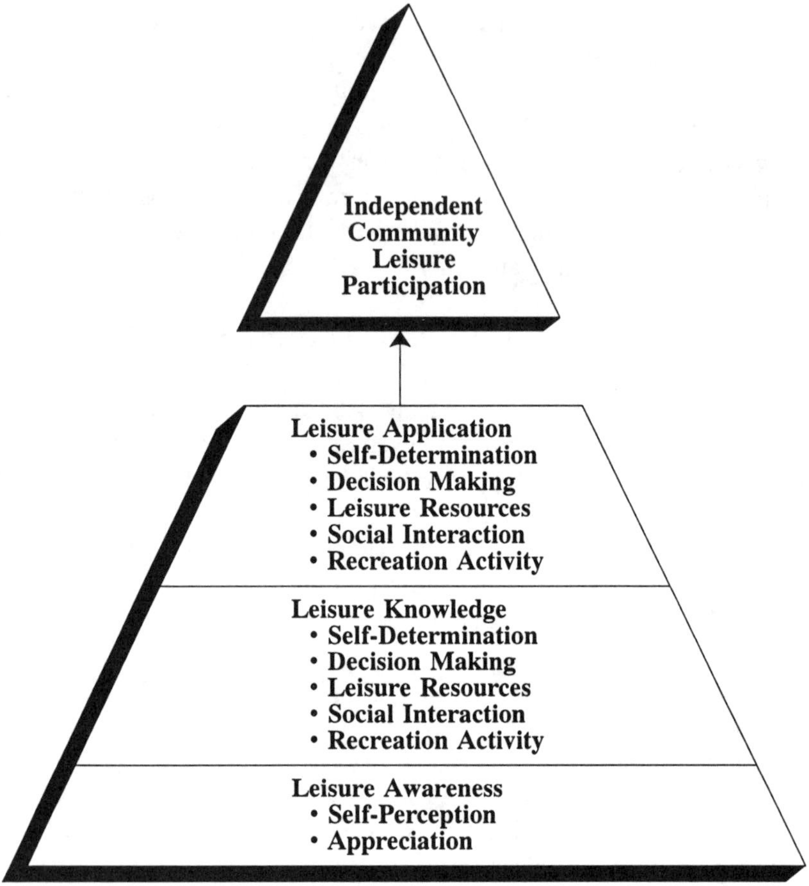

Figure 9.4 Content of the Leisure Education Model.

returning, each group could share the findings. Another learning activity might involve the use of equipment used with various recreation activities (e.g., baseball bat, ice skates, skateboard). Participants would be asked to choose equipment associated with their favorite activities. Opportunities for participation in those activities, characteristics of the activities, and previous experience with these activities could be explored.

Examination of personal attitudes toward leisure may provide individuals with information about their own barriers to leisure participation. One way to have individuals examine their attitudes is to place them in a forced-choice situation. For example, a room can be divided in half with one half of the room representing one way of approaching leisure participation and the other half of the room representing a different approach (e.g., exciting vs. relaxing, outside vs. inside, alone vs. with others). Participants must go to one side of the room or the other as the leader places large poster-board pictures associated with these concepts on each side of the room. When they arrive at their chosen destination, examination of the implications of their choices should occur.

Reflecting on past leisure pursuits may permit people with disabilities to gain insight into skills they possess. Frequently, analyzing individuals' current leisure involvement will assist them in identifying activities they enjoy as well as determining barriers they would like to overcome. Professionals should also encourage people with disabilities to look beyond their past and present leisure participation patterns and begin to consider areas for future discovery to enhance motivation for leisure participation.

To help individuals focus on what makes them happy and could make them happy in the future, a learning activity could be conducted requiring participants to identify as many enjoyable recreation activities as possible. They could identify these activities by pointing to them in a book, verbalizing them, or drawing them. After they have completed this task, materials associated with one activity chosen by each person should be gathered. The participants can be encouraged to observe or join each individual participating in a chosen activity. Following demonstrations, participants' desire to learn any of the activities presented should be assessed. Exploration of what activities they have yet to master but are motivated to learn about is often helpful.

Appreciation of leisure. To gain an awareness of leisure, it is useful for people with disabilities to develop an understanding of the concepts of leisure and leisure lifestyle. When people understand these concepts, abilities to participate in recreation activities resulting in satisfaction and enjoyment will be enhanced. For example, one way to help individuals gain an understanding of the difference between work and leisure may be achieved by dividing participants into two groups. One group is given paints and brushes and required to paint a specific object on a large piece of paper (e.g., a car). The other group can be provided with the same equipment and permitted to paint anything they like. After 10 minutes, have the groups switch tasks. Questions and statements can be made about the differences between the activities and the role freedom plays in leisure participation. By focusing on leisure awareness, people with disabilities should begin to develop a sensitivity for the uniqueness of leisure.

Because many people with disabilities have been overprotected, their abilities to take personal responsibility for leisure involvement may be reduced. Attempts at leisure education for people with disabilities should include teaching individuals to take responsibility for their leisure. It is crucial to stress that the individuals are capable and responsible for their own leisure and that they can change and improve their present leisure status (Luken,

1993). For example, to encourage development of a sense of responsibility within individuals, leisure education sessions can be divided into two parts. One portion of the session could involve instruction to teach individuals how to participate in specific recreation activities (e.g., table games). The following portion would permit them to engage in socially acceptable activities of their choosing. During this time they would be in control and responsible for their participation. The amount of time individuals are placed in this situation would vary according to their skills.

Self-determination in leisure. After reviewing the literature on leisure education, Bambara and Ager (1992) reported that professionals are advocating a broad-based agenda for leisure education, one in which the development of choice and the facilitation of self-directed activity are emphasized along with direct skill instruction in recreation activities (Dattilo, 1991). Unfortunately, choice and self-determination have been rarely addressed when facilitating leisure for people with disabilities.

Witt, Ellis, and Niles (1984) emphasized the need to provide leisure education services promoting an individual's perception of leisure control, leisure competence and intrinsic motivation to facilitate the person's sense of freedom of choice. This recommendation was based on arguments presented by many contemporary theorists for inclusion of choice in definitions of leisure (Csikszentmihalyi, 1975; Iso-Ahola, 1980).

Therefore, as detailed in the previous chapter, attempts should be made to incorporate opportunities for choice into leisure education programs for people with disabilities. The demonstration of choice through selection encourages spontaneous initiation of activity, engagement with elements of the environment, and the assertion of a degree of control over one's surroundings (Dattilo & Barnett, 1985). Development of a sense of self-determination facilitates the ability of individuals to make choices and sets the stage for acquisition of more complex decision-making strategies. Some people with disabilities typically need to be taught to make choices and experience a wide range of leisure options.

In an attempt to address the unmet leisure education needs of people with disabilities, Wuerch and Voeltz (1982) developed a leisure training project for these individuals. The program was designed to provide people with opportunities to learn and make choices during their free time. The three major goals of the project were to:

(a) develop leisure skills that are age-appropriate;
(b) encourage self-initiated enjoyable leisure skills; and
(c) facilitate cooperative leisure planning.

Leisure education should be designed to encourage self-directed, freely chosen, healthy and pleasurable choices (Luken, 1993). According to Luken, for leisure education to be effective it must encourage participants to go beyond mere leisure awareness and instill the ability and confidence to take personal action and choose to participate independently in meaningful experiences.

Decision-making skills. Some individuals with disabilities encounter difficulty in making decisions related to many aspects of their lives. This problem is evident in relation to their leisure lifestyle. Based on observations that persons with disabilities frequently fail in their attempts to adjust to community living as a result of inappropriate use of free time, Hayes (1977) recommended instruction in decision-making and encouraged selection of, and participation in, recreation activities by persons with disabilities. Making a decision related to leisure participation is facilitated by individuals' awareness of themselves relative to leisure and an appreciation of the concept of leisure as well as their development of a sense of self-determination about leisure involvement.

McDowell (1976) identified the importance of individuals using rational problem-solving and decision-making techniques to promote independent responsibility of making wise decisions about leisure involvement. According to McDowell, successful decision-making can be enhanced by:

(a) assessment of leisure interests and attitudes;
(b) identification of realistic leisure goals;
(c) determination of needs met through goal attainment;
(d) identification of barriers preventing leisure involvement;
(e) development of strategies for overcoming barriers;
(f) identification of leisure alternatives for each goal; and
(g) establishment of a plan for leisure participation.

A potential plan for leisure participation for people with disabilities may involve development of problem-solving skills. Gordon (1977) identified the following six steps that can be taught to encourage people to solve their problems:

(a) define the problem;
(b) generate possible solutions;
(c) evaluate the solutions;
(d) make decisions;
(e) determine how to implement the decisions; and
(f) assess the success of the decision.

One way to facilitate the development of decision-making skills for persons with disabilities is to place a large piece of collage paper on a table. A variety of pictures that participants cut from magazines representing different types of recreation activities could be used. The concept of a collage as a collection of pictures placed together on paper to communicate a theme or idea could be presented. Participants can be given a specific theme (e.g, camping, water sports, self-improvement) and instructed to decide which pictures are appropriate for inclusion in their collage and to glue them to the paper. Results of their collages can be discussed, reviewed with each participant, presented to others, and posted.

Knowledge and utilization of leisure resources. According to Overs, Taylor, and Adkins (1974), difficulty in making appropriate leisure decisions may result from people's lack of knowledge of leisure resources. A factor in people with disabilities failing to adjust to community living is their lack of awareness of recreation resources and their inability to use those resources of which they possess knowledge (Ashton-Shaeffer & Kleiber, 1990). Knowledge of leisure resources and the ability to utilize these resources appear to be important factors in establishing an independent leisure lifestyle (Peterson & Gunn, 1984). Therefore, Dattilo and Murphy (1987) recommended teaching individuals not only how to participate in an activity but how to answer questions such as:

(a) Where can one participate?
(b) Are there others who participate?
(c) How much will participation cost?
(d) What type of transportation is available?
(e) Where could one learn more about a recreation activity? and
(f) What equipment is required?

One way to help people with disabilities learn about the equipment needed for participation is to have them participate in a matching game that will stimulate their memory and concentration, and provide information on recreation activities and equipment. Two sets of cards, one with names and pictures of activities and one with names and pictures of equipment, are placed face-down on a table. The number of cards varies according to participants' skills. The object of the game is to match an activity with the equipment used in the activity by turning over the related cards. A discussion regarding the equipment needed could then occur after each match is made, accompanied by exposure to the actual equipment and activity whenever possible.

Joswiak (1979) developed a leisure education program for persons with disabilities emphasizing development of an awareness of leisure resources within the home and community. Anderson and Allen (1985) conducted an investigation incorporating Joswiak's leisure education program with 40 people with disabilities. Upon completion of their study, the investigators concluded that participation in the leisure education program emphasizing knowledge of leisure resources appeared to enhance frequency of activity involvement.

In addition to the need for people with disabilities to acquire knowledge of community leisure resources, utilization of these resources encouraging active participation in community life is crucial (Richler, 1984). To encourage utilization of leisure resources, families, friends, and human service professionals must also be made aware of the leisure resources available within the community.

Social interaction skills. One major deficit preventing many people with disabilities from developing a satisfying life is related to social interaction skills. Handleman and Harris (1986) identified interpersonal responsiveness and social development as two major problems for persons with disabilities. Absence of social skills is particularly noticeable during leisure participation (Marlowe, 1979) and frequently leads to isolation and an inability to function successfully (O'Morrow, 1980). Therefore, the development of social skills used in leisure situations appears to be critical for people with disabilities because acquisition of these skills facilitates integration (Keogh, Faw, Whitman, & Reid, 1984).

Development of effective social interaction skills can be taught through systematic leisure education programs. For instance, people with disabilities can be instructed to participate in an activity to help them practice how to introduce themselves to a group. In turn, participants will communicate to the group their first name, and for 30 seconds share with the group positive information about themselves (e.g., accomplishments, desirable personal traits, friendships). Participants will be instructed to communicate only positive information about themselves during this time. Leisure education learning activities such as this are designed to encourage social integration.

According to Schleien and Ray (1988), successful social integration of participants into recreation activities may be determined by collecting information on such behavior as:

(a) social interactions;
(b) eye contact;
(c) physical proximity;
(d) physical contact;
(e) sharing of equipment/materials;
(f) cooperating; and
(g) developing friends.

Recreation activity skills. If we believe choice is a critical aspect of leisure participation and choice involves options and alternatives, then, according to Peterson and Gunn (1984), it appears logical that a repertoire of recreation activities and related interests should exist for individuals to experience meaningful leisure. Based on recommendations by Peterson and Gunn, people with disabilities should be encouraged to select and develop recreation skills having the most potential for enjoyment and satisfaction. Selection of recreation activity skills should be contingent on needs, interests, motivations and aspirations of the person (Howe-Murphy & Charboneau, 1987).

Howe-Murphy and Charboneau (1987) reported that recreation activity skill development can provide physical and emotional support assisting participants, family members, friends and community professionals to overcome fears of the unknown and failure. Reduction of fears associated with leisure participation should reduce hesitancy of people with disabilities to become active participants in community life as well as develop support systems comprised of family members, friends, and professionals. Determination of which recreation activity skills a person is taught should result from participants' preferences, their ability to engage in the recreation activity in the near and distant future, the availability of activity involvement within their home or neighboring community and individuals' available resources (e.g., money, recreation equipment, clothing).

Conclusion

A primary purpose of services designed for people with disabilities must be to meet their leisure needs. The ability of professionals to meet the needs of persons with disabilities is impaired without the development of effective service delivery systems. Currently, many people with disabilities are not experiencing satisfying leisure (Dattilo, 1990). The intent of this chapter was to identify the need and rationale for including leisure education in transition services for people with disabilities. Information was presented to provide support for people with disabilities having difficulty experiencing meaningful leisure. The leisure education model is intended to encourage participants to acquire characteristics indicated in Figure 9.5 that facilitate successful transition into community life for people with disabilities.

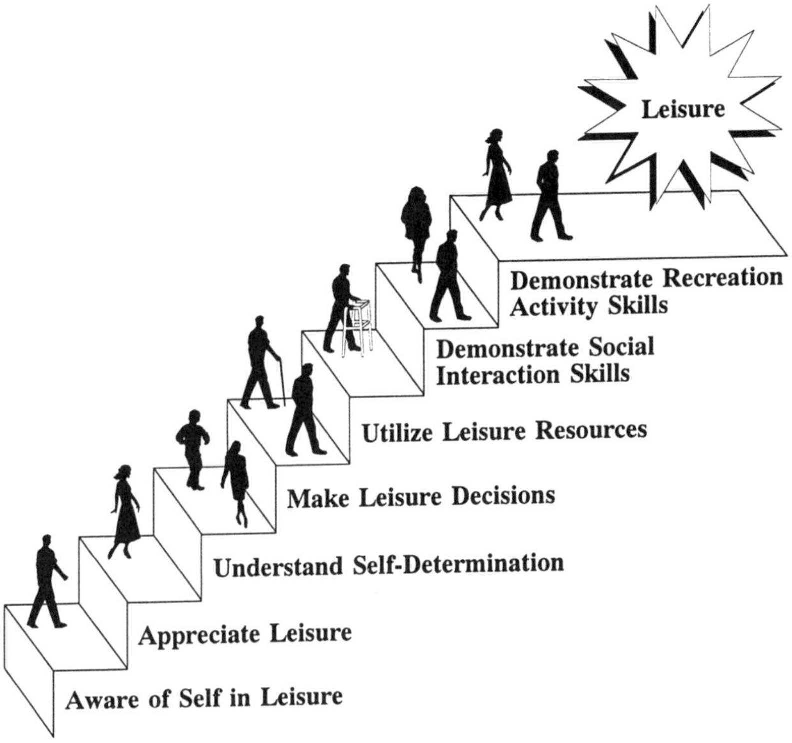

Figure 9.5 Characteristics of a person prepared through leisure education.

Discussion Questions

1. What are at least four benefits discussed in this chapter that can be derived from a leisure education program?
2. What are the three major goals of a leisure education program?
3. How would you go about developing a course on leisure education?
4. What are the primary responsibilities of a leisure coach?
5. How could you involve family and friends in leisure education?
6. Why is it important to do follow-up after leisure education?

7. What is meant by awareness of self in leisure?

8. How could you instill an appreciation of leisure in the people attending a leisure education program?

9. Why is self-determination an important component of a comprehensive leisure education program?

10. What are some components of the decision-making process?

11. What are some questions relative to leisure resources that are important for people to be able to answer?

12. What are some examples of important social interaction skills?

13. What are some guidelines to follow when teaching recreation activity skills?

Chapter 10

Facilitate Accessibility

All the world's a stage, and all men and women are merely players:
They have their exits and their entrances.
—William Shakespeare

Orientation Activity: Test Architectural Awareness

Directions When Alone: On a separate sheet of paper write the numbers 1 to 14 down the left-hand side. As you read each statement below, write the letter "T" next to the corresponding number if you think the statement is TRUE and the letter "F" if you think the statement is FALSE. Once you have finished, read the debriefing to check your answers.

Directions With Others: Move about the room and find another person who has completed the sheet. Introduce yourself to the person and find out the person's name. Share with the person one aspect related to accessibility that you have learned. Once you have finished talking to this person, move on to another person. Continue this process until a signal to end the activity has been given.

1. Ramps are easier for everyone to use than stairs.
2. Most guide dogs stop at intersection curb cuts.
3. Barrier-free buildings should have heat-sensitive elevator controls (touch the number and it lights up).
4. The color indicators used on stairs are a frequent cause of stairway accidents for people who are older.
5. Most people with visual impairments can understand direction signs in Braille.
6. Even short-nap carpets can cause barriers for wheelchairs.
7. Public bathroom signs marked "Ladies" and "Gentlemen" may pose barriers to some people with mental retardation.
8. If a door is wide, and has no threshold, it is accessible to wheelchairs.
9. A person with epilepsy should have many bathroom grab bars.
10. Many older adults and people with disabilities should have a telephone in their bathrooms.

11. Some people experience heat stroke in their shower or bathtub.
12. Rooms for people with limited mobility should be furnished with soft, overstuffed furniture.
13. Round doorknobs are generally the most difficult kind to use.
14. A dark sign with light lettering is generally easier to read than a light sign with dark lettering.

Debriefing

This Design Awareness Test has been adapted from an exercise developed by Interface, Human Factors Design Consultants, Raleigh, North Carolina. Answers to the statements listed above are presented on the next page.

1. ***False.*** Some people prefer stairs and can use them more easily than ramps.

2. ***False*** Dogs are trained to stop at curbs; they may lead their masters into traffic if a curb ramp is in their direct line of travel.

3. ***False*** They are nearly impossible for people who are blind to use; they may be especially deadly if used for wheelchair evacuation during a fire. Raised buttons must be placed on elevators to be accessible to persons with visual difficulties. They must be placed at a height that is accessible to people of small stature, and to those using wheeled assistive devices.

4. ***True*** Low-contrasting colors can trick the eye and are the cause of numerous stairway accidents.

5. ***False*** At least 90 percent of persons who are blind cannot read Braille.

6. ***True*** Some short-nap carpets have a tendency to pull wheelchairs to one side as they roll.

7. ***True*** Some people are taught to distinguish between restroom facilities by the length of the word on the door; short word means MEN, long word means WOMEN.

8. ***False*** Doors can have many barriers: door handles may be difficult; doors may close too fast and too hard; doors may be too heavy to push open.

9. ***False*** Grab bars may be a dangerous obstruction during a fall. Cushioning the fall would be more effective.

10. True The bathroom is the most dangerous room in your house and phones are often used to call for help.

11. True The heat from bath or shower water can cause heat stroke, especially in elderly persons. This may be prevented by lowering the hot water thermostat.

12. False Soft furniture does not support the spine adequately; it may be nearly impossible for some people to get up.

13. True Lever handles require much less hand and wrist action.

14. True That is why most interstate freeway signs are dark green or blue with white letters.

Introduction

The writings of George Alderson, a respected syndicated columnist and a strong advocate for the rights of any oppressed group, especially people with disabilities, were consulted frequently during the development of this chapter. His writings contain a great deal of information intended to increase access for people with disabilities.

During an average day, most people give little thought to how they get around in their environment. Merlo, Staniszewski, and Sarrett (1990) reported that mobility concerns arise, however, when people are confronted with a personal limitation or external hindrance such as broken bones, sprains, pregnancy, carrying heavy packages or using a baby stroller. At some point in their lives, most people will experience a temporary or permanent limitation and when this occurs, the issue of accessibility or usability suddenly becomes prominent (Merlo et al., 1990).

> If one considers recreation the right of all people, including those with disabilities, then the right to recreation services should include the rights of choice and access (Bedini, 1990, p. 16).

Know Which Access Standards to Follow

Cangemi (1992) reported that during the past two decades, changes in both federal and state laws have indicated an increased societal commitment to the rights of persons with disabilities. These laws led to development of standards and the creation of agencies charged with implementing the legislative mandate for access (Cangemi, 1992). However, Cangemi warned that recreation professionals should:

(a) always check federal, state and local requirements, and adhere to the more rigorous, specific standard;
(b) evaluate the regulations for a given accessibility item; and
(c) implement the regulation that provides the greatest amount of accessibility.

The **Architectural Barriers Act,** passed in 1968 by Congress, states that all facilities receiving direct or indirect federal funds must provide access to all people. It is considered the first federal policy directed toward protecting the rights of people with disabilities. In 1973, Congress passed the **Rehabilitation Act** that focused on the rights of all people to have equal access to jobs, education, housing, transportation, and all programs which directly or indirectly received federal funds. Section 504 of this act provided that no "otherwise qualified" person with a disability can, solely by reason of his or her disability, be:

(a) excluded from participation in;
(b) denied the benefits of; or
(c) subjected to discrimination under any program or activity receiving federal money or administered by a federal agency.

The Architectural Barriers Act of 1968 dealt with facility access and the Rehabilitation Act of 1973 addressed program access. Unfortunately, neither of these two federal acts covered facilities and programs not receiving federal funds. According to Cangemi (1992, p. 7):

> It wasn't until the enactment of the **Americans with Disabilities Act** on July 26, 1990, that the federal mandate for access to public accommodations and programs was extended to the private sector.

The American Transportation Bureau Compliance Board issued a comprehensive set of federal standards in 1981 entitled *Minimum Guidelines and Requirements for Accessible Design* after considering the American National Standards Institute accessibility criteria. These standards, and those contained in the Uniform Federal Accessibility Standards and the Americans with Disabilities Act Accessibility Guidelines, serve as the major sources of accessibility criteria for recreation facility planners (Cangemi, Williams, & Gaskell, 1992). Agencies must follow the Uniform Federal Accessibility Standards to assure compliance with federal accessibility legislation and comply with state and local building codes, where applicable. The development of the Uniform Federal Accessibility Standards reflects the legislative mandate for equal access for persons with disabilities to public accommodations, facilities, and programs (Cangemi, 1992).

The Americans with Disabilities Act Accessibility Guidelines (ADAAG) for Buildings and Facilities are of public record and located in the Federal Register, Volume 56, No. 144, posted on Friday, July 26, 1991, under Rules and Regulations and identified as Appendix A to Part 36—Standards for Accessible Design. ADAAG provides information on the purpose of the guidelines, general consideration, and specific instructions and definitions. In addition, ADAAG contains specific recommendations in providing accessible elements and technical requirements under the following headings:

application
exterior facilities (new construction)
accessible buildings (additions)
accessible buildings (historic preservation)
accessible route
ground and floor surfaces
curb ramps
stairs
platform lifts (wheelchair lifts)
doors
drinking fountains and water coolers
toilet stalls
lavatories and mirrors
shower stalls
bathrooms
shower rooms
storage
grab bars
controls and operating mechanisms
detectable warnings
telephones
assembly areas
dressing and fitting rooms
accessible sites
accessible buildings (new construction)
accessible buildings (alterations)
space allowance and reach ranges
protruding objects
parking and passenger loading zones
ramps
elevators
windows
entrances
water closets
urinals
bathtubs
toilet rooms
bathing facilities
sinks
handrails
tub and shower seats
alarms
signage
fixed or built-in seating and tables
automated teller machines

The description of accessible elements and spaces is followed by detailed guidelines for: restaurants and cafeterias, medical care facilities, business and mercantile, libraries, accessible transient lodging, and transportation facilities.

Learn Definitions Related to Access

Webster's dictionary defines **access** as "freedom or ability to obtain or make use of" or "ability to enter, approach, communicate with, or pass to and from." Access also has social connotations and involves total experiences. These experiences are influenced by positive or negative feelings and attitudes.

Accessibility or usability of a facility is the degree to which a person with limitations can get to, enter and use a building or area surrounding the facility (American National Standard A117.1-1986). The term **"barrier"** implies that there is an obstruction which impedes an individual's progress. A single stair can allow an individual to move from one level to another level with ease. However, that same stair can deny a person using a wheelchair or a parent with a child's stroller the right to enter that facility.

Understand the Types of Access Barriers

When many people think of access they often think of physical access, installing a ramp or renovating bathrooms for wheelchair users. But access does not end there. Consider the next situations presented by Laird (1992):

> What about the person who is deaf or has a **hearing impairment**? They can enter a building, but once they are inside, the information being transmitted when a leader is giving directions, a play is performed, or information discussed at a meeting is inaccessible to them because a sign language interpreter or an assistive listening device has not been provided for the occasion. What about the person who is blind or has a **visual impairment**? Once again the person can enter the building, but if it is a meeting in which information is being distributed on paper and must be read, then the meeting is inaccessible to this individual. Why? Because the information has not been produced in an alternate format such as Braille, large print, or on a cassette tape. What about the person who has **mental retardation**? This person may require the assistance of a support person to participate in community activities.

Two external forces faced each day by people who have disabilities are architectural and attitudinal barriers. Although much of the discussion in this chapter will focus on physical access, the aforementioned barriers, which prevent people with disabilities from participating in activities on a daily basis, can be eliminated if the barrier of negative attitudes is removed. Laird (1992) suggested that if people could change their attitude—from one where implementing changes to structures, or producing or providing information in alternate formats is considered to be "special treatment" to an attitude that says by making these changes the whole community benefits because everyone is involved—then the other barriers will begin to fall one by one. "All it takes is a willingness for communities to get active to make our communities accessible for all its citizens" (Laird, 1992, p. 8).

Architectural barriers usually consist of structures constructed by humans which present an obstacle for people who have a mobility, visual or sensory disability. Architectural barriers not only inhibit people with disabilities, but also affect many others, including the elderly, parents with carriages and people with temporary disabilities.

Attitudinal barriers tend to be the most difficult to identify and therefore are more difficult to overcome. As discussed in Chapter 1, an attitude is a way of thinking or feeling. Thinking or feeling negatively about a disability or a person who has a disability, creates an attitudinal barrier. Attitudinal barriers often arise from fear, lack of knowledge about a disability or lack of communication. In order to rectify this problem, people must start looking at an individual's ability first and not the disability and focus on people's potential, not their limitations.

Take Action to Increase Access

Cangemi and colleagues (1992) suggested that recreation professionals should consider adopting several strategies that can greatly improve the process of removing barriers to accessibility. As indicated in Figure 10.1 (see page 167), among those that Cangemi and colleagues described were for recreation professionals to:

(a) incorporate barrier-free design into the planning process;
(b) acquire knowledge of the laws and accessibility standards;
(c) include people with disabilities as planning team members;
(d) include an accessibility specialist on your planning team;
(e) exceed standards whenever possible;
(f) extend accessibility beyond the parking lot;
(g) incorporate accessibility into outdoor environments;
(h) plan for a continuous path of travel;
(j) consider aesthetics/environmental values when planning; and
(k) ensure materials comply with governmental standards.

Realize the Impact of Access

The following letter was printed in *Parks and Recreation Magazine* in an article written by Oestreicher (1990). The letter helps illustrate the importance of accessible recreation environments.

Dear Playground Director:

I was told about the playground you want to build for kids like me and regular kids, and that you were looking for ideas from handicapped kids. We really need a place to play, and maybe, if I tell you about my normal day in the summer, you will understand.

I lie in bed an hour to an hour-and-a-half, after I wake up, while Mom makes breakfast. I can help Mom make breakfast. I just don't do it as fast as Mom, and with two brothers and sisters, I "get in the way."

After breakfast, I roll out to the sun porch, while Mom cleans the house, or does the laundry, I could help with the cleaning, but Mom can do it faster, and . . . I "get in the way."

Most days, I go outside in the backyard and play by myself, or with our dog. We have a basketball hoop on the garage, and I'm pretty good, especially my hook shot. I know I could play with my brothers and their friends, but I slow down the game, so most days I sit in the backyard reading, or playing with the dog. It seems to me, we are both put out here so we won't be in the way. The only difference is the dog can run off and play with his friends when he wants . . . I can't . . . Deep down inside I know I can do just about anything anyone else can do, just a little different, just a little slower. It just seems I don't get a chance very often . . . or at all.

For a week every summer I go to camp for special kids. It's fun, but it's only for a week a year, and even when I enjoy playing and winning against another handicapped kid, it would be much better to play and win against a regular kid.

So Mr., I'm sorry I don't know how to spell your name . . . it's too long, but if you build a playground where I can go anytime and can play with regular kids, and not be in anyone's way, I'll play in it and I'll buy you a "Big Mac" with cheese and a Coke.

I won't sign my name, because it might hurt my family a little, and they do love me, very much . . . so do your best please.

Yours truly,

A friend from Springfield

The letter written by the friend in Springfield is a very powerful statement that helps illustrate the need for access. Another example reported in the pamphlet entitled "Fair Play" produced by the Regional Rehabilitation Research Institute on Attitudinal, Legal, and Leisure Barriers also illustrates the importance of access. Dana went to a basketball game with her husband who uses a wheelchair. She accompanied her husband to the "wheelchair section"

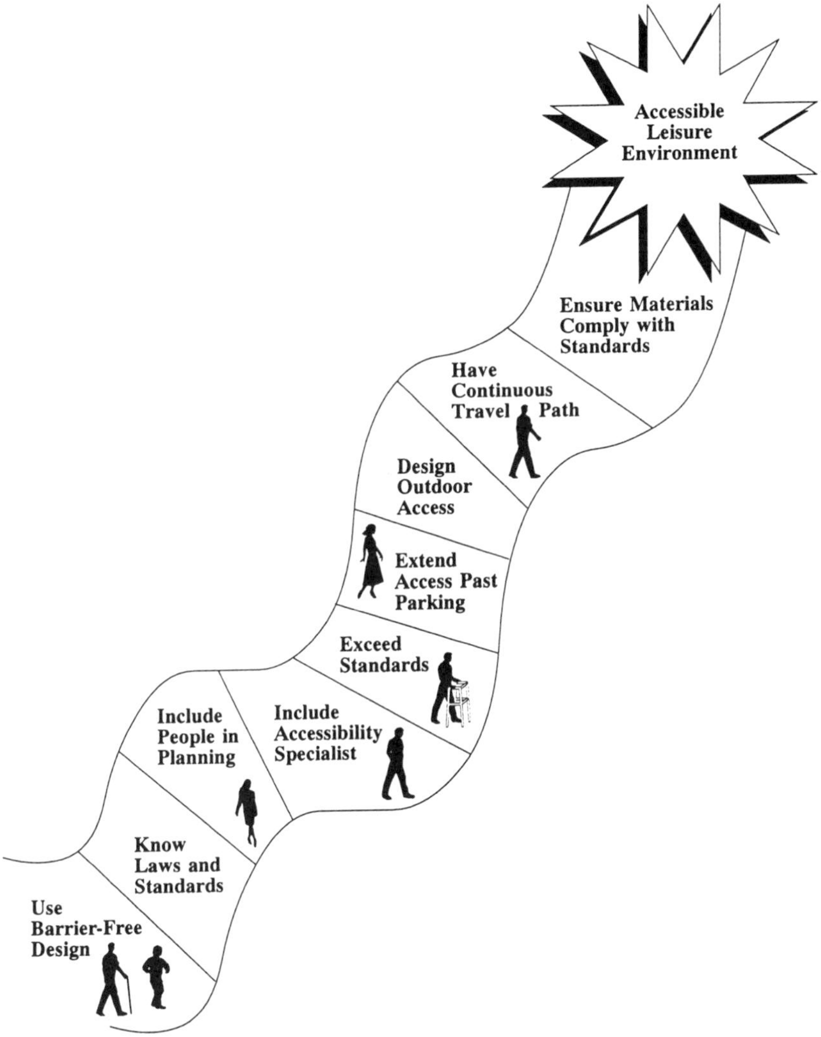

Figure 10.1 Suggestions to remove access barriers by Cangemi, Williams, and Gaskell.

and was told by the attendant that she could not stay there. The area was reserved for people in wheelchairs. This situation is repeated all too frequently at coliseums, sports arenas and stadiums. Making a facility accessible means more than just providing an entrance ramp and a section with seats removed to accommodate wheelchairs. Often these sections are situated in areas with the poorest view of the event. This practice also segregates people, separating them from their friends and setting them apart from the other spectators. Seating sections should be arranged so as to provide people a choice of seating locations and ticket prices. Portable chairs should be used in these sections to allow people with and without disabilities to enjoy the event together.

Consider The International Symbol of Access

Webster states "A symbol is a sign by which one infers a thing, (an object used to represent something abstract)." The International Symbol of Access, as presented in Figure 10.2 (a), represents the hope of independence and mobility to people with disabilities and, wherever it is displayed, people who depend upon it can be assured that they will not be barred by thoughtless obstacles or prohibited from participating in the mainstream of society (Alderson, 1985).

The use of signs to convey information to visitors and participants is an important consideration in the provision of access. The International Symbol of Access is often used in parking lots to indicate reserved stalls and in buildings to indicate accessible bathrooms. It can also be used in conjunction with directional symbols or a written message such as "Ask for Information Here," which tells the visitor that there are other services available. Such services may include interpretive cassettes, the availability of a wheelchair for loan, accessible transportation services, and other such accommodations.

The Symbol should also be used in informational materials such as maps, program announcements and information, and registration brochures, to indicate accessibility. Care should be taken in the use of these symbols. For instance, a building which has an accessible entrance should not have the access symbol displayed unless the facilities and services inside the building are also accessible.

During the 1975 Assembly of Rehabilitation International meeting, the following policies to govern the use of the International Symbol of Access were presented:

(a) the Symbol shall always be used in the design and proportions approved by the Assembly, reproduction of which shall be disseminated with this resolution;
(b) the colors used shall always be in sharp contrast and, unless there are compelling reasons to use other colors, the Symbol and its background shall be reproduced in either black and white or dark blue and white;
(c) no change in or addition to the design shall be permitted; and
(d) the Symbol shall be used only to mark or show the way to facilities that are accessible to persons whose mobility is restricted by disability.

To preserve the meaning of the Symbol of Access, to maintain the dignity of individuals for whom the Symbol was designed, and to avoid confusion to the general public, Alderson (1985) stated that the Symbol of Access must be displayed correctly and properly at all times. Any organization is permitted to display the Symbol in published material relevant to services for people with disabilities. The Symbol must be clearly identified as the International Symbol of Access, and it must always face to the right. The Symbol may face left, however, when it is meant to be a directional signal.

According to Alderson (1985), the Symbol of Access was not intended to identify a person who is disabled, and it should not be used in that manner. It is intended for the purpose of marking facilities that are accessible to and usable by persons who happen to be disabled. The Symbol of Access tells people that they can enter a building or facility without fear of being blocked by architectural barriers. To use the Symbol of Access for reasons other than to denote an accessible building or facility for use by persons with disabilities is prohibited.

While the International Symbol of Access is most commonly recognized for barrier-free access, the U.S. Architectural and Transportation Barrier Compliance Board (1992) reported the Symbol of Access for Hearing Loss is becoming known as the indicator for communication accessibility. According to the Department of Justice (1991), this symbol, presented in Figure 10.2 (b), may represent volume controlled telephones, text telephones, assistive listening systems or communication assistance.

(a) (b)

Figure 10.2 (a) The International Symbol of Access and (b) The International Symbol of Access for Hearing Loss.

Follow Access Guidelines When Planning Special Events

Recreation professionals who are planning conferences, workshops and special events must recognize the need to plan ahead for the attendance of persons with disabilities. McCarty (1991) recommended including people with disabilities when planning services and events. Alderson (1985) suggested that, while keeping the audience in mind, examine the premises closely and attempt to answer important questions: How much reserved parking is available for people with disabilities? How accessible are the rooms and baths? Are all the dining, social and conference rooms accessible? If there is more than one floor, are there elevators? Are public bathrooms marked with the Symbol of Access? Are public phones accessible to people who use wheelchairs? Are menus available on cassette tape or in Braille? Are elevators marked in Braille? How accessible are nearby stores, restaurants, theaters, lounges or amusement parks?

When visiting the potential location, Alderson suggested that professionals:

(a) make certain doorways are wide enough to accommodate wheelchairs;
(b) check for handrails and raised toilet seats in the bathrooms; and
(c) look for ramps, parking spaces, fire alarms in both audio and visual as well as any other items that may be required by the participants.

Using an accessibility guide, McCarty suggested asking the following questions:

(a) Have architectural and communication barriers been removed?
(b) Are common areas and meeting rooms designed to provide the most integrated setting? and
(c) Are auxiliary aids and services available?

Alderson (1985) also encouraged professionals to consider travel arrangements and ask the following questions:

(a) Is there a lift-equipped van service available for transportation from the airport to the conference location?
(b) What are the local taxi services' policies about transporting passengers with disabilities?
(c) Will these services transport people who use wheelchairs? and
(d) Will they assist the passenger who is disabled?

Prestige is added to any organization when attention is given to planning that increases comfort and ease for people with disabilities (Alderson, 1985). According to Alderson (1985), excessive accessibility is never a problem; too little accessibility can be a disaster. Accessibility means more than entering a building or the area; it means being able to use all the services usually available for all people in attendance.

Appraise Access Concerns for Specific Types of Disabilities

People with Visual Impairments

The following suggestions reported in the *AFB News* (1991) should be considered when encouraging access for people with visual impairments:

(a) signs in public areas should be available in large print on non-glossy surfaces, and should maintain a clear contrast between the letters and background;
(b) signs on elevator panels and for rooms and facilities should be marked in Braille;
(c) all information on Automatic Teller Machine screens and panels should be accessible via speech and/or telephone access and Braille and tactile markings;
(d) stairways in all facilities must be well-lit and have a handrail that runs the entire span of the stairway;
(e) a textured material that can be felt underfoot should be placed at the leading edge of stairways;
(f) the leading edge of each step should be marked with a paint or nonskid material in a high-contrast color;
(g) curb cuts should be marked with a textured material (that can be felt underfoot) that is placed along the line where the blended sidewalk and roadway meet to contrast clearly with the sidewalk and extend 36 inches back from the roadway; and
(h) the edges of rail and subway boarding platforms should have tactual markings (textured material that can be felt underfoot) that span the length of the platform and extend at least 36 inches back from the platform edge.

Examples of Access

A Student Can Make a Difference

This example was contributed by Stephanie Evans, previously a student of recreation and leisure studies, illustrating how people are striving to help change and improve the lives of people who have disabilities. This example deals with the subject of the Symbol of Access. Stephanie had the idea of using the accessibility sign in the Yellow Pages of a phone book to show that a building or place is accessible. One day Stephanie was talking to her brother, who worked for the United Phone Book Advertisers Inc., and suggested to him that they should use the accessibility sign in their Yellow Pages. He did not seem to take her too seriously at that time, but something must have stayed with him. About a week later, he called and told Stephanie that he spoke to his supervisor about it, and during that week they had decided to include the accessibility sign in the company's phone books. At the time, United Phone Book Advertisers had phone books in eleven cities across the nation. This experience is an example of how much one person can do just by speaking up. It shows that things are happening and access is changing for individuals with disabilities.

A Park Ranger Can Make a Difference

The Pennsylvania Constitution states that:

> "The people have a right to clean air, pure water and the preservation of the natural, scenic, historic and aesthetic values of the environment. Pennsylvania's public natural resources are the common property of all people, including generations yet to come. As trustees of these resources, the Commonwealth shall conserve and maintain them for the benefit of all people."

Based on the Constitution, the following projects have been completed:

(a) accessible railings for beach areas;
(b) accessible pathways and ramps to family cabins and park offices;
(c) accessible bathrooms and picnic tables;
(d) an accessible boat launch and fishing docks; and
(e) provision of a phone number on all brochures for information on access.

A Commercial Recreation Vendor Can Make a Difference

The following information was presented in the *Miracle Recreation Equipment Company Catalog.* The ADA is not specific in its approach to public playground design. The law does, however, mandate that all new or altered public or tax-supported playgrounds be accessible to people with disabilities. The term "accessible," as used in conjunction with playgrounds, can be interpreted to mean that a playground can be approached, accessed or entered (actually getting on the play structure) and used by people with disabilities. Similar sensations shall be available to people with and without disabilities, such as swinging, climbing, or sliding. The design of accessible equipment is very important, and personnel at Miracle are prepared to provide the design assistance needed to comply with ADA. All units that are accessible are identified in their brochure with an International Access Symbol.

The Forest Service Can Make a Difference

Within the Grand Teton Mountains, accessible camping experiences are designed in a variety of scenic and rustic settings. The Landers Forest Service, Challenges Unlimited, and others, work to provide accessible design at each campsite, providing various amenities and levels of accessibility for camping experiences. The several campsites located near main travel roads offering a lesser degree of physical challenge are equipped with accessible tent pads, restrooms and picnic tables to provide basic camping experiences. For people seeking camping opportunities in a more remote setting, mountaintop campsites provide accessible resources such as accessible picnic tables, tent pads, restrooms and electrical hookups, accessible boat ramps and fishing stations give campers the opportunity to canoe and fish at mountain lakes. Campers seeking even greater physical challenges can access camping facilities provided at one of the Grand Teton's most pristine sites. A two-hour drive up a 1,300-foot mountainside stretch provides a panoramic view of the valley floor. The road level reaches a meadow which serves as host to the accessible campsite, providing a rustic camping experience. The project offers integrated accessible camping in diverse settings.

A Parks and Recreation Department Can Make a Difference

Zertuche (1993) reported on "Fantasy Landing," designed, researched and constructed by the Dallas Park and Recreation Department, which was created in 1989 for *all* children, including youth who use wheelchairs, braces, crutches, or who possess any variety of disabling conditions. According to Zertuche, the park provides the following characteristics with the intent of minimizing differences between children playing on the playground:

(a) subtle changes in elevation and resilient rubber surfacing, allowing for more accessibility for participants who enter the multiplay units;
(b) ramps, rather than steps, were installed to enhance accessibility into the play area; and
(c) concrete paths connect the play units.

An executive that assisted with the development of the park stated that, "Our intent was to create an inviting playground environment where physically challenged and able-bodied children, who may even be from the same family, could play side-by-side."

Conclusion

Some professionals argue that they rarely, if ever, observe people with disabilities in their community accessing their facilities. Therefore, they conclude that even if they made their facilities and programs accessible, people with disabilities would not attend. The information presented in this chapter was intended to encourage professionals to promote access and thereby create opportunities for people with disabilities to engage in community leisure pursuits. Many people with disabilities agree with the whispers heard in the movie *Field of Dreams*: "If you build it, they will come."

Discussion Questions

The following questions can be used as a general guide when surveying a potential meeting site for accessibility. This form has been adapted from Alderson (1985).

1. Are parking spaces available for individuals with physical disabilities?

2. Are the parking spaces near to the building entrance? (Travel distance should not exceed 200 feet.)

3. Are the parking spaces easily accessible to the front entrance by level or ramped path at least four feet wide and free of obstructions?

4. Is the surface of the parking lot area smooth (but not slippery) and hard (not sand, gravel, etc.)?
5. Are walks leading to the facility level or nearly so?
6. Are there curb-cuts at crossways?
7. Is at least one primary entrance usable to individuals who use wheelchairs?
8. Do all doorways have a clear opening of at least 32 inches?
9. Are the doors operated by a single effort and is the pressure of the door light enough for the person who is disabled to open?
10. Are sharp inclines or abrupt changes in level avoided at thresholds?
11. Are ramps provided where there are stairs?
12. Do the ramps conform with the standard of no greater than one-inch rise in 12 inches of length?
13. Do the ramps have a surface that is firm, fixed and nonslip, with a 32-inch handrail on at least one side?
14. Are guest elevators accessible and usable by persons who are physically disabled?
15. Are all elevator controls 48 inches or less from the floor?
16. Are tactile identifications located beside all elevator operating buttons?
17. Do all bathroom doors provide a minimum of 32 inches of clear opening?
18. Is the bathroom floor the same level as the floor outside of the bathroom?
19. Does the bathroom contain a floor clearance area of at least 5 feet by 5 feet to permit a person in a wheelchair sufficient turning space?
20. Is there at least one bathroom stall usable by a person who uses a wheelchair?

21. Are sinks, mirrors, dispensers and disposal units within reach and usable by a person who uses a wheelchair?

22. Are there conveniently located public phones 48 inches or less from the floor?

23. Do public telephones have volume control devices?

24. Are TT's available?

25. Are water fountains available and have a clearance of 28 inches?

26. Are any of the guest rooms designed especially for persons who use wheelchairs?

27. Do all doorways have a clear opening of 32 inches?

28. Are there handrails in the toilet and shower area?

29. Is there sufficient turning space and maneuvering in the bath for a wheelchair?

30. Are hanging rods for clothing located within 48 inches of the floor?

31. Are all booths and tables (conference, social and dining) able to be converted to wheelchair use, with a clearance of 28 inches from the floor?

32. Is the meeting space accessible and usable by persons with disabilities?

33. Will a person who uses a wheelchair be able to exit and return to the conference area with minimum effort?

34. Are all common areas accessible to all people?

35. Is help available for those who might need any type of assistance?

36. Who can be called if assistance is needed?

37. What is the general attitude of all personnel towards persons with disabilities?

Chapter 11

Encourage Integration

"A candle loses none of its light by lighting another candle."
—Taylor

Orientation Activity: Plan for Integration

Directions When Alone: Choose an agency with which you are familiar or simply imagine an ideal job you might have and consider the agency for which you work. On a separate piece of paper, list at least 10 different ways you could prepare this agency to accept people with disabilities into recreation programs. Next, list at least 10 different ways you could facilitate the integration of a person with a disability once they have arrived at the agency.

Directions With Others: Move about the room, find a person, introduce yourself and ask the person's name. Discuss one idea for integration preparation and one idea for integration facilitation. Once you have discussed the information move to another person. Continue this process until you have shared all the items on your list.

Debriefing

If given the choice, most people with disabilities want to participate in integrated recreational activities (Oestreicher, 1990). People with even the most severe disabilities can be successfully included in programs and settings with peers who do not have disabilities. Through such initiatives, inclusive recreation settings and programs are not only feasible, but can be mutually beneficial to participants, both with and without disabilities (Ray & Meidl, 1991). The following questions, adapted from a list by Ray and Meidl (1991), could be asked when evaluating if a program is promoting integration:

1. Does this program teach participants skills that can be applied in "real life" situations?
2. Are participants learning skills that make them less dependent on others?
3. Does this program serve as an avenue to opportunities that will help participants to grow, develop, and enhance inclusion?

4. Do the activities in which the participants are engaged enhance their acceptance, value, and appreciation among their peers?
5. Do participants really like this activity and are they having a good time?

Introduction

Decker (1987) characterized integration as full participation in community life. According to Langlois (1990), **integration** means that people with disabilities:

(a) use the same community resources used by other people;
(b) participate in the same community activities as other people;
(c) live, learn, and enjoy life in contact with other people;
(d) develop friendships and relationships with other people; and
(e) reside in typical homes in proximity to community resources.

Wolfensberger (1972, p. 45) stated that integration needs to be achieved by "obtaining services from generic agencies which serve the general public, rather than from specialty agencies which serve only or primarily groups of individuals perceived as deviant." Later, Wolfensberger (1983) emphasized that **social role valorization** is a critical aspect of effective integration efforts. According to Wolfensberger, if a person holds a valued social role, that person will be given the respect that typically is given to people fulfilling that valued social role and, in turn, be less vulnerable to being devalued. Integration, therefore, includes a strong social component that involves participation of people with disabilities in social interactions and relationships with people who are not devalued in ordinary settings and contexts (Wolfensberger & Thomas, 1983).

Integration, by its very definition, includes relationships as its core element (Hutchison & McGill, 1992), and involves the process of people who have been devalued receiving support as needed to establish relationships with valued members of their community (Langlois, 1990). Flynn and Nitsch (1980) reported that for people to have access to valued social roles, they need to be supported to grow and learn with their peers and develop close relationships with valued members of their communities. Dolnick (1993, p. 43) reported that:

> Historically, advocates for every disabled group have directed their fiercest fire at policies that exclude their group. No matter the good intentions, no matter the logistical hurdles, they have insisted, separate is not equal. Thus buildings, buses, classes, must be accessible to all;

special accommodations for the disabled are not a satisfactory substitute. All this has become part of conventional wisdom. Today, under the general heading of "mainstreaming," it is enshrined in law and unchallenged as a premise of enlightened thought.

However, many people who are deaf do not support the application of integration and mainstreaming principles toward people who are deaf. According to Dolnick (1993, p. 43), some people object to integration because they believe that even well-meaning attempts to integrate people who are deaf into a society that hears "may actually imprison them in a zone of silence." Therefore, it is important for leisure professionals to keep in mind the statement by Helen Keller that, "Deafness cuts people off from people," and make every attempt to enhance communication efforts with people with hearing impairments attempting to access leisure services.

Since there are increasing numbers of people with disabilities living in the community, community park and recreation agencies must assume responsibility for providing leisure services for people with disabilities (Fico, 1992). Fico (1992) reported that perhaps now our purpose has become greater than trying to overcome and eliminate discrimination and segregation; that is, to provide recreational opportunities for people with disabilities to interact and develop relationships with their peers.

Schleien and Green (1992) suggested that as a result of a growing preference of people with disabilities and their families for integrated recreation programs, and recent legislation supporting and mandating services for people with disabilities in integrated community environments such as the Americans with Disabilities Act, all recreation professionals must be prepared to provide services to people with disabilities in integrated settings along with their peers. Unfortunately, despite research showing the benefits of integration, implementation has been slow and has sometimes been met with resistance (Dreimanus et al., 1992). Rynders and Schleien (1991) reported that the majority of people with disabilities currently participate in segregated recreation services, if they participate at all.

Know the Benefits of Integration

Some people assume that the benefits of integration are experienced only by people with disabilities. However, the benefits of integrated recreation participation can be also significant for people without disabilities. According to Galambos, Lee, Rahn, and Williams (1994) the benefits of integrated recreation experiences are mutual for people with and without disabilities. People with disabilities have increased choices and opportunities for recreation participation and people without disabilities learn new ways to solve problems and increase acceptance. Oestreicher (1990) suggested that integrated recreation prepares people with disabilities for life in an integrated society, and, just as importantly, prepares society to accept individual diversity.

People with Disabilities

Cultivate friendships. People with disabilities can develop real friendships with other participants when involved in integrated community recreation programs. For example, Dwane and Marcia reported that as a result of developing friendships during participation in a community recreation program, their daughter, Sasha, was invited to birthday parties, received telephone calls from friends, and had friends come over to her house to play. Since having friendships is important to the quality of every person's life, people with disabilities learn best when learning what their friends are learning.

Produce a sense of affiliation. Hultsman (1993) reported that activities that permit interaction with a person's peers provide:

(a) opportunities for shared interests;
(b) a sense of accomplishment and belonging; and
(c) personal identity and mastery over the environment.

Sable (1992) reported that integrated recreation experiences break down barriers and create a forum for emerging relationships. In fact, Dreimanus and colleagues (1992) observed that children with disabilities are no more likely to be rejected than their peers when participating in an integrated environment.

Develop life-long skills. The presence of appropriate integrated recreation options promotes the development of life-long functional recreation skills. People with disabilities can learn appropriate "interdependent" behaviors (e.g., asking for assistance as needed) by experiencing challenges that are part of integrated community life. Enjoyment associated with recreation participation can reward different levels of ability, if professionals encourage valuing each individual's contribution.

Acquire social skills. People with disabilities are more likely to develop social skills needed to develop relationships when participating in integrated recreation opportunities. For example, Cole and Meyer (1991) reported that children with severe disabilities in integrated learning environments showed gains in social competence, whereas those in segregated settings did not. Carefully planned integrated programs result in increased learning opportunities for people with disabilities (Hanline, 1993).

Increase social interactions. Sable (1992) reported that youth with and without disabilities were able to develop spontaneous friendships that emerged out of the shared interests as a result of an integrated recreation experience. Guralnick and Groom (1988), after observing play groups that contained children with and without disabilities and groups that contained only children with disabilities, concluded that integrated play groups facilitated peer interaction, whereas segregated play groups constrained peer interaction and promoted adult-child interaction. In addition, Dreimanus and colleagues (1992) reported that children with severe disabilities interacted more often with other children when they were in integrated environments, and that preschoolers with disabilities exhibited more socially advanced skills in integrated settings. Schleien, Ray, Soderman-Olson, and McMahon (1987) also observed that social behaviors and interactions of children with disabilities increased during an integrated art education program.

Enhance image. Storey, Stern, and Parker (1991) examined the attitudes of college students towards a woman with disabilities participating in either Special Olympics or in typical recreational activities within an integrated setting. The researchers reported that in the Special Olympics presentation, the woman was regarded as younger and more in need of segregated treatment settings than in the typical activities presentation. This investigation lends support to the belief that the image of a person with disabilities is higher with integrated participation as opposed to segregated participation.

Provide role models. Integrated recreation environments can provide role models that promote age appropriate participation patterns for people with disabilities. For example, Stainback and Stainback (1987) reported that participants without disabilities provided models of age-appropriate dress, language, gestures, and social behavior for their peers with disabilities. Integrated play opportunities stimulate and motivate children with disabilities, offering them opportunities to imitate and model play behaviors of their peers without disabilities (McGill, 1984).

In summary, when participating in integrated recreation programs, Galambos and colleagues reported that people with disabilities experience:

(a) increased options and choices;
(b) a chance to learn skills in ways typical of their peers;
(c) development of positive relationships and friendships;
(d) enhanced self-concept and self-esteem;
(e) risks to learn from failures and successes;
(f) enhanced personal growth and development; and
(g) a valued place among a network of people.

People without Disabilities

Develop positive attitudes. The benefits of an integrated leisure opportunity extend beyond recreation services providers and the participants with disabilities. People who are not disabled often positively alter their attitudes about individuals with disabilities as a result of joint participation in selected activities (Hamilton & Anderson, 1991). For example, Schleien, Ray, Soderman-Olson, and McMahon (1987) reported that after participation in an integrated art education program, the attitudes of children without disabilities toward their peers with disabilities changed positively. Carefully planned integrated programs result in positive developmental and attitudinal outcomes for young children without disabilities (McLean & Hanline, 1990).

Encourage acceptance. By encouraging and facilitating integrated leisure opportunities for all community members, recreation professionals can contribute to the acceptance of people with disabilities by people without disabilities. According to Schleien (1993), recreation professionals can take an active role in reducing social stigmas associated with persons with disabilities by emphasizing similarities rather than differences. Brown and colleagues (1989) concluded that long-term heterogeneous interactions between people with severe disabilities and people without disabilities facilitate development of skills, attitudes and values that will prepare both groups to be sharing, participating, contributing members of complex communities.

Experience personal growth. As a result of participation in integrated leisure opportunities, many people report that they experience personal growth and increased social sensitivity, including improved capacity for compassion, kindness, and respect for others. Others report that they develop skills and attitudes needed to live harmoniously in communities that include people with and without disabilities.

Increase understanding. According to Schleien and Green (1992), exposure to integrated recreation services results in a greater understanding and acceptance of individuals with varying backgrounds and ability levels creating the potential for integration to have a positive impact on the social development of all individuals. Enjoyment of recreation and education opportunities that reward different levels of ability can occur when people value each individual's contribution. When involved in integrated programs, people without disabilities become more accepting of differences and begin to appreciate the capacities of persons with disabilities (Ray & Meidl, 1991).

The following quotations from the Georgia Advocacy Office (1992) illustrate the benefits people without disabilities receive when participating in integrated programs:

> Our world includes a vast array of people who, we believe, are more alike than different. We have watched education become more and more exclusive in the definition of which students "belong" in the regular classroom. We believe that what children learn from each other about difference and acceptance is equally as important as the technical education that they receive. We all need to learn how to live and work together (p. 4). Students develop more fully when they welcome people with different gifts and abilities into their lives and when all students feel secure that they will receive individualized help when they need it (p. 9).

Facilitate Integration

According to Schleien (1993), although recent laws mandate agencies to accommodate individuals of varying abilities both architecturally and programmatically, often these agencies have only removed architectural barriers. Unfortunately, as Schleien elaborated, physical accessibility and physical proximity between people with and without disabilities does not, in and of itself, ensure positive results. Without programmatic access, participants without disabilities continue to view their peers with disabilities and integration efforts negatively (Schleien, 1993). Many programmatic strategies can be used to encourage the integration of people with disabilities into community recreation programs. As depicted in Figure 11.1 (see page 184), this section of the chapter highlights six such strategies to help encourage integration. As part of regularly scheduled in-services, all employees (i.e., clerical, maintenance, administration, service providers) should be educated on the agency's commitment to integration.

Prepare for Integration

Provide ongoing opportunities for staff training. Possible topics for training could include a presentation on the rationale for inclusive leisure that addresses:

(a) benefits for people with and without disabilities;
(b) legislative mandates that support inclusion, and
(c) philosophical underpinnings of inclusion.

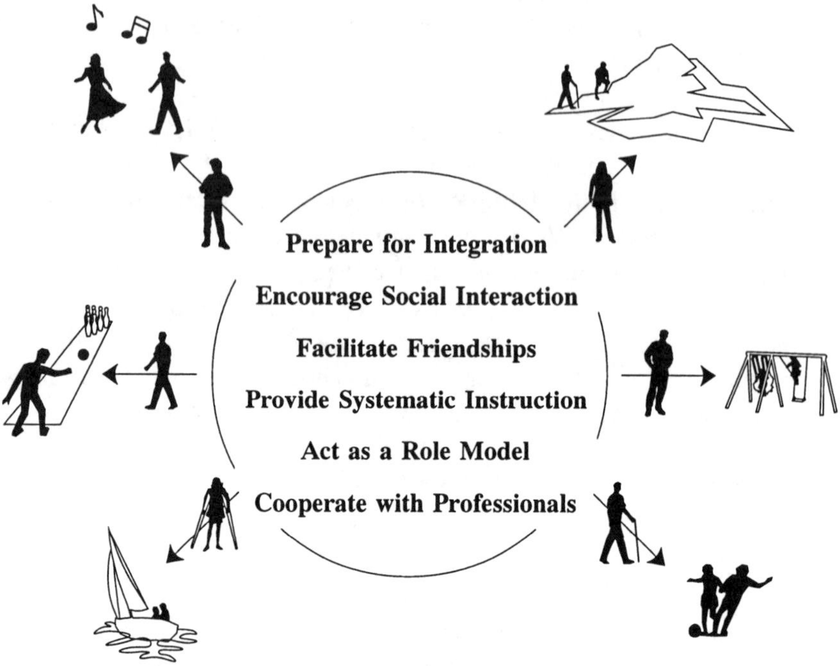

Figure 11.1 Some strategies for facilitating integration.

Training should describe the roles and responsibilities of people who can contribute to integrated services such as parents, participants, advocacy groups, schools, and various other recreation professionals. It can be helpful to highlight strategies for inclusion such as:

(a) encouraging accepting attitudes among staff;
(b) implementing program methods to attract and support individuals;
(c) evaluating and soliciting feedback on efforts; and
(d) developing networks and resources.

Assess participant interests. To discover people's needs and interests it may be useful to avoid relying solely on surveys but also to observe participants' expressions and unique ways of communicating. Professionals may wish to provide participants with repeated opportunities to choose between two or more activities to establish a preference profile. Once preferences are identified, professionals can assist people to act on their interests and provide opportunities to learn and to practice leisure skills in various settings. Dreimanus and colleagues (1992) reported that grouping children by mutual interests helped increase acceptance of children with disabilities by their peers.

Include people in planning and decision making. It is valuable to involve people with disabilities and their families on boards and advisory committees. The act of soliciting feedback on programs offered previously can facilitate integration. Some professionals have found value in involving participants and families when designing modifications that promote participation in integrated programs. An invitation to people with disabilities and their family members to assist in staff development can be effective. The designation of a staff person to act as facilitator of inclusive experiences may be useful. One approach involves including statements in promotional literature on policies of inclusion giving potential participants someone to contact.

Design cooperatively structured activities. Activities that require cooperative efforts can facilitate integration. A cooperative learning structure can create an interdependence because completion of a task by a group requires that everyone contribute in some way. Each person should encourage all other participants to achieve group goals that are realistically attainable. Participation in joint activities may result in peer acceptance and interaction between children with and without disabilities (Ballard, Corman, Gottlieb, & Kaufman, 1977). For example, Green and DeCoux (1994) reported that modified rules of a basketball league promoted the inclusion of a child using a wheelchair. Rynders and Schleien (1991) recommended that to facilitate cooperative interactions:

(a) provide prompts for positive interactions when these behaviors are not occurring;
(b) reinforce positive interactions as they occur; and
(c) redirect behaviors if participants get off task.

Encourage Social Interaction

Divide participants into small groups. After reviewing the literature, Chandler, Fowler, and Lubeck (1992) reported that peer interaction typically occurs more often in small groups that contain two or three people. As the number of people becomes smaller, the opportunity for expression is typically enhanced, and thereby creates situations conducive to social interaction.

Promote development of peer companions. Peer companions can promote positive social interactions between people with and without disabilities. The relationship between two peers should be viewed by all concerned as being relatively equal. Goldstein, Kaczmarek, Pennington, and Schafer (1992) reported that peer-mediated intervention has been one of the strategies used successfully to increase social interaction between children with and without disabilities in integrated settings. According to Goldstein and colleagues

(1992), in these interventions, peers with and without disabilities are taught ways to interact with each other. Peer-mediated intervention strategies attempt to increase the social behaviors of people by teaching peers to:

(a) initiate interactions at an increased rate, thus providing more opportunities for interactions; or
(b) respond to the social initiations of others.

Provide a small area for participation. A small area in which activities are enjoyed can stimulate interaction and integration. Small areas can result in more peer interaction than large play areas (Brown, Fox, & Brady, 1987). Speigel-McGill and colleagues (1984) reported that peer interaction occurred more often when children with disabilities were within one or two feet of each other than when they were 10 feet apart.

Choose equipment that promotes interaction. After reviewing the literature, Chandler and colleagues (1992) reported that specific types of toys (e.g., cars, games, gross motor equipment, and socio-dramatic materials) may promote peer interaction, whereas other toys (e.g., small manipulatives, clay, books, and puzzles) often inhibit social interaction. Limited numbers and varieties of materials tend to promote sharing and positive peer interaction (Skellenger, McEvoy, McConnell, & Odom, 1991).

Facilitate Friendships

Be aware of isolation. People with disabilities are most often isolated from their peers without disabilities if interactions are left to chance (Hutchison, 1990). Hanline (1993) reported that children without disabilities tend to:

(a) communicate with other such children more often than they communicate with peers with disabilities;
(b) choose other such children as playmates and friends more often than they choose children with disabilities; and
(c) prefer to sit next to peers without disabilities in group activities.

Typically, people who have limited social networks usually spend their free time either alone, with family, with friends of family, or in structured group activities with other people with disabilities (Hutchison & McGill, 1992). Therefore, Hanline (1993) suggested that professionals encourage interactions and help people without disabilities at a very young age to understand and respond to the unique behaviors of peers with disabilities so that they may develop meaningful friendships.

Realize the benefits of friendships. Coleman and Iso-Ahola (1993) reported that the impact of leisure participation on social support is likely to be significant for those who have limited friends or few social contacts, such as some people with disabilities. Heyne, Schleien, and McEvoy (1993) identified strong agreement that friendships serve many important functions, such as:

(a) learning social skills;
(b) encouraging children's separation from parents;
(c) developing a sense of autonomy;
(c) enhancing self-esteem;
(d) instilling a sense of belonging to a community;
(e) achieving feelings of intimacy;
(f) being assured of being valued and loved; and
(g) enriching their quality of life.

Larson, Zuzanek and Mannell (1985) concluded that regular social contact through engagement in leisure activities helps overcome a considerable deficit in perceived social support for people who are isolated. By engaging in some of the many leisure pursuits that are conducive to social interaction, Coleman and Iso-Ahola (1993) suggested that people are more likely to make friends and develop closer friendships. Hamre-Nietupski, Hendrickson, Nietupski, and Sasso (1993) reported that:

(a) true friendships between people with very severe disabilities and their peers without disabilities are possible;
(b) friendships benefit both people with and without disabilities; and
(c) people with severe disabilities must learn, live, and plan in integrated environments to develop and maintain friendships.

Facilitate the leisure experience. Leisure is an excellent social context for the development of friendships and for the expression of social identities (Kleiber & Rickards, 1985). Friendships developed and fostered through leisure participation and perceived availability of social support generated by leisure engagement help people cope with stress as well as maintain or improve health (Coleman & Iso-Ahola, 1993).

According to Coleman and Iso-Ahola (1993), friendships may be facilitated by situations characterized by perceived freedom and intrinsic motivation (i.e., leisure). As an example, Rook (1987) suggested that choosing to be with a companion in free time communicates to the companion the existence of a close relationship. In another example, Larson, Mannell and Zuzanek (1986) reported that the ability of friends to generate positive feelings is partly associated with a greater rate of active leisure activities with them.

Integrated leisure participation can play an important role in facilitating the development of friendships. According to Gold and Crawford (1989), the leisure context can encourage friendships because it gives people something to do together, a reason for spending time together, and a way to get to know one another through shared experiences.

Provide Systematic Instruction

Consider the individual. As discussed in Chapter 1, many stereotypes about people with disabilities exist because people lack awareness and understanding. All participants are unique and require a specific individualized approach that recognizes their uniqueness. Recreation programs that promote inclusion through systematic attempts at integration should be designed to support each person's participation and to enhance success and enjoyment.

Teach social interaction skills. It is helpful to encourage individuals to learn from being together during the years when their attitudes and perceptions are most pliable (Antia & Kreimeyer, 1992). Placing children in the same physical environment without any assistance does not necessarily lead to social interaction or social acceptance between children with and without disabilities (Odom & McEvoy, 1988). Programs that teach children with disabilities social skills or how to initiate and respond to peers' social contacts can promote positive peer interactions (Odom, Hoyson, Jamieson, & Strain, 1985). It appears that systematic efforts to allow children to interact frequently with a small, stable group of peers is likely to lead to some increase in interaction between children with and without disabilities (Antia & Kreimeyer, 1992).

Act as A Role Model

Foster age-appropriate behaviors. The presence of a disability may not have an influence on whether the person can successfully participate in a given recreation program. Ray and Meidl (1991) encouraged professionals to treat participants with disabilities as they would others their age by expecting them to be as independent as possible, encouraging others to interact with them, supporting and assisting only when necessary and encouraging accomplishments. It is helpful to compare a participant's abilities to what is expected of all participants and, if there are aspects of the activity that a person cannot perform independently, problem-solve to determine what types of supports are needed (Ray & Meidl, 1991). Using age-appropriate materials and methods, accommodating for individual patterns of development, learning through interacting with peers, and teaching within natural environments and meaningful routines are emphasized when providing services that include people with disabilities (Hanline & Fox, 1993).

Encourage participants to learn. To accomplish this task, recreation professionals should provide needed supports. Supports can range from incorporating volunteers, providing helpful reminders, assisting people with equipment, and providing help during some aspects of participation. According to Ray and Meidl (1991), regardless of the level of support, participants should have every opportunity to learn and become as independent as possible in recreational activities.

Cooperate With Other Professionals

Develop networks. Schleien and Ray (1988) encouraged practitioners to set the stage for integrated recreation by developing communication links between persons and agencies concerned about community leisure services. This process is known as **networking.** Networking involves establishing and maintaining connections with professionals and paraprofessionals from various disciplines and organizations—including community members, families, and consumers who share a common interest and concern regarding the provision of leisure services in the community at large and for persons with disabilities in particular (Hamre-Nietupski et al., 1988). The process of networking ensures the transition of participants into community organizations by individualizing, coordinating, and ensuring relevance of leisure services (Carter & Foret, 1994).

Identify "key players." One way to enhance networking and ensure ongoing, accessible, and integrated leisure services is to identify all "key players" and their roles and responsibilities within the community leisure service process (Schleien & Ray, 1988). According to Dattilo and Schleien (1994), these individuals may include family members, care-providers, consumers with and without disabilities, teachers, therapeutic recreation specialists, advocacy group members, commercial recreation professionals (e.g., health clubs, ski areas), youth and family service organization professionals (e.g., YMCA, Scouts, 4-H, Jewish Community Center), professional and educational resource people (e.g., universities, consultants), and community leisure professionals. Each of these players assumes a significant role by providing potential participants with leisure environments and by making pertinent information about individual participants available to community leisure professionals.

Assume responsibility. To meet the needs of individuals with disabilities, leisure professionals, educators, and families must work together to improve and expand leisure services. If tasks are distributed among too many agencies, however, it is possible that no one organization will assume responsibility for their completion. Other undesirable outcomes of such a situation are lack of communication among agencies and duplication of or gaps in services.

Consider the entire support system. Although shared responsibility appears the natural approach to providing comprehensive leisure services, such practice is fairly uncommon due to the complex communication and shared-resource networks it necessitates. Schleien and Werder (1985) suggested that future integrated leisure programming include:

(a) a delineation of networks across agencies to reduce duplication of services and complement resources;
(b) expansion of activity offerings;
(c) encouragement of integration of individuals with disabilities into leisure services with participants who do not have disabilities;
(d) generation of support for increasing the number of specially trained personnel across agencies; and
(e) improvement of access and availability of community leisure opportunities.

Examples of Successful Integration Efforts

Fitness and recreation for everyone. Weirs (1988) reported that people with and without disabilities were encouraged to participate in integrated recreation activities during a special event entitled "Recreation and Fitness for Everyone." This event lasted for three hours and featured activities led by university athletes, people with disabilities and members of Hand in Hand. Hand in Hand is a nonprofit organization designed to promote community awareness and integration for individuals with mental, physical, social and emotional disabilities. Activities included:

(a) aerobics, led by two women, one who happened to have a hearing impairment;
(b) wheelchair games, in which people tried their skill maneuvering a wheelchair;
(c) soccer, coordinated by a man with mental retardation in conjunction with a player from the university's women's soccer team;
(d) beeper ball, a baseball game featuring a noise-making ball that permits people with low vision or blindness to participate, was led by Hand in Hand members; and
(e) a sing-a-long, performed by people with and without hearing impairments.

An information table was provided where people registered to volunteer for future Hand in Hand events, and obtained information about people with disabilities.

Bankshot. Miller (1991) reported on "Bankshot," a modified version of basketball that allows participants with and without disabilities to compete with one another. The "nonexclusionary" basketball contest was developed so that entire families can play. Although the configuration of the ball and rim is not modified, the rim has been lowered to eight feet from the floor, different backboards have been designed, and running and jumping is not permitted. "The result is a game that is a mix of basketball, billiards, miniature golf and even fine art" (Miller, 1991, p. 5). The format is similar to miniature golf, with 18 stations plus a tie-breaker in an area approximately half the size of a tennis court. The stations have uniquely shaped backboards that require different types of shots. At each hoop, the shooter takes aim from three different circles on the ground. A complete circuit usually takes approximately 45 minutes. Points are determined by distance and difficulty of the shots. Bonus points are gained by hitting from all three circles at any given station. Bankshot is being played at miniature golf courses and parks in over 60 cities across the United States and in Israel.

Every-Buddy. Ledman, Thompson, and Hill (1992) reported that in 1989, a cost-effective program, the Every-Buddy Program, was developed to provide supervised, after-school services to children with multiple disabilities. The participants were integrated directly into the YMCA programs by adding trained staff to three of the YMCA's after-school program sites. These personnel provided individualized support needed by children with disabilities to participate in the program alongside their peers. Children with disabilities were then integrated at those preselected sites. Parents strongly agreed that:

(a) the environment was safe;
(b) children were eager to attend the program and were participating in activities;
(c) the needs of families and children were being met; and
(d) they enjoyed telling others that their children were attending the program.

The YMCA staff felt that both the children with and without disabilities benefitted from the integration effort and that there had been no negative response to the program from the parents of children without disabilities; to the contrary, the parents of the children with disabilities reported that they were frequently approached by the other parents who expressed not only acceptance of the children with disabilities but gratitude that their children had the opportunity to be with people with disabilities.

Shared interests at home. Montgomery (1992) reported that when young children meet a child who is different, they are naturally curious and may ask uncomfortable questions. The child without the disability may not have the experience to handle the situation, and the child with the disability may not have had much experience meeting new people. A parent reported that the quickest way to help young visitors connect with her son was to suggest that he show them his room. Once there, his model horse collection—rather than his disability—usually became the center of attention. As interests are shared, or skills identified, acceptance and integration is enhanced. A child with a disability who knows sign language can teach some simple signs to new friends or a child who is competent with the computer or card games might invite guests to play.

Acting Together. Miller, Rynders and Schleien (1993) reported on the results of a project entitled "Acting Together," a drama class incorporating theater games and improvisational acting experiences for children. According to the authors, "Acting Together" demonstrated the value of creative drama as an approach to promote the integration of people with and without disabilities. Miller and colleagues (1993) stated that:

> Drama is essentially a social art; it does not exist in the absence of an audience nor in the absence of a society of players (actors). This quality may make it a particularly useful medium when participants have very limited repertories of social skills.

Conclusion

Dreimanus and colleagues (1992) reported that despite lagging attitudes, it appeared that the focus of the debate about integration is shifting from determining whether or not integration is a sound educational practice to how to implement it properly. The research appears to indicate that making integration work calls for the following strategies (Dreimanus, 1992):

(a) give professionals a chance to interact with people with disabilities before integration;
(b) teach social skills to people with disabilities in the setting where they are expected to use these skills;

(c) give people without disabilities information about the interests of people to be integrated;
(d) help people without disabilities to see those with disabilities as similar to them;
(e) get others to interact with them in an ongoing way;
(f) make use of cooperative learning strategies;
(g) use peer tutors carefully to improve progress; and
(h) have people with and without disabilities participate in structured interactions together.

Discussion Questions

The following questions have been adapted from Hutchison and Lord's (1979) integration questionnaire. They are presented here to assist the reader in reviewing the information presented in this chapter. Similar to the directions provided in the orientation activity, choose an agency with which you are familiar or simply imagine an ideal job you might have and consider the agency you work for.

1. How have you adopted integration as part of the philosophy of your agency?

2. What financial commitments have been made in your agency for integration?

3. Who has been delegated responsibility for coordinating integration?

4. What has been done to ensure open communication with advocacy associations?

5. Do you have an integration planning group which includes representatives from: (a) agency staff and administrators, (b) volunteers, (c) advocacy associations, (d) community resource persons, (e) participants with disabilities, and (f) participants without disabilities?

6. Do the following clearly defined planning stages exist for integration: (a) contact potential participants, (b) evaluate interests of participants, (c) assess community resources, (d) develop specific objectives, (e) develop and implement strategies, and (f) evaluate services?

7. How is input and feedback from participants solicited?

8. Is evaluation ongoing?

9. Do staff and volunteers understand and support the need for integration?

10. Is staff development related to integration promoted through: (a) availability of current material, (b) in-service training, and (c) use of community resources and workshops?

11. Is there time at meetings for staff to share feelings and concerns regarding integration?

12. Are you aware of the number of people with disabilities in your area?

13. Have you identified attitudinal and architectural agency barriers to integration?

14. What are you doing to eliminate barriers?

15. How do you assist participants who require support?

16. How can you help participants understand and support participants with disabilities?

17. What changes have been made to enhance services for people with disabilities?

18. Are programs designed for people of similar ages?

19. What support or "enabling" services do you provide which facilitate integration?

20. Are there opportunities for people to upgrade skills in individualized programs?

Chapter 12

Make Reasonable Adaptations

"The more things change, the more they are the same."
—Alphonse Karr

Orientation Activity: Be Flexible and Make Adaptations

Directions When Alone: On a separate sheet of paper record the name of a recreation activity that requires materials or equipment for participation. Keeping this recreation activity in mind, answer the following questions to help encourage you to make adaptations to your programs.

Directions With Others: Record your activity on a card. Attempt to find other people who chose the same recreation activity as you. If there are more than four people who have chosen the same recreation activity, divide into smaller groups not less than two and not to exceed four. If no one else identified your activity, find another person who has identified an activity that is similar to yours. Once groups have been formed, share your ideas about making adaptations with the other people or person in your discussion group. After a specified time, discuss the highlights of what you have learned with the entire group.

1. What materials or equipment could you change to meet the needs of some people with differing abilities?
2. What aspects of the activity itself could you change to meet the needs of people with differing abilities?
3. What aspects of the environment could you change to meet the needs of people with differing abilities?
4. What could you change about the way you are teaching participants that might meet the needs of people with differing abilities?

Debriefing

When attempting to adapt existing recreation programs to meet the unique needs of current participants, many facets of a given program can be considered. For the purposes of this chapter, identification of possible adaptations of recreation programs are divided into five major areas:

(a) materials that are used;
(b) activities;
(c) environment in which the activity is conducted;
(d) participants; and
(e) instructional strategies employed by practitioners.

These five areas are not necessarily mutually exclusive and are intended to help organize suggestions on adaptations. As you reflect on the orientation activity, respond to the following questions:

1. What is the value of making adaptations for people with disabilities that provide them with the opportunity to participate in community recreation programs with their families and friends?
2. What can you do in your current or future position to help encourage personnel to make adaptations that facilitate participation by people with disabilities?
3. What can you do to maintain the enjoyment of all participants when making adaptations for one person or only a few people?

Introduction

This chapter, devoted to adaptations, is intended to encourage current and future practitioners to adapt the information presented in their programs as necessary. When needed, these adaptations should permit the leisure services professional to meet the varying needs and abilities of the people receiving recreation services. The suggestions for adaptations are not intended to be all-inclusive. They are, however, intended to communicate some options available to practitioners to make adjustments that can facilitate active leisure participation for people with disabilities. Material from this chapter was adapted from Dattilo and Murphy (1991).

General Considerations

Place Emphasis on the Person First

Individualize adaptations. A key to adapting recreation programs is to consider the individual needs of each participant. Therefore, adaptations must be tailored as much as possible to each participant. Because many people possess differing levels of skills, and experience a variety of consequences as a result of different disabling conditions, practitioners should individualize their adaptations.

Focus on abilities. A person-first philosophy also requires practitioners to focus on participants' abilities rather than on their disabilities. Too often, assessments are conducted that initially identify what participants can *not* do. Next, practitioners design adaptations to accommodate this limitation. Perhaps a more useful procedure may be to initially focus on the skills and abilities of participants and then make adaptations building upon these skills. When people's abilities become the focus of attention, practitioners are more likely to allow participants to be as independent as possible; therefore, they will tend to avoid stifling these people by making unnecessary adaptations that fail to capitalize on their skills.

Match challenge and skills. Each recreation program contains learning experiences that possess a certain degree of challenge. In addition, prior to conducting a recreation program, practitioners should systematically assess the skills and interests of the people for whom the program is designed. Then, when conducting programs, practitioners will be in a position to better achieve the delicate balance between the challenge of specific activities and skills of the participants. If an imbalance exists between the degree of challenge of a program and the participants' skills, barriers may be created to leisure participation. As discussed in previous chapters, if a specific activity is too easy for participants, boredom often results. However, if an activity is too difficult, frustration can occur. One way to reduce these barriers is through adaptation. Adaptations can permit modification of the challenge associated with participation to meet the abilities of the participants. Once adaptations are made, they must continually be adjusted to meet the changing skills of the participants. A summary of the suggestions to help place emphasis on the person is presented in Figure 12.1 (see page 198).

Encourage Participant Autonomy

Facilitate independence. Since part of any leisure service should be devoted to increasing participant independence, practitioners should adopt the goal of independence when attempting to adapt their programs. Therefore, modifications should decrease the ability of participants to rely on others for assistance and provide people with disabilities with increased opportunities to actively participate in leisure as independently as possible.

Determine necessity of adaptation. Because many people with disabilities experience barriers to leisure participation, some practitioners may be quick to change a recreation program. In addition, changes may be readily made to a given program because recreation professionals are often skilled at

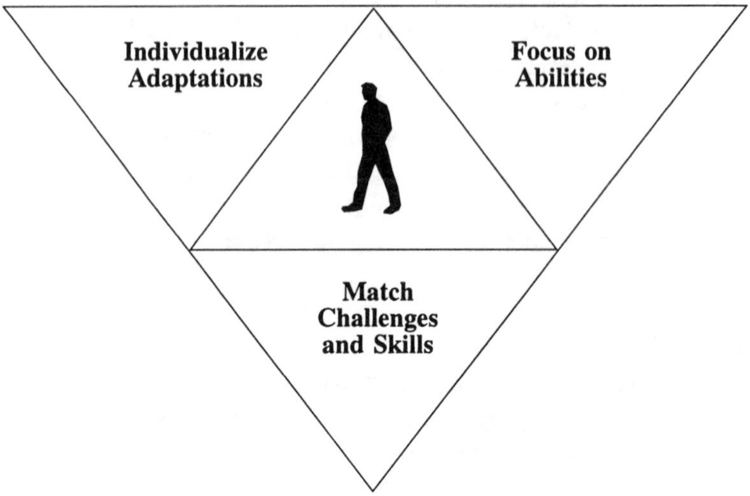

Figure 12.1 Place emphasis on the person first when making accommodations.

making modifications. Sometimes these changes are made with the knowledge of the general characteristics of a group of individuals rather than with explicit information about the specific participants. Although this practice may be practical in some situations, it may also create a problem. Some aspects of recreation programs may be changed when, in fact, they need not be. Therefore, it is important for practitioners to examine each adaptation and determine if it is actually necessary. There is a strong similarity between many people with disabilities and their peers without disabilities. Smith (1993) reported on similarities in:

(a) motivation to participate;
(b) perceptions of important aspects of athletic events; and
(c) psychological profiles.

He suggested that recreation professionals do not need to modify programs extensively in order to meet the needs of constituents with disabilities.

View adaptations as transitional. Adaptations can permit active participation for persons with a wide range of knowledge and skills. The very nature of leisure services implies that individuals will learn and change. As people learn and change, their skills and knowledge fluctuate. Therefore, if an adaptation was made at one time, it may no longer be appropriate because the individual has now acquired the ability to participate without any adaptations. At that point, the adaptations may impair, rather than encourage, leisure participation. Other people participating in recreation programs may possess degenerative or progressive conditions that require continual modifications. A previous slight adaptation to a particular activity may be insufficient later to provide the person with the opportunity to participate. In any case, practitioners must be willing to adopt the view that any adaptations they make to a given situation may need to be altered in the future. A summary of suggestions to help encourage participant autonomy is presented in Figure 12.2.

Involve Participant in Adaptation Process

Discuss adaptations with consumers. In almost every aspect of planning, practitioners are encouraged to consult with consumers regarding their opinions and desires (Smith, 1993). A critical task in motivating participation by people with disabilities is to encourage them to perceive that they have input into the chosen program. Active involvement in shaping a recreation program can provide individuals with a sense of investment that may increase their motivation to initiate and maintain participation. This principle applies as well

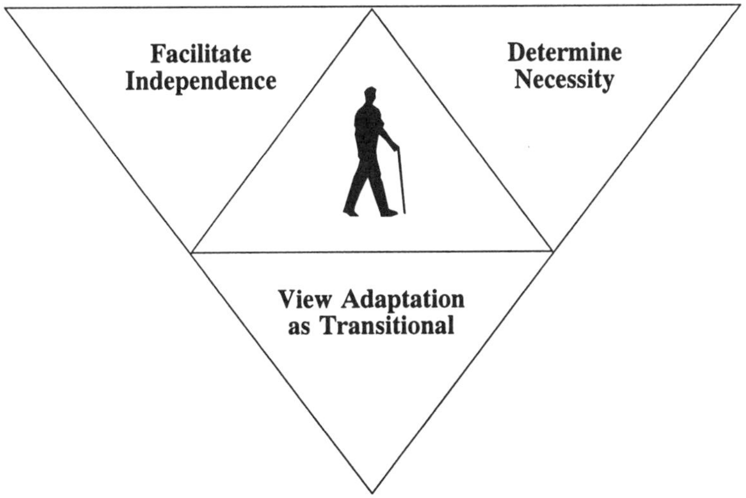

Figure 12.2 Encourage participant autonomy when making accommodations.

to adapting aspects of the recreation program. Discussions with participants may provide practitioners with valuable information about methods to adapt the activity and instill feelings of control and commitment by the participants. When participants do not currently possess the skills to effectively communicate their feelings and ideas toward an adaptation, then observations can be used to obtain input from these consumers.

Determine feasibility of adaptation. Involving participants in the process of adapting recreation programs can provide practitioners with a means to determine the feasibility and usability of the adaptation. If participants feel that the adaptation detracts from the program, their motivation may be reduced. Therefore, asking participants their opinions and encouraging them to make suggestions can enhance the ability of practitioners to make feasible adaptations. Sometimes, practitioners may go to great lengths to adapt a specific learning activity, only to find that people are no longer interested in participation as a result of the adaptation. Discussion with consumers prior to and during adaptations can help encourage active leisure participation following adaptations.

Ensure safety of adaptations. The most critical element to remember when making changes to any recreation program is safety. Commercially available equipment, materials, games and many other aspects of a recreation program typically have been tested and re-tested to determine their safety for potential participants. Anytime an adaptation is made, the previous research conducted by the manufacturers is compromised and associated safety claims change. Therefore, practitioners must examine and evaluate any program they adapt and consider the safety of participants. One strategy to help evaluate the safety of an adaptation is to actively seek participants' input regarding ways to ensure and increase the safety associated with a given aspect of a recreation program. A summary of ways to involve participants in the adaptation process is presented in Figure 12.3.

Evaluate Adaptations

Conduct systematic observations. When adaptations are made to specific aspects of a recreation program, continuous observation of individuals participating in the program is suggested. Observations of individual participation should allow practitioners to determine if the adaptations are achieving their intended goals. These observations provide practitioners with the ability to examine unanticipated difficulties participants may be experiencing relative to the adaptations. Continuous observations put professionals in a position to be able to understand the effectiveness of the adaptations.

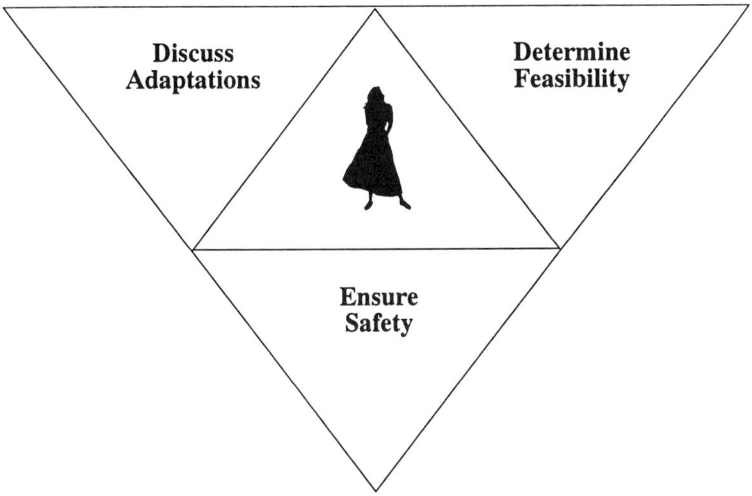

Figure 12.3 Invoke participant in adaptation process.

Make necessary adjustments. Observations provide practitioners with the opportunity to discover problems with adaptations. When problems are identified, practitioners must then be willing to respond to any difficulties associated with adaptations. This willingness to change an adaptation must stem from the belief that even if a great deal of time and energy is put into a given task, it may need to be altered to permit active leisure participation for persons with disabilities. A slight adjustment to an aspect of a recreation program may make the difference between active and meaningful participation or failure.

Consider resemblance to original task. Each time an adaptation is made, that aspect of the program becomes less like the original task. Therefore, adaptations can tend to limit the ability of individuals to participate in different programs that do not contain such adaptations. Practitioners should attempt to keep aspects of the program as close to the original program as possible to encourage participants to generalize their ability to participate in the activities in other environments and situations. A summary of considerations for evaluating adaptation is presented in Figure 12.4 (see page 202).

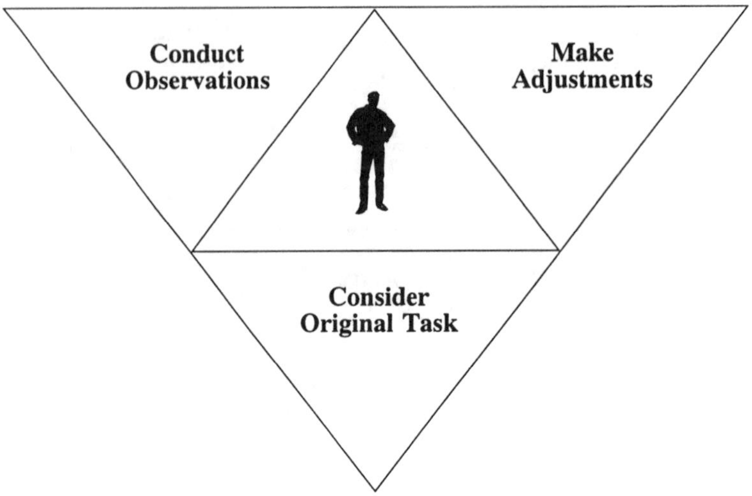

Figure 12.4 Evaluate adaptations.

Areas of Adaptation

The intent of the following information is to encourage professionals to consider a variety of aspects of the recreation programs when attempting to make adaptations facilitating leisure participation. The materials used during a recreation program can be adapted to meet the needs of the participants. In addition, the specific requirements associated with the learning activities may be changed. The environment provides another adaptation alternative for practitioners to facilitate active involvement for participants. Efforts toward adaptation can be focused on the participants themselves to increase the likelihood of their success. Finally, practitioners are encouraged to turn their focus of adaptations inward and examine possible ways to modify instructional strategies to teach persons with disabilities about leisure. The descriptions related to these five areas are not intended to be all-inclusive, but are designed to assist practitioners in developing plans for adaptations for recreation programs. Examples given in many of the following situations are made with recreation activities to provide instances that enable visualization of the suggested adaptation.

Materials

Many aspects of materials used in recreation programs can be adapted. Some examples of possible methods for adapting materials are presented below relative to the following areas:

(a) size;
(b) speed;
(c) weight;
(d) stabilization;
(e) durability; and
(f) safety.

Size. The size of materials can be adjusted for participants by making objects (e.g., puzzle pieces) larger for those having difficulty grasping small objects. Tape can be wrapped around handles to increase their size and permit manipulation. Conversely, other people may have difficulty grasping larger objects (e.g., felt-tip markers) so smaller ones could be used. Decreasing the size of objects that are intended to be inserted into an opening (e.g., a basketball) can increase success, while making the opening larger (e.g., a basketball hoop) may also lessen the requirements of an activity. Large, colorful cards can assist individuals with visual problems in playing table games designed to teach about leisure. If individuals are participating in racquet sports, the racquets can be shortened for more control or lengthened to allow participants to cover more ground.

Speed. Some individuals with disabilities may experience problems associated with gross motor coordination. A coordination problem can be quickly observed as individuals respond to moving objects. One way to increase the success of persons responding to objects is to reduce the speed of the moving object. Air can be removed from a ball so when struck it will move at a slower speed. Wedges can be placed under any angled surface to reduce the incline on which a ball may be placed to slow the ball (e.g., pinball) or increase the angle of a ramp (e.g., bowling) to increase the speed of the ball.

Weight. The weight of objects can be adjusted to meet the strength of the participants. Wooden and metal materials can be exchanged for those that are made from plastic or rubber. For instance, plastic balls, sponge balls and balloons can be substituted for heavier balls in some situations, while lighter plastic or Nerf™ bats can be used in lieu of heavier metal or wooden bats.

Stabilization. Sometimes people who have unsteady movements may be prevented from using some expensive technology because they are likely to break the equipment. Suction cups and clamps can be used to stabilize the material (e.g, a tape recorder). In this way, the person can use the material without fear of accidently damaging it. People participating in craft projects who possess grasping skills with only one portion of their bodies can be assisted by securing the project to a board or table (e.g., tape paper to a desk for drawing or painting).

Durability. Material for recreation programs should be made durable so that the material will last as long as possible. Duct tape is often helpful in reinforcing many different pieces of equipment. Game boards and playing cards should be laminated to increase the ability of the objects to withstand regular use. Velcro™ can also be used to secure objects that need to be removed at different times.

Safety. When making any adaptations to objects it is critical to continuously evaluate each adaptation in reference to safety. Any substances that are added should not be toxic. If changes to objects occur, they should be examined and any sharp edges removed. Possibilities of ingestion of objects and suffocation should be considered and prevented. In all cases, problems should be anticipated and steps taken toward prevention of any injuries.

Activities

Many traditional recreation activities can be adapted to facilitate more active participation by individuals with disabilities. Some examples of possible methods for adapting activities are presented below relative to the following areas:

(a) physical aspects;
(b) cognitive requirements; and
(c) social conditions.

Physical aspects. Individuals receiving recreation services vary a great deal relative to their physical strength, the speed at which they move, their endurance, energy level, gross motor coordination, eye-hand coordination, flexibility, agility and many other physical skills. To adapt a physical requirement of a program, the typical *number of people* associated with a game can be changed. For instance, the number of people participating in volleyball can be changed from six to 10 people for persons with limited speed and agility.

People with limited endurance and strength may benefit from making the requirements to complete an activity less strenuous by reducing either the *number of points* needed (e.g., need to score 8 points to win a table tennis game rather than 21) or the *length of time* a game lasts (e.g., change the length of time to complete a recreation learning activity from 30 to 15 minutes).

While learning some activities, the *physical movements* can be changed by requiring participants to walk instead of run (e.g., basketball). For those individuals who have impaired mobility, changing the required *body position* from standing to sitting may provide opportunities for participation (e.g., throwing Frisbee™). Some people receiving recreation services may possess limited physical endurance; therefore, practitioners may wish to provide more *opportunities to rest* during a particular event, such as hiking.

Cognitive requirements. People with disabilities may encounter problems associated with cognitive requirements as a result of many disabling conditions. For example, people may have impaired cognitive functioning because of a trauma due to a head injury, neurological disorders such as cerebral vascular accident, the developmental disability of mental retardation, learning disabilities due to dyslexia, mental health problems such as depression, or from the side effects of medications taken for physical illness. To accommodate these individuals' reduced cognitive functioning, the *rules* associated with different games can be changed. For instance, if short-term memory appears to be a problem for persons with head injuries, the number of cards used in a card game can be reduced (e.g., rather than using all cards in a deck in a game of concentration, only the face cards can be used).

People who do not yet possess counting skills may be able to play a game by substituting matching of colors, instead of requiring the recognition of numbers or words to move game pieces. If the requirements for *scoring* during an activity are too difficult for participants, changes can be made such as having people with mental retardation initially keep track only of the number of bowling pins they knock down, rather than using scoring procedures associated with calculating spares and strikes.

Some individuals with learning difficulties may require some minimal assistance with reading cards used for a table game. Practitioners may wish to change the game from requiring individuals to play alone to participation with *partners*. Often, teams of participants can be developed that allow the individual team members to complement each others' skills and abilities. In addition, friendships may be developed from the team interaction.

Social conditions. Many people receiving recreation services are doing so because they may be experiencing barriers to their leisure involvement. Frequently, these barriers are related to problems encountered in a social context. Some individuals may be intimidated by activities requiring larger groups. A reluctance to participate in larger groups may be a result of previous experiences associated with failure and perhaps ridicule. To assist people in gaining the confidence needed to participate in large group activities, practitioners may initially choose to *reduce the number of people* required to participate in an activity and begin instruction and practice of an activity in small groups or, if resources are available, on a one-to-one basis. For instance, social skills instruction related to learning how to make friends may be conducted initially with a few individuals.

As participants acquire the social skills, the context could be expanded to include more participants. The pressure involved in some activities involving direct competition against another team may be extremely threatening for some people with disabilities. A person's failure to perform may result in the entire team losing to an opponent. This failure can decrease confidence and self-esteem and contribute to a reduced motivation to participate. One approach to adapting an activity could be changing the activity so *cooperation is emphasized* and direct competition against another team is eliminated. To accomplish this cooperative atmosphere, practitioners may decide to eliminate the opposing team. The opposing team would be replaced by a series of established goals to be achieved by the team. For instance, in lieu of the traditional game of basketball, one team could participate by establishing goals related to making a basket (e.g., begin at the opposite end of the court, require all five team members to dribble the ball as it is brought down the court, attempt to make a basket in the least amount of time).

Environment

The environment can play an important role in the ability of individuals to actively pursue leisure involvement. Practitioners may be in a position to adapt the environment in which leisure participation is intended to occur or to make recommendations for changing the environment. Because practitioners are attempting to provide recreation in a variety of contexts, possible adaptations to the environment are suggested in this section that relate directly to:

(a) sensory factors; and
(b) the participation area.

Sensory factors. Participation can be enhanced for some individuals by simply manipulating the *sounds* occurring within the environment during participation. For instance, when playing a recreation game, some people who are easily distracted may have difficulty concentrating when the game is being played in a multipurpose room with other people present talking to one another as they engage in other activities. Moving the recreation game to a small, quiet room where only people participating in the game are present may facilitate more active participation for some individuals. In addition, some people using hearing aids can experience difficulty when participating in a gymnasium because of the echoing effect that can occur. Placement of drapes and sound absorbing tiles near the ceiling may muffle some distracting sounds and provide persons with hearing impairments the opportunity to attend to directions more easily.

Providing an environment that permits people to see as much as possible is important when attempting to teach people. Therefore, practitioners should examine the context of an activity and determine if adequate *lighting* is available. Completion of craft projects engaged in at a table may be enhanced by simply placing a lamp on the table. Some people's vision, however, may be substantially impaired as a result of glare. Therefore, recreation professionals must consider the angle of the lights and realize the possibility that some lights may be too bright and inhibit, rather than enhance, participation.

Participation area. The area in which an activity is played can be adapted to facilitate more active participation. To accommodate individuals with reduced mobility, the *playing area* used for an activity can be changed. This can allow participants with limited speed to successfully participate. For instance, rather than using an entire baseball field to play kick ball, participants can be required to keep the ball in play within the infield. In softball, participants can be required to hit to one side of the pitchers mound allowing more individuals to cover a small area.

Boundaries designating the end of the playing areas can also be changed to make people more aware of these designations. Wider chalk marks can be used on soccer fields to allow people to see more clearly when they are approaching an area designated as out-of-bounds. Ropes can be placed along a walking trail to permit individuals with visual impairments to follow the trail and maintain their awareness of boundaries associated with the walking trail.

The *surface area* can also be changed to permit some people to more easily access activities. A person who uses a wheelchair may be able to join a hiking expedition when some firm foundation has been applied to a trail. Changes in textures on the ground and adjacent walls of playgrounds can indicate to children with visual impairments that they are moving toward different equipment.

The *facility* where the activity is conducted may be also changed. For instance, ramps may be placed in a swimming pool to permit access by persons with limited mobility. In addition, the water in the swimming pool could be lowered to only two or three feet to initially accommodate those people with significant fears associated with water.

Participants

When considering adaptations, the changes previously mentioned in this chapter (changes associated with materials, activities and the environment) often come to mind. If, however, adaptations are viewed as changes that are made to facilitate active leisure participation, then another category for making adaptations may be established. The participants themselves may actually be altered to encourage active participation in those experiences that bring them joy and satisfaction. This section of the chapter provides suggestions on how to make some of these adaptations to the participants. Modifications can dramatically influence participants' level of participation, and such modifications may include the way individuals are:

(a) *positioned;*
(b) aided with *prostheses* and *sensory aids;*
(c) provided with opportunities for increased *mobility;*
(d) able to *communicate;* and
(e) using participation *skills.*

Positioning. The optimal condition in which individuals learn and actively participate is the "ready state." That is, participants should be sitting or standing as erect as possible, not in discomfort, able to reach materials and objects associated with an activity, and facing in the direction of the activity. Pillows, foam wedges and support belts can be used to help individuals prepare for activity involvement.

If individuals who have limited muscle control wish to read a book, a triangle wedge can be placed under their chest with the larger side close to their neck and the smaller side near their stomach. The book can be placed on the floor and can be controlled with their hands.

In another situation, a person using a wheelchair can be securely fastened into the chair and provided access to toys by placing them directly on a lap tray attached to the chair. For the activity of swimming, life jackets can be used to support individuals as they learn to swim. If people using wheelchairs wish to actively contribute to the development of a mural that is being painted, they can be positioned sideways to the wall or easel to allow them to reach the mural.

Prosthesis. Many people's participation in recreation activities can be enhanced by providing prosthetic support for the individuals. For instance, people may encounter difficulty grasping a fishing pole because of severe weakness associated with their wrists. A brace may be used to help support the wrist when holding the fishing pole.

Some participants involved in a nature walk may have a limited range of motion. This reduced range of motion would typically limit their ability to bend at the waist and collect samples of leaves, bark and other items used for debriefing sessions following the walk. Providing them with a scooping device attached to an extended handle would permit them to participate more actively in the walk and accompanying discussion. In addition, people who have limited grasping capabilities can paint, if a paint brush is strapped to their hand by using Velcro.™

Sensory aids. If practitioners notice that participants appear to have difficulty seeing demonstrations or responding to other visual cues used to facilitate participation, they should check to determine when the person was last seen for an eye examination. If there has not been a recent eye exam, the practitioner should recommend one. The eye exam may result in the prescription of *corrective lenses or contacts,* which would then promote more active participation.

In addition, some participants may not respond quickly to verbal instructions. At times, they may seem confused or inattentive. These characteristics may be indicative of a hearing loss. Records should be checked to determine the most recent audiology examination. Again, if a recent evaluation has not been performed, practitioners should make a recommendation for the person to have a hearing examination completed. The examination may result in people using some form of *hearing aid* to enhance their ability to hear and thus reduce barriers to leisure participation.

Method of mobility. Some individuals receiving recreation services may have reduced mobility as a result of many different conditions. For instance, mobility may be limited because of a degenerative disease, such as multiple sclerosis; a traumatic accident resulting in injury to the central nervous system, such as a spinal cord injury; or from an orthopedic disorder resulting in reduced range of motion, such as arthritis. In response to this reduced mobility, people may find assistance in their mobility by using a variety of aids (e.g., wheelchairs, crutches, walkers, braces).

Although their primary means of ambulation may be effective in the majority of situations across their life experiences, they may be able to participate more actively in some recreation activities with a different variation of the mobility aid. For children who use wheelchairs and are participating in activities in a gymnasium, a *scooter board* can inject fun and increased speed into the activity. For instance, when playing kick ball, children could use scooter boards to move about. This adaptation could be made in conjunction with an activity modification by establishing the rule that participants use their hands to hit the ball and then move to the bases quickly on the scooter boards.

Some people's personal wheelchair may be the most appropriate for their daily experiences. There are, however, many commercially available *sport wheelchairs* designed specifically for the requirements associated with particular types of sports. For instance, there are chairs designed for activities that require a great deal of rapid turning. These types of chairs may be used when participating in activities such as tennis, basketball, and racquetball. Other people may be interested in participating in races on or off the track. These individuals frequently use chairs designed for speed and movement in a forward direction. Practitioners should examine the participation patterns of persons experiencing reduced mobility and consider variations to their typical mode of transportation that could enhance leisure involvement.

Mode of communication. Many individuals with severe disabilities cannot meet their communication needs through standard forms of spoken communication (Vanderheiden & Yoder, 1986). Therefore, practitioners must be willing to modify the required response mode for a particular activity. These individuals may require augmentative and alternative communication (AAC) systems to fulfill their needs.

AAC systems include those which are unaided (e.g., gestures, sign language, finger spelling), nonelectronic aided systems (e.g., communication boards or books containing symbols, words or pictures) and computer-based assistive technology producing speech synthesis and/or word printouts. AAC systems vary considerably according to message storage and retrieval systems, communication speed, and communication-aid output capabilities (Vanderheiden and Lloyd, 1986).

People who use AAC systems typically acquire their disabilities from congenital physical disabilities (e.g., cerebral palsy, mental retardation), acquired neurogenic disorders (e.g., closed head injury, cerebral vascular accident), progressive neurological diseases (e.g., multiple sclerosis, muscular dystrophy) and temporary conditions such as those resulting from shock, trauma, or surgery. There is a large range of competencies and abilities across individuals using AAC systems (Kraat, 1985), resulting in an extremely heterogeneous population (Light, 1988) of ACC users. Practitioners must be open to these alternative forms of communication and be willing to change the required mode of communication for a specific activity to permit active participation by persons using communication systems other than speech.

Skills. As stated previously in this chapter, if an imbalance exists between the degree of challenge of a program and the participants' skills, barriers to leisure participation may be created. The majority of this chapter has focused on adaptations that can permit modification of the challenge associated with a recreation program to meet the abilities of the participants. Practitioners, however, possess another option when attempting to assist individuals in matching the requirements of an activity. Recreation is designed to *teach people skills and knowledge* that facilitate their ability to meet the challenges encountered when attempting to experience leisure. For instance, if people do not possess the skills to access public transportation to go to a fitness club, instruction related to use of public transportation will increase the ability of individuals to meet the challenges associated with enhancing their physical fitness.

In addition, *systematic instruction* may need to occur within the facility with professionals and persons with disabilities to provide the opportunity for independent participation in community recreation programs. Through systematic instruction, practitioners can encourage individuals with disabilities to increase their skills and knowledge. In the most general sense, a change has been made in the individuals. The people have adapted themselves to meet the demands and challenges associated with a particular experience.

Instructional Strategies

The four areas for making adaptations previously mentioned have required practitioners to focus their attention away from themselves and onto the participants, activity, materials and environment. The fifth and final area of consideration presented is intended to encourage professionals to consider examining their practice of recreation.

If people receiving recreation services are not developing leisure skills and knowledge at a rate consistent with their potential, there may be ways to modify the instructional strategies employed by the professionals to allow individuals with disabilities to more effectively and efficiently meet their needs. The next section will address the following considerations related to instructional strategies:

(a) establish objectives;
(b) develop instructional steps;
(c) implement practice;
(d) include instructional prompts;
(e) apply reinforcement; and
(f) consider personnel.

Establish objectives. At times, consumers of recreation services may encounter difficulty achieving preestablished objectives. Practitioners may continue to focus on the inability of individuals to achieve their objectives and thus create further difficulty. A possible problem may have occurred during the establishment of objectives, resulting in tasks that may be too difficult to master. If this occurs, practitioners should be willing to reassess the objectives and change them to meet the needs of participants. This is not to say that practitioners should develop objectives that are not challenging. In fact, they should be monitored closely for the possibility of having objectives that are too easily completed by participants. Rather than create frustration for both participants and practitioners as with overly rigorous objectives, the development of objectives demanding too little of individuals can create an environment conducive to boredom and apathy.

Develop instructional steps. An extremely useful tool in the provision of leisure services for people with disabilities is task analysis. Task analysis involves the segmenting of a task into components that can be taught separately. The instructional components can then be sequenced together to allow individuals to complete an identified task. The procedure of task analysis is used when attempting to teach a multifaceted task that may appear complex for participants. Although task analysis requires identification of components that, when accomplished in sequence, permit completion of the task, the number of components identified for any given task may vary considerably. For instance, in one situation the act of swinging a table tennis paddle to hit the ball may be divided into four steps, while in another circumstance the task may be divided into 10 components.

The skills of individual participants should determine the level of specificity associated with a task analysis. Therefore, if people are encountering difficulty learning a skill, practitioners should examine the components being taught. They should determine if further delineation is needed for those individuals stagnating on a particular component or if some components should be collapsed to accommodate people who feel they are not being sufficiently challenged.

Implement practice. To educate people with disabilities about leisure, practitioners develop content and then attempt to present this content in a systematic fashion. Sometimes people enrolled in recreation programs fail to progress at the rate practitioners expect. One reason people may not acquire skills and knowledge associated with a particular aspect of recreation is that they may not have received sufficient opportunity to practice the information presented in the program. Another way to adapt the instructional strategy is to change the amount of practice associated with a particular objective.

If participants are not acquiring the skills and knowledge, they may benefit from increased opportunities for practice. Repetition through practice can allow individuals to integrate the newly acquired knowledge and skill into their existing leisure repertoire. Continuous practice of previously learned skills can increase the likelihood that individuals will maintain the skills over time. When planning practice sessions, practitioners should be creative and make these opportunities as interesting and fun as possible. Frequently, people do not acquire an understanding of a concept the initial time they are presented with the idea. Practice provides experiences that permit repetition of concepts and ideas that enable people to retain that information more easily.

Include instructional prompts. As practitioners provide instruction, they may observe that participants are not responding to their directions. Therefore, they may wish to consider the use of prompts to assist participants. Prompts can provide auditory cues for individuals, typically through verbal instructions. There are, however, other forms of prompts that can be used. Environmental prompts can encourage participant involvement by simply manipulating the context in which an activity is provided. For instance, one way to encourage use of recreation table games in a recreation lounge may be for the practitioner to place the games on tables in the room or open the closets where they are stored so that participants entering the area will see the games.

Additional visual cues may be provided to stimulate participation. Modeling appropriate behaviors and providing systematic demonstrations may allow participants to more clearly see the desired leisure behavior. In addition, hand-over-hand physical guidance may permit individuals to feel the specific movements associated with participation and thus increase their ability to correctly perform the skill. Because people may respond differently to various prompts, practitioners must examine their procedures and be willing to modify the way they are prompting participants to learn and apply new leisure skills.

Apply reinforcement. Practitioners often provide individuals with a reinforcer: an object or event to encourage the acquisition of leisure skills and knowledge. The object or event, however, may not be perceived by the participant to be a reinforcer. Dattilo and Murphy (1987b) reported that reinforcers differ from one person to another. According to the authors, "selection of an object or event to serve as a positive reinforcer must be person specific; that is, it must be something that will effectively influence that individual's behavior" (p. 54). Therefore, practitioners must monitor the participants' responses to a consequence in order to determine if it is truly a powerful enough reinforcer to influence behavior. If, over time, behaviors do not increase in response to administration of a specific item or activity, practitioners should be willing to make adaptations. Testing various items and activities until reinforcers are identified may provide practitioners with a systematic procedure for identification of reinforcers.

Consider personnel. Interaction between participants and practitioners is a highly complex process. Some participants may respond to some practitioners more energetically than to others. Failure of some program participants to progress at an anticipated rate may be significantly influenced by the professionals who are delivering the services. Practitioners should closely monitor their interactions with participants as well as other personnel delivering recreation services. In-service training can be provided in an attempt to improve skills of practitioners. In addition, adapting schedules to accommodate both staff and participant needs may also encourage more effective implementation of recreation programs.

Conclusion

This chapter focused on ways to make adaptations. These adaptations should permit practitioners to meet the varying needs and abilities of the people attending recreation programs. The suggestions were intended to communicate some options available to practitioners to make adjustments needed to facilitate active leisure participation for persons with disabilities. General considerations were initially presented in the chapter to provide guidelines to follow when making any adaptation intended to promote leisure involvement. The remaining portion of the chapter was devoted to providing suggestions on adaptations related to materials that are used, the activity, environment in which the activity is conducted, participants, and instructional strategies employed by practitioners.

Discussion Questions

1. What are five major areas of adaptation to recreation programs?

2. What are the three general considerations in emphasizing the person first?

3. How can you encourage participant autonomy?

4. What are the three ways discussed in this chapter to involve the participant in the adaptation process?

5. What are the three steps suggested to evaluate adaptations?

6. Describe six possible methods for adapting materials that are used in recreation programs.

7. How can activities be adapted to best facilitate recreation participation by people with disabilities?

8. How does the environment play an important role in the ability of individuals with disabilities to participate in recreation activities?

9. How can you adapt the environment to facilitate recreation participation for individuals with disabilities?

10. What is a "ready state?"

11. What are seven ways of altering the participants to facilitate their participation?

12. Describe the six instructional strategies that may be modified as presented in this chapter.

Chapter 13

Advocate for Services

"On an occasion of this kind it becomes more than a moral duty to speak one's mind. It becomes a pleasure."
—Oscar Wilde

Orientation Activity: Go Ahead and Be an Advocate

Directions When Alone: Identify 10 of the following advocacy actions that you would like to adopt as personal goals by writing the numbers associated with the 10 statements on a separate piece of paper. Prioritized these 10 actions, assigning the number 1 to the most important and 10 to the least important.

Directions With Others: With your paper in hand, move about the room and find another person who chose one of the same activities as you. Introduce yourself, find out the person's name and discuss why you each choose the item. Once you have finished, find another person and continue the process.

1. Invite people with disabilities to attend programs.
2. Ask adults with disabilities to serve as leaders.
3. Organize a People with Disabilities Awareness Day.
4. Survey architectural barriers and share results.
5. Write articles about barriers facing people with disabilities.
6. Advise people with disabilities of community recreation and support services.
7. Talk with people with disabilities to learn more about them and their disability.
8. Discuss the problems architectural and attitudinal barriers create.
9. Volunteer to record materials for people with visual impairments.
10. Urge radio and television stations to donate service time to the topic of barriers.
11. Develop public service announcements for radio and television stations.
12. Contact organizations for ideas concerning their work with citizens who have disabilities.

13. Write letters to local newspaper editors urging removal of barriers from facilities.
14. Plan exhibits to create awareness and dispel myths about people with disabilities.
15. Ask people with disabilities to appear on local speak-out programs.
16. Learn about building codes and laws concerning access.
17. View a film on problems that people with disabilities face.
18. Do research on people with disabilities and share the results.
19. Teach awareness activities to community groups.
20. Keep the media informed of successes obtained by people with disabilities.
21. Campaign for the display of the Access Symbol where appropriate.
22. Learn requirements for displaying the Access Symbol and check buildings for compliance.
23. Conduct a poster contest related to the removal of barriers.
24. Volunteer at an agency serving people with disabilities.
26. Learn about injuries that can disable people and then visit a rehabilitation center.
27. Develop a babysitting course for teens to sit for children with disabilities.
28. Form an advocacy committee to work on removal of barriers.
29. Meet with a legislator and learn about policies and laws.
30. Compliment TV stations that show people with disabilities in a positive manner.
31. Encourage community groups to sponsor sign language courses.
32. Invite a person with an auditory impairment and an interpreter to talk to your agency.
33. Learn to sign a song and teach it to your friends.
34. Sponsor an idea exchange among people with disabilities and other agencies.
35. Discuss ways to involve people in community activities and how to remove barriers.
36. Give a disability quiz and lead a myth-slaying discussion.
37. Read children's stories and discuss how people with disabilities are portrayed.
38. Identify transportation for people with disabilities.
39. Learn about technology that assists people with disabilities.
40. Record a favorite recreation activity, assign a disability and determine necessary accommodations.
41. Interview people with disabilities at work in the community.
42. Speak about recreation opportunities to parents of children with disabilities.

Debriefing

Most attempts at advocacy, by and on behalf of people with disabilities, have been to urge opportunities for all people to participate as fully as possible in community life, and to end discrimination based on disabilities. The demands for community inclusion, integration, and civil rights, have been widely recognized as just (for example, Americans with Disabilities Act).

Advocates are needed not because people with disabilities are inherently weak and incapable, but because they are members of an unfavored minority group. People with disabilities should receive community services because they have a right to them. The services are provided because people with disabilities are citizens. If disabilities interfere with citizens' rights, then society must make the changes that will enable them to enjoy those rights—regardless of costs. Ultimately, people with disabilities should be their own advocates. The aim of the advocate should be to step aside and let the people manage their own affairs. As you reflect on the orientation activity consider the following questions:

1. What is an advocate?
2. How can you begin to advocate for people with disabilities today?
3. Why is advocacy necessary?

Introduction

At times, people with disabilities are socially isolated and disconnected, and therefore have difficulty getting their voices heard by the community. They are devalued in our society, and are often cut off from social roles which bring power, status, influence and opportunities. According to Gill (1994), people without disabilities often have difficulty accepting people with disabilities as equal members of society. Some people with disabilities do not have the skills to communicate their wishes effectively and may need a spokesperson. Many people with disabilities need services and supports to facilitate participation in society. Unfortunately, the systems to provide these are often complex, segregated, and controlling. Anthony (1985) stated that advocacy is an important means to facilitate inclusion of people with disabilities because it is concerned with securing rights, encouraging full participation, promoting access, and empowering people.

Learn Terminology Related to Advocacy

To **advocate** means to recommend, to be in favor of, to plead for. An advocate is a person who advocates a policy, or proposal and pleads on the behalf of another. An advocate is generally defined as one who pleads the cause of another or gives support to a particular cause. The word "advocate" is derived from the Latin *avocare,* "to summon." The advocate is one who is called upon to provide assistance.

According to Hutchison and McGill (1992), advocacy is required when ordinary actions have been unsuccessful in ensuring that a person's rights are being met. To illustrate this point, the authors used writings from Perske (1979) and Wolfensberger (1977) to develop a list of characteristics that distinguish between advocacy and other everyday activities, in that advocacy:

(a) involves in-depth feelings and commitment to a cause;
(b) calls for doing more than what is done routinely;
(c) involves risk (advocates' actions are open to criticism); and
(d) must be structured to be free from conflict of interest.

As stated in the previous chapter, a **barrier** is any obstacle or obstruction, natural or man-made, that impedes progress but is not necessarily impassable. An **architectural barrier** is any feature of the man-made physical environment which impedes or restricts the mobility of people to the full use of a facility. An **attitudinal barrier** is a way of thinking about or perceiving a disability in a restrictive, condescending or negative manner.

To **empower** someone is to give power or authority to that person. All people have the right to live life to the fullest and experience leisure, but many people with a disability face barriers which prevent them from doing so. These barriers may be in the form of limited access to facilities, transportation, information, programs or job opportunities. Whatever the reason for the barrier, advocacy, the process of speaking up and working for changes in policies, opportunities and attitudes, can help.

Advocate for People with Disabilities

One way to become an effective advocate is to take time to prepare a strategy for advocacy, follow some guidelines when advocating, and evaluate attempts at advocacy. Suggestions related to these three strategies are presented below.

Prepare for Advocacy

Establishing advocacy goals, becoming informed about people with disabilities and listening to people with disabilities are all helpful ways to prepare for advocacy. Figure 13.1 identifies these techniques.

Establish advocacy goals. Professionals are encouraged to formulate goals specific to advocacy and develop an effective strategy to meet those goals. Prioritize the goals you have established. Be persistent, and realize change may take time. Many advocacy efforts can take years to come to fruition.

Become informed. Professionals that become informed about the rights and desires of people with disabilities are taking an important step toward advocacy. Credibility is lost when you are unable to answer pertinent questions. Failing to be aware of significant events relating to the issue being pursued can be equally problematic. However, an honest response that a topic has not been studied and that the answer is not known can be disarming—and helpful. There is not a need to become an expert, just the desire to be resourceful and know where to find information.

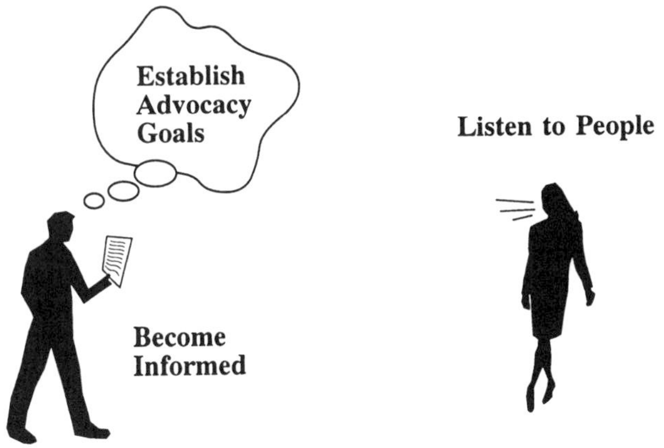

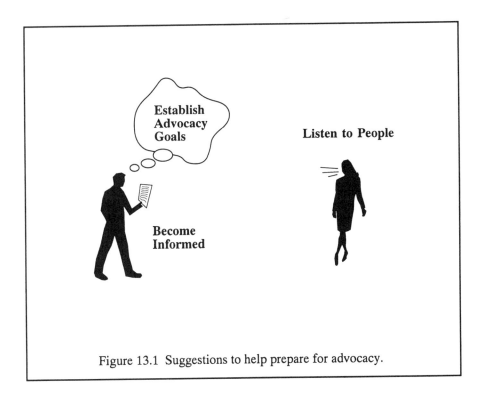

Figure 13.1 Suggestions to help prepare for advocacy.

Listen to people's perspectives. It is critical that advocates listen to other people's perspectives about integration, disability, and providing a supportive environment for people with disabilities. Resistance to including people with disabilities into services may be an indication of negative feelings or fears. Respond by actively listening to feelings in order to keep communication open.

Engage in Advocacy

Presenting information which is clear, tactful and contains humor may be useful when advocating for people with disabilities. In addition, professionals may attempt to provide people with suggestions to help improve their approach to interacting with people with disabilities. These techniques are illustrated in Figure 13.2.

Present information. Professionals are encouraged to present information regarding the rights and desires of people with disabilities to other people. An informal discussion emphasizing how integration can benefit all people is often a good beginning. Provide examples of successful attempts at integration which you have achieved within your agency or program.

Be clear. Based on basic principles of communication, it is helpful to be clear about whose interests you are representing. It is important to talk with people with disabilities to verify if they agree with your perspective of certain issues. Define and present the issue in a way that is comfortable to you.

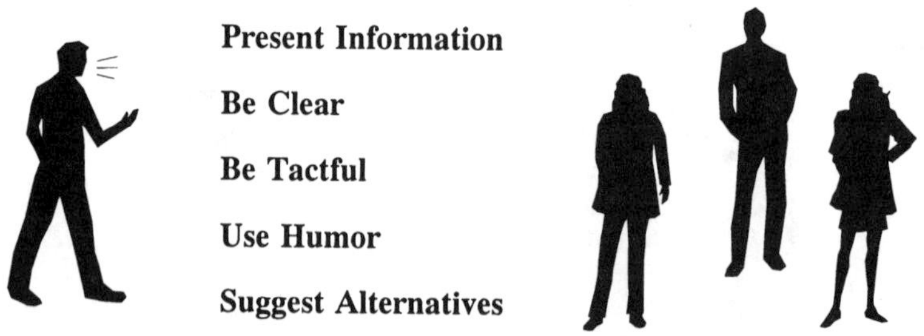
Present Information
Be Clear
Be Tactful
Use Humor
Suggest Alternatives

Figure 13.2 Suggestions when engaged in advocacy.

Make attempts to be tactful. When serving as an advocate, avoid being unnecessarily confrontational but be consistent with your beliefs. It is necessary to present facts accurately. Demonstrate your appreciation to people and organizations who are helpful and are willing to listen to you. Show concern for problems, and enthusiasm for solutions. When addressing other people, demonstrate the belief that they will provide assistance if they are aware of the problems and understand methods for remediation. Offer to show others how to comply with legislation, while generating public approval.

Use humor. Advocates and individuals with disabilities who have gained acceptance often are able to use playfulness and humor effectively. If done appropriately, humor can dissipate tension and lead to common understanding. Playfulness primarily involves changing the context in which people are used to functioning.

Suggest alternatives. Sometimes direct information or responding to feelings is not enough to break through rationalizations. Suggest alternatives to people after initial dialogue and negotiations. Alternatives to time and financial constraints are often appreciated.

Evaluate Attempts at Advocacy

Leisure services providers often take pride in their ability to effectively evaluate their services. Evaluation of advocacy efforts that include analyzation of the content presented, examination of the presentation style, and identification of successful advocacy attempts may be useful. These techniques are presented in Figure 13.3 (see page 224).

Analyze informational content. It is helpful for advocates to examine closely the content of the information you presented. Consider if people seemed to understand what you were attempting to convey. Determine if other, more helpful information may be available.

Examine the process. Examine the way in which the information was presented. Consider the limitations, as well as the strengths, of the different advocacy approaches that were used. Consider the effectiveness of reaching the intended audiences.

Identify successful advocacy attempts. Professionals engaged in advocacy should celebrate their successful attempts at advocacy. Reward yourself and others associated with these efforts. Use these successes as examples in future advocacy efforts.

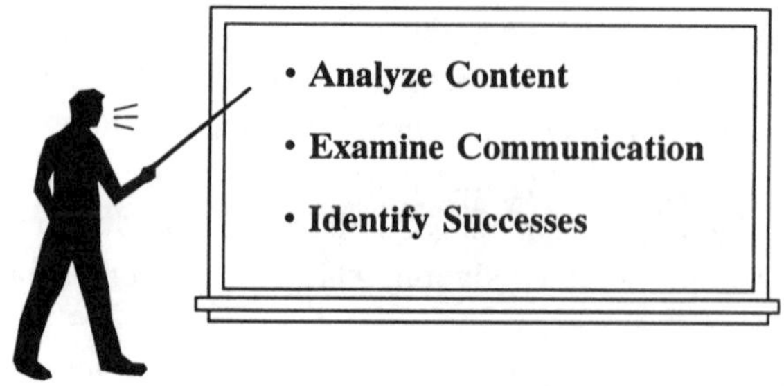

Figure 13.3 Suggestions to help evaluate advocacy efforts.

Encourage Self-Advocacy

Advocacy has traditionally meant speaking on behalf of others. In recent years the term **self-advocacy** has been coined to refer to individuals and groups who have traditionally been powerless and largely voiceless, speaking up on their own behalf to try to change their social status and situation. The self-advocacy movement among people with disabilities has been very important and influential in improving opportunities.

Advocates and advocacy groups which act on behalf of others run the risk of becoming paternalistic—that is, of defining what the "best interests" of the individuals or groups are, and working for these without really stopping to ask the people what they want. To avoid this paternalism and to be authentically empowering, advocacy must be "instruction based." Parent (1993) reported that choices made by people with disabilities often are based on avoidance of undesirable alternatives rather than true preferences. The actions of advocates must reflect the expressed wishes of the individuals or groups they are representing, not upon what others believe is "best" for them.

It is usually best to initiate advocacy efforts with an honest, open, "common problem" approach, and to be willing to negotiate and to compromise where necessary. If, however, we are serious about empowering people who have been powerless, we need to recognize that a certain amount of confrontation, and a certain adversarial relationship with "the powers that be" will always be part of advocacy movements.

Empowering people inevitably means taking some power away from one person, or group, to give it to another. Neither individuals nor organizations typically relinquish power willingly. Some advocates will need to be adversarial, others cooperative. These two approaches complement each other, and are necessary for the social change that people with disabilities seek.

Many people with disabilities have formed self-advocacy groups. Self-advocacy groups began among people with disabilities who thought that together they could help each other become more independent, learn to speak for themselves, and gain a measure of self-respect and confidence that they had not had in the past. Self-advocacy groups do many things. They organize socials, learn social skills, learn about rights and responsibilities, acquire the skills needed for running meetings, and more. Regardless of what they do, the important thing is that the activities grow out of the needs of consumers, and they promote independence and the ability to speak and act for themselves.

The underlying assumption in self-advocacy is that dependence encourages dependence, and independence encourages independence. Thus, self-advocacy groups seek to provide peer support which can help break established patterns of dependency. People with disabilities become self-advocates because they want to become more independent. Parents, friends, and organizations often encourage self-advocacy because they recognize that as people with disabilities learn to make decisions and accept greater responsibility for their lives, everyone—disabled and nondisabled—benefits.

Examples of Advocacy Efforts

The Use of Toys

Mattel® formed a not-for-profit corporation called "For Challenged Kids" to produce and market toys specially designed for children with disabilities. All profits from the sale of these toys will be dispersed among organizations that work with children with disabilities. The first "For Challenged Kids" product line, "Hal's Pals," consisted of five, 19-inch soft-sculptured dolls, each with a different disability. Hal (one of the best skiers in Colorado) is a ski instructor with one leg. Bobby is an athletic little boy who uses a wheelchair for mobility. Suzie is an adventurous girl who is sight-impaired and uses her cane and guide dog to explore her neighborhood. Laura is a ballerina who wears hearing aids. Finally, Kathy is a little girl wearing a party dress, a big smile and leg braces. Mattel® believes "Hal's Pals" are really mainstream toys and not just for children with disabilities. Each doll portrays its disability in a familiar, comfortable way, focusing on ability and strengths. The dolls have been identified as useful educational tools, providing insight and improved understanding into what it's like to have a disability.

Reading the Newspaper and Writing Letters

In an editorial in a college newspaper, a person wrote:

> Have you seen what they're doing to Atherton Hall? They're destroying it. They are going to build up the front courtyard and level it off so that wheelchairs, etc., will be able to get to it easier. I'm not against the idea that buildings should be accessible to the handicapped, but Atherton is not the building to do it to. Every floor except the second has some levels which are connected by stairs. This means that the only places that a wheelchair could get to once it was inside the building was the lobby, the TV room, the second floor, and the parts of the others that the elevator is level with (and that elevator only goes to the ground, first and second floors). Another problem is the bathrooms. Every bathroom in the building has a step at the doorway that you have to step over to get in. Also, there are no handicapped toilets, showers or sinks. There is going to have to be a lot of work done just to make the University and a couple of senators or representatives who want to make this building accessible happy. Again, I'm not against the idea in general, but it is not a feasible option in the case of Atherton. Besides the monetary and time expenditures, there is the problem of a major inconvenience to the inhabitants of the dorm (e.g. noise, privacy, physical inconveniences of closing the front entrance when they rebuild parts of the interior) and even more importantly is the historical nature of Atherton Hall. It is one of the older and most beautiful dorms on campus. Its beautiful main entrance has greeted many dignitaries and honored guests of the hall and this "remodeling" will destroy the original landscaping and architecture of this building. After considering limitations of this project and the inconveniences and the problems it will cause, I have to conclude that the work currently being done to Atherton Hall is inappropriate, unnecessary and should be halted before any further destruction takes place.

The following is a response to the previous editorial entitled "All or None" that was prepared by three students majoring in Recreation and Leisure Studies.

> We would hardly refer to a building which is being altered for better accessibility as a building which is being, as you stated, "destroyed." You seem to only be concerned about the minor inconveniences that the inhabitants of the dorm will experience during the construction

period. You complain of the "physical inconvenience of closing the front entrance" to the building. Did you ever stop to consider the constant inconvenience people who use wheelchairs face daily because they can not get into a building that has only stairs as a means of entrance? Typically, it would only take a couple of months of "inconvenience" to make a building accessible, yet it would provide a lifetime of accessibility to people who use wheelchairs. You refer to the "many dignitaries and honored guests" that this hall has greeted. Speaking of dignitaries, do you realize that one of our presidents, Franklin D. Roosevelt, used a wheelchair? In addition, you also stated that you are "not against the idea that buildings should be accessible to the handicapped, but Atherton is not the building to do it to." Isn't this a bit contradictory? If you are going to support a cause, you must support the entire cause—it is not right to exclude a portion just because it may cramp your lifestyle for a brief time. This reminds us of those people who used to say, "I'm not against blacks riding buses, but not my bus." If your description of how making Atherton Hall accessible is accurate, it is possible that the University is not going about it in the most efficient manner. However, this does not suggest that Atherton Hall is not a feasible building to make accessible. We suggest that rather than focusing your efforts on condemning accessibility to Atherton Hall by people using wheelchairs, that you focus your efforts on examining the plan for accessibility. In the past few years considerable strides have been made which have provided individuals with disabilities access to buildings. These breakthroughs have enabled integration into the mainstream of society a reality instead of only a dream.

Discussion Questions

1. What is meant by the term "advocacy?"

2. What role does advocacy play in relation to barriers experienced by people with disabilities?

3. How does empowerment relate to advocacy?

4. What are methods you can use to help prepare yourself to be an effective advocate?

5. When presenting information to other people on behalf of people with disabilities, what should you consider?

6. What are some ides to consider when you are evaluating your ability to be an advocate?

7. What is the value in encouraging people with disabilities to be their own advocates when possible?

8. What is one action you could take today to advocate for people with disabilities?

9. Why is advocating for the rights of people with disabilities your responsibility?

10. Who benefits by advocacy efforts?

Section C

Consider Individual Characteristics

Chapter 14

People, Inclusion, and Physical Limitations

Jon Franks

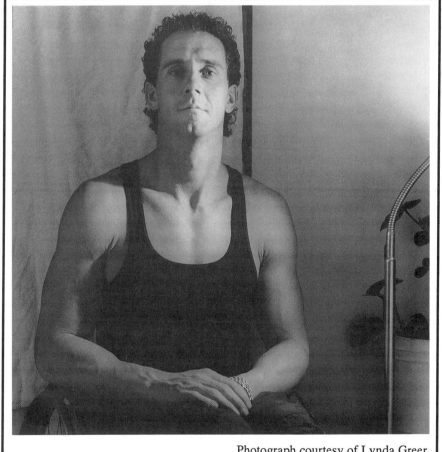

Photograph courtesy of Lynda Greer

Jon Franks is a chiropractor who owns a fitness center in Venice, CA. He sustained a spinal cord injury in a motorcycle accident in 1985. Jon is a triathelete who has raced all over the United States, in China, and the Virgin Islands.

Jon's Story

It was November, 1985. I was on my way to a UCLA basketball practice . . . I was working with the team . . . when the engine on my motorcycle seized up on me, doing a curve at about 40 mph; and I slammed into a utility pole. As a chiropractor I do know about the spine, so I knew right away what the score was.

Basketball and fitness have been part of my life since I can remember, so well-meaning people suggested that I go for wheelchair basketball. No way would I settle for less with a sport I excelled in on my feet. So in the hospital I set my mind on the triathalon. I've always been a competitor and the accident didn't kill that spirit. The triathalon is a grueling event . . . just what I wanted. Two months after the accident I was training 15 to 20 hours a week. I'm most competitive in the swimming and running events, weaker in the cycling division. For swimming I wear a wet suit and webbed gloves to give me power, and I do the backstroke . . . breathing's easier. For the run I use a lightweight chair and I use a hand-powered bike designed and built by my friend, Bruce Eikelberger. We're working to develop a better bike.

I love the challenge of racing. But it isn't just for me that I do this. I intend to change the image most adults have of people in chairs. And I'm doing it in an effort to raise bucks as well as consciousness. Attitude-wise I want to teach people that being in a chair isn't the most disabling thing; it's the attitude of others. Sometimes it's very difficult for athletes to participate in certain events. I've had my share of rejection because I'm in a chair and a pain in the butt to work around. This segregating athletic events along able-bodied/disabled lines has to stop. And I'm also racing to get sponsors to help raise money for research and technical advances. I believe I'll be out of this chair someday and that kids . . . anyone with a spinal cord injury . . . deserve the chance of complete recovery.

But as long as I'm in this chair I'm going to prove to others that people in chairs are really no different from them. A lot of people don't feel comfortable with wheelchairs . . . and that's got to change. Believe me, it will be better for everybody.

Latent abilities are like clay. It can be mud on shoes, brick in a building or a statue that will inspire all who see it. The clay is the same. The result is dependent on how it is used.
—James A. Lincoln

Orientation Activity

Directions: Read each of the following three situations. On a separate sheet of paper answer the questions posed at the end of the scenarios.

1. Mary, an accountant in your home town, would like to participate in a tennis program offered by the private country club of which she is a member. As the director of recreation for this country club, what might you do to facilitate participation by Mary, who has paraplegia, in the tennis program?
2. Michael, a college student, has expressed a desire to participate in a hiking expedition planned for a weekend adventure with a local community outing club. As a member of this club, what suggestions might you make to assist Michael, who has spina bifida, to successfully participate in the program?
3. You are the assistant coach of your child's softball team. Susan, a 12-year-old, would like to play on the team. Susan has muscular dystrophy and is still able to walk. What are some things you may wish to consider when coaching Susan and what is some information you may wish to discuss with Susan, the coach, and perhaps her parents?

Debriefing

To include Mary in the tennis program you must ensure that the parking lot and the path to the tennis courts are accessible to people using wheelchairs. Advertise that the tennis program is available to every member in the club. Modification to the rules as established by the National Foundation of Wheelchair Tennis will help assure success for Mary. For example, players who use wheelchairs are allowed two bounces of the ball. Ensure that she is able to participate with her friends. If she is a new member, arrange matches with peers of relatively similar ages. Identify other resources she could take advantage of to improve her skills. If Mary has limited strength and endurance, perhaps the use of a ball retrieving basket or a person to pick up the loose balls may be helpful.

To facilitate Michael's participation in the hiking expedition, first talk with Michael about his skill and experience as a hiker. The difficulty level of the trail should be obtained and matched with the skill level of the participant. You may want to hike the trail in advance conducting an environmental inventory to identify obstacles that will need to negotiated. Determine what the weight of his pack should be based on his endurance, strength and agility. As with any camping expedition, a communication device that can signal others if there is distress may be useful. Determine strategies to accommodate people on the expedition who move at slower speeds. Schedule breaks to allow participants who are moving more slowly than others to catch up and rest. Schedule meeting points along the trail to encourage the gathering of people on the expedition. If Michael is unsteady on his feet, he may wish to use a hiking stick, cane, or he may feel comfortable being paired with someone who can assist him as needed.

To encourage Susan's inclusion on the softball team, visit with Susan and her family to discuss her strengths as well as concerns for participation. Have her share with you any adaptations she has already made when playing softball. If Susan has difficulty running, you may suggest she hit and have another player run the bases for her. If she has difficulty moving, perhaps she may prefer to play the position of catcher, pitcher, or first base. She may be paired with someone playing other positions that could catch the ball, throw it to her, and then allow her to make the play. Rotating the entire lineup to avoid fatigue may be useful if endurance is a problem. For instance, players only play for two consecutive innings and then are rested for one inning. Consider the following questions as you think about the orientation activity:

1. How can you promote participation of individuals with physical limitations in your recreation program?
2. Why is it important for recreation providers to talk to new participants when they begin a program?
3. What are some considerations for the inclusion of participants who may have limited strength, balance, or endurance?

Meet Joan, Whose Interests Are Many

People describe Joan as a lifelong activist, committed to a wide range of issues and interests such as the peace movement and international affairs. Recently, she has become an activist for the rights of people with disabilities. "When you don't have something wrong, it's not part of your life," she said. "It didn't hit home until it hit me."

Joan's range of interests are obvious in even a quick visit to her apartment. The wheelchair ramp to the door is flanked by huge flower boxes made of railroad ties, overflowing with her flowers. The most prominent object in the living room is a loom—she says she made 10 sweaters one year as Christmas gifts. Delicate Japanese rice-paper cutouts, gifts from a friend, decorate the walls. And of course, there are the books and records.

Joan has no intention of slowing down. "I have to keep going—there's a lot left to do," she said. "There's so much—the homeless, the hungry . . . civil and social rights." She said, "We are not facing the needs of the poor, the homeless, the children . . . These are the problems we need to face as a country, a state, and as a county right down here in the local level." "I hate this flag-waving, this superficial patriotism," she said quietly. "It's just blinders to cover the real problems."

Joan has multiple sclerosis. The symptoms became noticeable during her freshman year in college, approximately 20 years ago. In addition to other physical traumas, the multiple sclerosis has weakened her legs so that she has used a wheelchair full time for the past 13 years. Joan said she has learned from her disability. "My aims and goals in life changed a great deal because of my illness. Things that were so important weren't important after all. You learn to smell the flowers, look at the trees. I'm really pretty normal—that's all part of our advocacy, to get people to see that persons with disabilities are just like anyone else."

About Multiple Sclerosis

Multiple sclerosis is a progressive disease affecting the central nervous system, which includes the brain and spinal column. "Multiple" means many or varying and "sclerosis" means scarring or hardening (Cornwall & Winn-Orr, 1991). There is no known cause of the disease. Multiple sclerosis typically affects men and women who are 15-50 years old; however, the average age of onset is 29-30 years (Sibley, 1990). Multiple sclerosis affects more women than men and Caucasians more than other ethnic groups (Smith, 1988).

Multiple sclerosis involves spontaneously appearing lesions at the nerve endings of the central nervous system and the disappearance of the protective nerve coverings. As the lesions heal, the sclerosis (scarring) occurs. The scars prevent neurological impulses from traveling to and from the brain. The result of these damaged transmissions include numbness and tingling of hands or feet, weakness of lower extremities, loss of voluntary movements of muscles, loss of vision in one or both eyes, and facial numbness (Sibley, 1990). Over half of all individuals with multiple sclerosis will also develop cognitive problems and affective disorders which result in personality changes, memory loss, and decreased planning and organizational abilities (Sanford & Petajan, 1990). The location and severity of the sclerosis will determine the degree of disability.

For most individuals, multiple sclerosis follows a course of **exacerbations** and **remissions** (Brooks & Matson, 1987). A new outbreak of lesions is called exacerbation and is characterized by increasing severity of the symptoms listed above. When lesions heal, relief of some symptoms may result. These episodes are known as periods of remission. At times, exacerbation is characterized by decreased motor ability and remissions by increased motor proficiency. Periods of exacerbations and remissions are unpredictable and depression is a common emotional response by individuals with this disease (Sanford & Petajan, 1990). As the disease progresses, the individual may need to rely upon a cane or wheelchair for mobility and may need increasing assistance. Currently, there is no known cure for multiple sclerosis (McQuillen, 1990).

Considerations for Inclusion

Since the skills of people with multiple sclerosis vary from time to time because of exacerbations and remissions, leisure services providers who are prepared to deal with fluctuations in performance may enhance the success of their programs. Some people may require the use of a wheelchair during times of exacerbations and then later be able to walk with assistance during a period of remission. The fluctuation in performance may be interpreted by some participants as a lack of effort or commitment to an activity. Being aware of this variation in abilities can allow the recreation professional to make accommodations for the person and facilitate positive interactions between participants. Finally, the fluctuation and reduction in participation skills, as well as the cognitive and affective changes, can be frustrating for a person having multiple sclerosis. The provision of support for this person and demonstration of sensitivity to the experience can help leisure services providers increase the likelihood that participation will be viewed as a positive experience by all participants.

Meet Chuck, Who Enjoys Lifting Weights

Fabbri (1991) reported that as a youth playing tackle football games between neighborhoods, Chuck awkwardly pursued running backs and took on blockers. He wore a pair of steel leg braces at his defensive line position. "The offensive linemen looked at me kind of funny and played me namby-pamby. But after the first couple of plays, they realized I could play and started taking clean shots at me." Chuck progressed from neighborhood noseguard to world champion weightlifter. He won the gold medal at the 1988 Paralympics in Seoul, Korea, and has won four world titles.

"I wanted to be a wrestler. When I was a sophomore in high school, I asked the wrestling coach if I could try out for the team. He told me that I couldn't come out because of the handicap, but he asked me if I wanted to be the damn equipment manager. I was disappointed big time," Chuck said. Another coach suggested he try the weight room instead. In six months, Chuck was bench-pressing 260 pounds. That year, he finished second in the national championships and two years later he was the national champion. His national bench-pressing record in the 165-pound division was 485 pounds and his world record was 462 pounds. Chuck fits his training schedule around a full-time job as a stockroom manager.

Chuck's participation and excellence in athletics may be viewed as unique by some people because he is paralyzed from the waist down by spina bifida. He can walk with the aid of braces and crutches and has been able to make many adaptations to recreation activities of interest allowing him to continue active participation.

About Spina Bifida

Spina bifida means cleft spine and is a congenital disability of the spinal column that occurs early in prenatal development, as the central nervous system is forming (NICHCY, 1991). The defect, usually located in the lumbar area, occurs when the covering of the spinal cord is displaced and forms a sac-like protrusion. The protrusion then causes improper formation of the vertebrae and results in externally exposing the abnormal protrusion. The effects of this congenital disability range from no noticeable effects to paraplegia.

Spina bifida occulta is a mild type in which "there is an opening in one or more of the vertebra (bones) of the spinal column without apparent damage to the spinal cord" (NICHCY, 1991). As many as 40 percent of Americans may have spina bifida occulta but never know it because they experience no difficulty and no treatment is needed.

Spina bifida meningocele is a more serious type in which the meninges (protective covering around the spinal cord) has pushed out through the opening in the vertebra in a sac called the meningocele (NICHCY, 1991). Although the spinal cord remains intact, surgical closure is required to prevent infection.

In the most severe form of spina bifida, **mylomeningocele,** a portion of the spinal cord itself protrudes through the back, sometimes exposing tissue and nerves (NICHCY, 1991). Seventy to 90 percent of children born with this form also have hydrocephalus, an enlargement of the head because of unabsorbed spinal fluid. A surgical shunting procedure can control hydrocephalus by draining the fluid into portions of the body that can dispose of the fluid. Without this procedure the pressure can cause seizures, blindness, and brain damage.

The effects of myelomeningocele may include muscle weakness or paralysis below the affected area of the spine, accompanied by loss of sensation and loss of bowel and bladder control. Children with this type of spina bifida often need mobility assistance in the form of crutches, braces, or wheelchairs. Furthermore, children with both spina bifida and hydrocephalus may have learning problems (e.g., attention, expressive and receptive language deficits) which can be alleviated with early intervention.

Considerations for Inclusion

People with spina bifida often have reduced sensation in their legs and may not be able to differentiate between temperatures. Care should be taken in activities to prevent burns from hot water or other sources of heat. In addition, with the loss of pain sensation, people with spina bifida may not feel the friction of their braces, resulting in pressure sores (decubitus ulcers). Keeping open lines of communication with individuals who have spina bifida will help alleviate possible problems.

Leisure services providers should speak with participants who have spina bifida to determine their interests and preferences. It is important to avoid being overprotective of participants with spina bifida and to make assumptions about their interests. For example, Zoerink (1988) found that many of the young people with spina bifida in his study preferred active and group-oriented leisure experiences and sports activities. Together the participant and the leisure services provider can explore ways to facilitate optimal participation with attention to safety and health.

Meet Marty, the "Family Man"

Marty is considered by his friends as a "family man." His wife, children and grandchildren are the most important aspects of his life. He takes great pleasure in spending time with them and talking about their accomplishments. In addition to his family, he has two major leisure pursuits.

Since his retirement, Marty volunteers at a local hospital, assisting nurses with office management tasks. Although the nurses appreciate his contributions to office operations and his strong work ethic, they value even more his friendship and sense of humor. They characterize him as a person who is playful and fun to be around while he accomplishes a great deal of work.

Walking is another one of Marty's passions. He rises early in the morning to complete a vigorous 30-minute walk. Marty views walking as an activity he enjoys and something that offers him a sense of accomplishment, including significant health benefits. Since developing osteoarthritis, Marty awakens in the morning stiff and in pain. However, after his morning stroll, the pain subsides and he is able to go about his day with increased range of motion and vigor.

About Arthritis

According to the Arthritis Foundation (1986), arthritis is a disease which occurs among one in seven people (children and adults) and one in every three families. It affects three times as many women as men (Goldenson, 1978). With over 100 different forms, it is the most common crippling disease in the United States (Rice, 1989). While many will not experience serious physical problems, more than 37 million people have arthritis that requires medical treatment (Arthritis Foundation, 1986).

The word "arthritis" is derived from the Greek word "arthros," which means "joint," and the suffix "itis," which is translated to mean "inflammation." Understanding the derivatives of this word help us define **arthritis** as a group of conditions that involve an inflammation of the joints. Most types of arthritis are characterized by inflammation of the joints, tissue, and bones, which results in stiffness, swelling, redness and pain. Two of the more recognized types of arthritis are osteoarthritis and rheumatoid arthritis.

Osteoarthritis is the most common form of arthritis. This form of arthritis affects people's joints and can result in swelling of the hands, feet, knees, and other joints of the body (Gall, 1992). Osteoarthritis is degenerative and, although milder than some other forms of arthritis, still creates stiffness, swelling and pain.

Rheumatoid arthritis is one of the more profound forms of arthritis, typically resulting in severe inflammation that "attacks primarily the joints, but can also affect the skin, blood vessels, muscles, spleen, heart, and even the eyes" (Goldenson, 1978). Individuals may report feeling "sick all over," with fatigue, poor appetite, fevers, weight loss, enlarged lymph glands, and excessive sweating or cold tingling hands and feet. It is a progressive type of arthritis that is characterized by unpredictable fluctuations in the degree of pain and stiffness.

Considerations for Inclusion

Since some people with arthritis may be in considerable pain, maintain open communication with them when participating in activities. Open lines of communication will increase the likelihood they will feel comfortable discussing with you their mobility limitations in certain situations. In addition, it is often useful to consider the existing weather conditions, because weather conditions can affect the extent of stiffness and pain associated with the joints. Typical treatment for many people with arthritis is rest, exercise and the use of nonsteroid anti-inflammatory drugs such as aspirin (Gall, 1992).

The Arthritis Foundation offers extensive written recommendations for activities and exercise programs tailored for people with differing forms and severity of arthritis. A consistent exercise program may help reduce pain and increase flexibility. Aquatic programs such as water walking, swimming, and water exercise are frequently recommended forms of exercise for people with arthritis. When people experience pain during periods of exercise, encourage them to take a brief rest. If affected joints are hot and inflamed, the activity may be too strenuous—recommendations that they discontinue the exercise at that time can be helpful. The goal for an exercise program should be mobility rather than strength. Moving the joints through their full range of motion at least twice daily can be a help in continued free movement.

Smith and Yoshioka (1992) demonstrated the benefits of making adaptations to recreation activities so that individuals with arthritis may continue to participate. Many adaptations require minor adjustments such as adding a Velcro™ strap to a lap pillow to help hold a book (Klein, 1992). Card holders can be improvised as simply as sticking cards upright in Silly Putty™ or Play-Doh,™ or standing them in a shallow box filled with sand (Levin & Enselein, 1990). Leisure services providers will find that buildings meeting the requirements of the ADA in regard to faucet handles, door openers, and ramps enable people with arthritis to move about with dignity and independence.

Meet Stacy and Jimmy, Who Are Quite in Love

Sleek, aerodynamic racing wheelchairs spin around the practice track, pushed by athletes intent on bettering a previous time. As he finishes his last lap, Jimmy rolls to a stop, panting, and gratefully accepts ice water from the coach. "Pretty good time," she says, consulting her stop watch. The coach is Jimmy's wife, Stacy. The two met at a track meet several years ago when Stacy was a student intern. They hit it off immediately. In one year, they were married. "My parents thought I was crazy," she admits. "They had that old-fashioned way of thinking that people in wheelchairs can't do a lot of things. They said 'You love scuba diving, dancing, sports—think of all the things you'll miss!'"

As they got to know Jimmy, Stacy's parents' fears dissolved. And from the many interests the couple shares, it appears that neither of them miss out on anything. "We're both very athletic, and training for wheelchair sports competitions keeps us pretty busy. Often when he's training for a race, I'll ride my bike alongside for exercise," says Stacy. The two introduced each other to new interests that they now share. Due to Stacy's love of scuba diving, Jimmy got his certification and the two go diving in the Florida Keys almost every year. Jimmy sparked Stacy's interest in deer hunting, and now they try to hunt together when time allows. Jimmy hunts from an all-terrain vehicle that he drives to the spot he chooses after he drops Stacy off at her chosen location.

Things weren't always this picture-perfect for Jimmy. "I was 23 when I was paralyzed in a car accident. After that, I went into seclusion for about a year. I didn't want to see my old friends because I didn't want them to feel sorry for me. I had been dating several girls, but I dropped them, too. I had no interest in seeing anyone. I thought, 'What would a girl see in me, in a chair?'" After he finally started getting out of the house and being active, his confidence returned. "You eventually realize you're the same person you were before. And as you meet people and find that they still find you attractive, your self-esteem comes back. You have to keep believing in yourself in order to be a likable person. No one's interested in being with someone who's having a pity party for himself! When I was injured, it was kind of like I ended one life and started another one. Of course, I'd love to walk again. But honestly, if the choice came down to giving up Stacy and wheelchair sports and going back to my life the way it was before, I'd choose to stay in a chair."

About Spinal Cord Injury

The spinal cord is contained within the vertebrae and transports impulses to and from the brain. Impairment of the transporting of impulses occurs as result of the extent and location of an injury to the spinal column. Impairment experienced from a **spinal cord injury** is permanent because the spinal cord is not able to regenerate.

The degree of disability is classified according to the level of the injury to the spinal column, as well as the severity of the injury. Spinal injuries are classified as complete (no sensation or movement) or incomplete (some sensation and/or motor function).

Paraplegia describes injuries to the sacral, lumbar, or thoracic areas. The sacral and lumbar regions of the spine are the areas below the waist; injury to this area may cause some paralysis, which can result in needing leg braces for mobility, and some loss of sensation in the lower extremities. People with injuries in the thoracic area (between the waist and shoulders) can typically live independently in a wheelchair accessible environment.

Injuries to the cervical (C) area or neck are the most serious and result in **quadriplegia,** which causes the greatest amount of disability. At the lowest level (C7), some individuals "can live alone, independently, with proper alterations to their homes" (Maddox, 1988, p. 29). At the highest level (C2-C4) individuals will be able to control some neck muscles. They can typically control their wheelchairs with the assistance of chin controls or sip and puff apparatus. They are able to control their environments or work a computer with a mouthstick, but need human assistance for daily care needs (Maddox, 1988).

Considerations for Inclusion

People with spinal cord injuries are characterized by having reduced mobility and motor strength. Therefore, some recreation activities that have extensive physical demands may need to be adapted. If an adaptation is required, it is valuable to work with the person to determine the most effective adaptation.

Individuals with impaired sensation will need to shift their weight when sitting to avoid developing pressure sores; therefore, inserting breaks into extended activities may be helpful. Many people must attend to bathroom needs on a strict schedule so it is important to have accessible restrooms near areas where programs are provided. Because individuals with spinal cord injuries are unable to regulate their body temperatures below the level of injury, it is necessary for leisure services providers to be sensitive and provide appropriate means for cooling and warming, such as water spray bottles or blankets.

When they are first injured, many people with spinal cord injuries think their lives are over. They think they will never be athletic again; they will never be able to work again; they will never fall in love again. During the rehabilitation process, these myths are stripped away one by one. They discover that there are many recreation activities available to them, that there are many jobs they are qualified for, and they learn that relationships can be as meaningful as they ever were.

An important contribution that leisure services providers can make to the lives of people with spinal cord injuries is to not set limits on them because of their reduced mobility. Whenever people think an individual with a spinal cord injury cannot participate in a given recreation activity, such as mountain climbing or hang gliding, people who happen to have spinal cord injuries prove them wrong and successfully participate in these activities. Recreation professionals are encouraged to make their programs available to all citizens and work with individuals to find ways to foster their ability to experience leisure.

Meet Jim, the Big-League Pitcher

Hersch (1991) wrote about the moment Jim had long strived. At that time, Jim was a 23-year-old left-hander who had started the baseball season by losing four games for the California Angels. His critics complained that he had no control, no off-speed pitch to confuse hitters, and no minor-league seasoning to draw on. The words missing were the ones Jim was most accustomed to hearing, the ones that said he could not succeed because he had no right hand. "It was all about pitching—this guy stinks. I thought, 'There it is. Finally. I've arrived.'"

After untold fastballs in Little League, three successful years at the university, stardom at the Olympics, award-acceptance speeches, and three seasons in the majors, Jim was at last being seen as he had always seen himself—simply put, as a pitcher. He was no longer the feature attraction of a media circus or the living embodiment of a made-for-TV movie; he was one-fifth of the Angel rotation. True, he is visible proof that what appears to some a limitation need not be. But he is equally notable for the commercial ventures he turns down and for the time he takes with the children with physical disabilities who flock to him. Interestingly enough, immediately following his disastrous start, he went on to win 14 games, losing only 4, and becoming one of the best pitchers in the American League.

For Jim, being born without one hand seems about as much of a hinderance as wearing a pair of sneakers would be for a basketball player. Since he was 5, Jim has practiced switching his glove from his left hand to his right arm and back again—a maneuver that is now as fluid and routine as a sleepy-eyed shave. He can do it in that instant before the bat meets the ball. Jim is living his dream, and he appreciates it. He is also living the dream of many others who aspire to overcome their disabilities, and he appreciates that, too. He still answers more than 300 pieces of mail a week, sometimes giving personal responses to writers who need encouragement or reassurance. In each city he goes to, Jim chats easily with youngsters who come to the park just to see him.

Description of Amputations or Congenital Absences

The absence of a portion of a limb is an **orthopedic impairment** that can occur in two possible ways. A person who is born with a portion of one or more of their limbs missing is identified as having a **congenital anomaly** (NICHCY, 1991). If, however, a person is born with all their limbs but experiences a trauma or infection that results in the need to remove a portion of a limb, then the person is identified as having an **amputation.** Sometimes individuals with amputations or people born without a portion of a limb will wear a **prosthesis.** Prostheses are customized to the person and, with growing children, will need to be changed periodically.

Considerations for Inclusion

In the case of amputation, changes in the residual limb may require adjustment of the prosthesis (Rice, 1992). Since prostheses are very expensive, care should be taken not to damage them (i.e., extreme heat or cold, dampness or wetness). Typically, prostheses are removed before entering a swimming pool area and may be covered when participating in recreation activities requiring active physical contact. Individuals with missing lower limbs or an amputation may choose to use a wheelchair for mobility and for sport and recreation participation.

Recreation participation is beneficial to all individuals because of its ability to increase flexibility and agility. Nissen and Newman (1992) reported that the inability to participate in recreational activities was the most restricted aspect of their patients' ability to reintegrate to normal living following amputation. They identified a specific need for mobility skills for walking on uneven ground during such activities as hunting and fishing (Nissen & Newman, 1992). People with amputations and those born without a portion of a limb should be permitted to receive these benefits as well by actively participating in recreation activities of their choosing.

Meet Darren, Who Loves to Travel

According to Gething (1992), Darren stated that "I use an electric wheelchair and my father looks after most of my daily physical needs. Movement is fairly restricted and I must rely on others to hand me things. This does not stop me going out or doing many things. It does mean, however, that activities must be planned in advance. I have gone out with a number of girls, but I have not had a long-term relationship. Nonetheless, I have lots of friends, I have traveled overseas a number of times, I frequently go out socially and I work part time. I really believe that you must live your life, do your best and experience as much as you can."

Darren, who has childhood muscular dystrophy, attributes much of his success to his parents' support. His motorized wheelchair allows him to be active within his community and facilitates his involvement in travel and tourism.

About Muscular Dystrophy

Muscular dystrophy is a general designation for a group of chronic, hereditary diseases characterized by the progressive degeneration and weakness of voluntary muscles (Goldenson, 1978). It is not typically painful. Three common forms of muscular dystrophy are classified by age of onset and affected muscle groups.

Childhood muscular dystrophy (Duchenne) is the most common type of muscular dystrophy, displays the most rapid progression, and has a poor prognosis. It occurs only in males (Goldenson, 1978). Typically, onset occurs prior to six years of age, with the pelvic musculature affected first (Hyser & Mendell, 1988), resulting in some loss of independence by age 10. The condition involves general weakening and loss of voluntary muscle control.

Limb girdle muscular dystrophy involves paralysis of the shoulder and pelvic musculature, typically occurring in early adulthood. With this form of muscular dystrophy, disability may be slight, and individuals may live to advanced age (Goldenson, 1978).

Another form of muscular dystrophy, **facio-scapulohumeral muscular dystrophy,** occurs during puberty and results in facial paralysis spreading to shoulders and upper arms. The course of this type is typically slow, with mild to moderate reduction in movement (Goldenson, 1978).

Considerations for Inclusion

Since common characteristics of muscular dystrophy include slowness and fatigue (Gething, 1992), leisure services professionals may consider making adaptations to activities requiring physical participation, and incorporate rest periods into prolonged activity. Because muscular dystrophy is progressive and not static in nature, it is helpful to observe participants frequently and make adaptations as skills deteriorate.

It can be useful to provide social support to help people with muscular dystrophy adjust to reduced skill levels. Attempts to make accommodations that permit continued participation with peers is critical to avoid the possibility of social isolation developed in response to recent reductions in physical skills. Development of skills associated with recreation activities which require limited vigorous physical exertion may provide additional avenues for individuals to experience leisure.

Meet Roberta, Who Enjoys Her New Image

Roberta was an active girl who was involved in many activities, including her high school cheerleading team. At the age of 16, the car Roberta was driving was hit by an intoxicated driver and she sustained a spinal cord injury that resulted in paraplegia. After months of intensive rehabilitation, she could walk again with the aid of crutches and long-leg braces. Roberta soon discovered however, that walking took considerable time and effort, and despite her early insistence about walking, she began to use a wheelchair for mobility.

Roberta's insurance company covered the cost of her wheelchair: a 40-pound, stainless steel chair with padded armrests. In 1974, this chair was state-of-the-art. By 1991, Roberta's wheelchair was badly worn: the armrests were torn and the broken vinyl covering scratched her arms. One footrest now dragged on the ground, impeding her mobility. Although Roberta had a good job at a hospital, she could not afford a new wheelchair. She was embarrassed to go out socially in her worn-out chair, which hindered her leisure lifestyle. Her only outlet now was a new performing arts group that included people with disabilities. This was her opportunity to be able to dance and act in a supportive environment. Dancing and acting were activities she had wanted to participate in since her accident, but had found acceptance in other groups difficult.

Through Roberta's participation in the performing arts group, she learned about a small grant that would buy her a new wheelchair. Roberta applied, and six months later she finally got a new wheelchair. She was ecstatic! She picked a bright red chair built for speed and agility. The new wheelchair only weighed 18 pounds, allowing her to transfer it into the car with much less effort than her old chair. Roberta loved her new-found freedom. She took up tennis, and even went out socially with her friends from work. She claimed, "Not only am I able to participate in recreational activities that were almost impossible with my old chair, I feel like I look better. I used to be embarrassed to leave my house, now I feel like a new person. This is better than a new car."

About Wheelchair Technology

The modern wheelchair has changed considerably from the "wicker chair on wheels" used earlier in this century. Wheelchairs today can be customized to meet individual needs and lifestyles. In addition, wheelchairs can be equipped with seating systems to accommodate individuals with specific positioning needs. Some wheelchairs are designed to be used for specific sports, such as those built for road racing, tennis or fishing.

Lightweight wheelchairs are most frequently used by individuals with paraplegia and lower-extremity amputations and disabilities. With aluminum, titanium, or composite frames, lightweight chairs are available with rigid frames and pop-off wheels (average weight 20 pounds), or folding frames with fixed wheels (average weight 26 pounds). Other optional features include swing-away or removable armrests; flip-up, swing-away, or rigid footrests; anti-tip casters; push handles, and mag wheels. The presence or absence of these features helps individuals tailor the chair to their work and leisure lifestyle. The lightweight wheelchairs are reviewed annually in *Sports 'N Spokes* using the American National Standards Institute's standards (Axelson, 1994).

Highly specialized sports chairs for use by athletes, both amateur and professional, came into popular use in the 1980s. Many racing wheelchairs feature aerodynamic, tri-wheel designs for greater stability, cornering, and speed. Court chairs are used for sports such as tennis and basketball, and some feature one central front caster to facilitate sharp turns and forward stability. In addition, one particular chair designed for fishing is suspensioned and has a quick dry, polypropylene seat.

The American National Standards Institute (ANSI) and the Rehabilitation Engineers Society of North American (RESNA), an interdisciplinary organization that promotes assistive technology for people with disabilities, have developed standards for wheelchairs (Axelson, 1993). The standards address seating (e.g., dimensions, upholstery, and optional cushions); structure (e.g., weight and frame material, casters); performance (e.g., minimum turn around width, camber); and safety (e.g., flammability, tip angles). According to Axelson (1993), these standards are voluntary and "designed to help consumers make more educated selections and purchases" (p. 34). The U.S. Department of Veterans Affairs partially funded the development of these standards and is the single largest purchaser of wheelchairs in the U.S. For additional information on assistive technology, refer to Chapter 17.

About Using a Wheelchair

Many people choose to use a wheelchair for a variety of reasons. Some people can walk with aids and use a wheelchair because they can conserve energy and move about quickly. However, other people require the use of the wheelchair to move about freely. Consider Jynny, who stated, "I feel distinctly affectionate toward my wheelchair. I did a lot of falling down and hurting myself and wasting a lot of energy using canes and crutches. When I see a visual image of myself in my wheelchair, I see a handsome, accomplished woman instead of the 'fearful-of-falling-down' woman I was when I was struggling to remain standing. Would I be happier if I could suddenly walk and not need the chair anymore? Only if I could keep the attitude toward it that I have gained up until this time as a result of being a wheelchair user. Only if I didn't lose the spiritual growth I have experienced working as a person with a disability. Without this continued growth I could not be happy."

One concern common among individuals with obvious disabilities is the fear of being viewed as "an easy target" by individuals looking for someone to victimize. Retzinger (1990) quoted Larry, who realizes that defending oneself on the street is more necessary today than ever before. "You hear about muggings every day. People with visual impairments knocked down and robbed while they lie helpless on the ground. Purses snatched from people in wheelchairs as they go about their daily errands. Many people using wheelchairs would go out more if they had some form of self-defense knowledge. To go out by yourself, you must develop confidence that, if confronted with a situation, you can defend yourself. I've always had a strong desire to help other people who use wheelchairs feel that they're not vulnerable or easy targets for muggers. Through wheelchair karate, this has become a reality."

Jerry, a fourth-degree black belt in karate who runs a karate school, suggested to Larry that a wheelchair did not have to prevent him from protecting himself. Together the two developed a wheelchair karate system. After extensive discussion and training, the two discovered that some techniques would work on the street and others would be important in developing speed and accuracy. Wheelchair karate techniques use various movements involving wheelchair maneuvers, enabling people to defend themselves against possible assailants.

Considerations for Inclusion

Speak directly to the person in the wheelchair and not to someone nearby as if the person in the wheelchair did not exist. If the conversation lasts more than a few minutes, consider sitting down, squatting, or kneeling to get on the same level as the person. It is fine to use expressions like "running along" when speaking. It is likely that the person expresses things the same way. Avoid discouraging children from asking questions about the wheelchair, because communication helps overcome negative attitudes. It may help to describe physical obstacles that could impede travel when giving directions to an individual who uses a wheelchair.

Avoid classifying people who use wheelchairs as sick because, as stated earlier, wheelchairs are used for a variety of reasons. Do not assume that using a wheelchair is a tragedy; it is a means of freedom that allows independent movement. Therefore, it is important to remember that when a person "transfers" out of the wheelchair to a chair, car, swimming pool, or bed, do not move their wheelchair out of reaching distance.

Children can begin to use a wheelchair for independence as early as 3 or 4 years of age. One wheelchair manufacturer even has a club for children, featuring T-shirts, a newsletter, and summer camping opportunities. Children's wheelchairs come in child-pleasing colors ranging from cotton-candy pink to neon green, and in manual as well as power (see the chapter on technology for information on power chairs).

Conclusion

The following passage is adapted from the verse entitled "Other People" by an anonymous author.

> I don't think anybody's ugly. I think that something ugly always has something beautiful in it. I don't judge a person of ugliness and prettiness in their faces, in their figure. I don't judge a person like that. I judge a person by talent, by their personality, how they think about other people. A beautiful person smiles.
>
> I appreciate people that try to help me. But sometimes they want to help too much. Mostly, I can do everything for myself. Going downstairs, for instance. Some people try to carry me all the way. But I can do that mostly by myself unless it's too high. People that know me and are around me often, they know what I can do and can't do for myself. But people that I'm just getting to know, they want to treat me different so I try to tell them. I try to explain what they could do for me, what I appreciate. For example, if I'm getting to know somebody and the ice cream truck comes, they go "I'll buy it for you." I try to explain, "That's okay, I could do that."
>
> The way I was raised was to do things for myself. My mother is a very strict woman. I got polio when I was four-and-a-half. She always taught me to do all I could for myself and not to depend on

everyone else. It makes me feel useless when people think I can't do nothing myself. I don't like them to treat me nice, or any special way. I like them to treat me like any other kid running around—just like a regular kid."

Discussion Questions

1. What is spina bifida?

2. Describe the three types of spina bifida.

3. Which of the disabilities discussed in this chapter are caused by a disease process?

4. Which disabilities discussed in this chapter are congenital?

5. List and describe five physical changes that can result from a spinal cord injury?

6. Why is the level of a spinal cord injury significant?

7. What is hydrocephalus?

8. Describe the three types of muscular dystrophy discussed in this chapter.

9. Describe osteoarthritis and rheumatoid arthritis. Which is the most common?

10. What are two reasons individuals who can ambulate might choose to use a wheelchair.

Kate Gainer

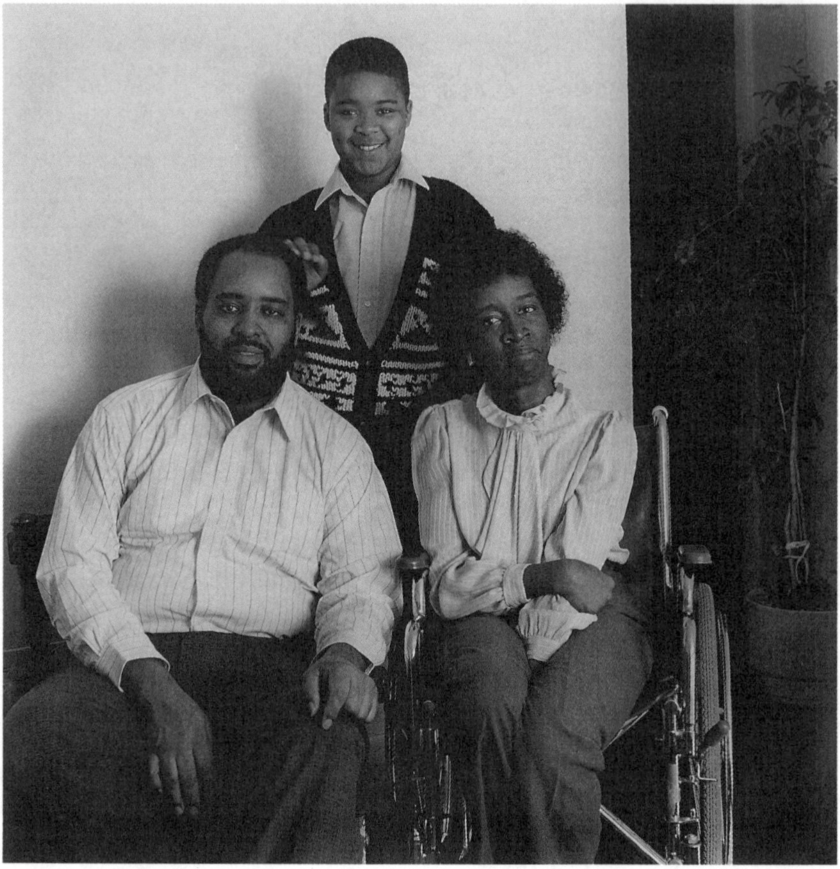

Photograph courtesy of Lynda Greer

Kate Gainer, pictured with her husband, Willie Smith, and their son, Michael, was born with cerebral palsy. Kate is an active advocate for people with disabilities, serving as a volunteer member of various commissions and advocate organizations. She also works for the Atlanta Center for Independent Living.

Kate's Story

I guess I was one of the pioneer children in special education in Atlanta. In 1953, when I was four, the first special education class for black children opened up. It was funded by Easter Seals and 16 of us were selected by doctors at a clinic in Atlanta. When my mother learned of the program she pushed hard to see that I got in; she wanted her baby to go to school. When I went to the elementary program, the teacher from pre-school went with us. Mrs. Muscia White was the only black teacher in the city with a background in special ed. More important than her background, though, was her belief that her "babies" deserved the best. She exposed us to a lot of things other kids didn't get . . . all kinds of field trips . . . to a farm . . . the symphony. After all this time she still keeps up with her "babies." This was a very important time in my life; it was during this period that Kate was formed.

In the sixth and seventh grades I was mainstreamed on a partial basis. It was great! Those kids treated me like one of the gang. These same kids were my classmates at Booker T. Washington H. S., the first black high school built in Atlanta. So I had a support system already. The only real problems I had were architectural barriers.

By the time I got to college those barriers weren't a problem. I wanted to go into marketing. I've always had strong writing skills and wanted to use them in the area of marketing. One of my professors told me that he didn't think I'd make it in marketing because the business world wasn't ready for a severely disabled person who made strange involuntary movements and talked what I call the "C. P. dialect." And he was right. For every interview I had I got a ridiculous reason I couldn't have the job. None of them had anything to do with my professional ability. I was shocked and angry. Up until college I believed that if a person is smart enough and works hard enough, disability doesn't make any difference.

So I decided I was going to save the world . . . at least for kids with disabilities that would come along later. The first thing I did was serve on the accommodations committee for Federal Section 504 funding qualifications. Since then I have served on a lot of committees, councils, etc. to secure a better life for people with disabilities. The most frustrating thing is that it should be so simple. The basic level of accessibility to life . . . jobs, transportation, housing . . . should be there for all of us without such a struggle. But that's not the way it is. And until that's the way it is, Kate Gainer will be out there, WORKING!

Chapter 15

People, Inclusion, and Cognitive Limitations

Peter Thornburgh

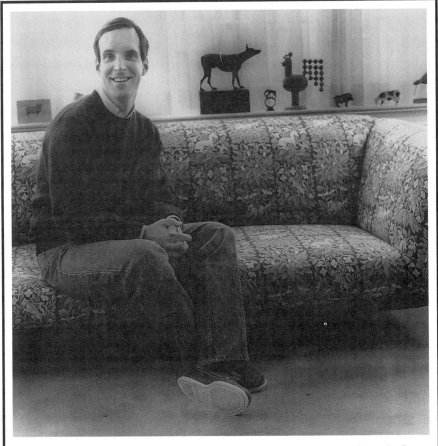

Photograph courtesy of Lynda Greer

Peter Thornburgh lives in Harrisburg, Pennsylvania, and works in nearby Mechanicsburg at the Center for Industrial Training. Peter sustained brain injury when he was in an accident at the age of 4 months. This portrait was made in Washington, DC, at the home of his parents, Dick and Ginny Thornburgh.

Peter's Story

I'm 31 years old. I live in Harrisburg in a house with Brian, Todd and Ron, Michael and Tim. Four people come in to help. They don't live there. They help plan, remind people about things . . . just help out. Everyone who lives in the house works.

I work in Mechanicsburg at C.I.T. (Center for Industrial Training). I like my work . . . I pack boxes, sweep, help people. I have good friends at work. I take four buses to work . . . two over and two back. I like taking buses. I know how to take buses in Pittsburgh, Harrisburg, and Washington. I take Greyhound buses, too. I like to fly.

My church is the Linglestown Church of God. I go every Sunday. The church van picks me up. At church I sit with Carol Grauel. Her husband is Jim. He sings in the choir. They are my church family. I love going to church. I love God. He is in Heaven, so is Jesus. And my first Mom. Mom (Ginny Thornburgh) is my second Mom.

I want to live somewhere else . . . with more room, not so many people. I want more friends my age. I want to do more things . . . shopping at malls and stores, baseball games . . . the Phillies . . . I like the Pirates, too . . . hockey games and the Hershey Bears.

I know how to get up by myself. I know when to pack my lunch. I know how to take a bus. I do a lot for myself. Sometimes I do need staff. Sometimes I don't need staff at all.

Recognizing our common humanity opened all of us to further learning.
—K. E. Eble

Orientation Activity

Directions: Read the following two situations. On a separate sheet of paper write a paragraph describing your reactions to the situations.

1. Bill is a 28-year-old man with Down's Syndrome. He is not feeling well and decides to call his doctor. Dr. Goodman says, "Billy, come into my office. Be a good boy and we will see what's the matter with you." Bill is hurt and angry. He does not like being called Billy or being considered a "good boy." He thinks of himself as a man. He works, lives in an apartment, and has a girlfriend. He doesn't enjoy being treated or talked to like a child. He wishes Dr. Goodman would treat him just like any other patient. Bill cannot understand why he is called "Billy," while every other man is called "Mr." in the doctor's office.
2. Sandra enjoys bowling and went one night after work with a few women from her office. Afterwards, a bowler told Sandra that she would be better off joining the bowling league sponsored by the local Association for Persons with Mental Illness, because all her "friends" would be there. Sandra was very hurt. She just wanted to bowl and meet new people. The bowler's remark made her feel different—like she didn't belong.

Debriefing

For years both professionals and the general public believed that people who experienced some disruption in their cognitive process, including mental retardation, cerebral palsy, epilepsy, traumatic brain injury, mental health problems and similar conditions, should be "with their own kind." This belief created many of the problems we are now trying to remedy: institutionalization, segregated education, and lack of communication with those who have cognitive impairments. As leisure service providers, we must include people in programs even though they may not think, learn, act, or respond to situations in typical ways. We must begin by getting to know people with cognitive impairments, learn a little about their conditions, and be prepared to include them in our programs. As you reflect on the learning activity consider the following questions:

1. How should you talk to recreation participants who have cognitive impairments?
2. Why is it important to treat all recreation participants in a similar manner?
3. How can you facilitate inclusion of individuals with cognitive impairments into recreation programs?

Introduction

The brain is the master organ of the body. It controls autonomic functions such as heart rate, body temperature, respiration and other vital functions. These functions are automatic and do not require any conscious thought. The brain also controls voluntary functions, those actions that require us to think before acting, such as speaking, walking, and reaching (Girdano, Everly, & Dusek, 1990). Damage to the brain can affect either or both autonomic and voluntary functions, depending on the location and severity of the injury.

Damage to the brain can occur at any point in the life span: prenatally, during childhood and adolescence, or at any time during adulthood. Howell (1978) reported that damage can be caused by toxic agents (alcohol, carbon monoxide, lead), brain tumors, infection (AIDS, encephalitis, meningitis, rubella), disease processes (hypertension, sickle-cell anemia, Tay Sachs disease), and trauma (brain surgery, concussion, skull fracture). This chapter will describe impairments caused by damage to the brain throughout the life span.

Meet Nancy, Who is a Strong Advocate

When Nancy received her high school equivalency diploma, it was like getting a key and an eraser. The diploma was a key to further education and a career in a helping profession and it helped erase the label that has dogged her for most of her 34 years: "retarded." As a child, she was diagnosed as mentally retarded: that colored the image her teachers, classmates, and even her parents had of her. Teachers' low expectations for her became evident to her when in high school she was still reading from the same textbook she had in fifth grade.

Working in a series of nursing homes, Nancy realized that older adults were also victims of labeling and she decided to pursue a career in geriatrics. She entered an Adult Basic Education program, and passed the battery of tests for her General Educational Development (GED) diploma. "I loved it," she said, adding that having the GED helped dispel negative stereotypes that have stood in her way. "I feel I was definitely improperly labeled. I know I'm slow, but I don't feel I am retarded."

Nancy plans to pursue an education in human services and obtain a job helping others overcome their labels. As a vocal advocate for people with disabilities, she has had practice doing that. Nancy is a leader of a chapter of People First, an organization promoting the rights of people with disabilities. "We want people to see us as people first and not our disability, she said. "Label jars, not people" is the message on her People First T-shirt. Nancy has testified before her state legislature on bills related to people with disabilities, and traveled to various states to help organize People First chapters. Through People First, she has worked to eliminate outdated language in state laws which refer to "idiots," "morons" and "imbeciles"—labels which she considers archaic and harmful. The lobbying has been an educational experience for both speakers and listeners, she said. "It shows that people with a disability can speak for themselves, and it also teaches us that we can do it."

About Mental Retardation

Mental retardation is associated with more than 200 known medical entities, including genetic defects, chromosomal disorders, infections during pregnancy, accidental poisonings and injuries, metabolic disorders, and central nervous system infections (Gottlieb, 1987). However, Carter, Van Andel, and Robb (1985) identified research indicating that the present known number of causes, nearly 300, represents only one-third of those possible. According to the authors, there is rarely one cause or simple explanation of mental retardation.

Schalock and colleagues (1994) observed that since 1983, when the last terminology classification manual was produced by Grossman (1983), there has been a change in the conception of mental retardation not as an absolute trait expressed solely by the person, but as an expression of the impact of the interaction between the person and the environment. The change in the way mental retardation is conceptualized stipulates that services are provided in typical integrated environments that contain necessary supports based on the capabilities of the person with the purpose of empowering the individual to function within our society (Smull & Donnehey, 1993).

The American Association on Mental Retardation (AAMR) (1992) reported that the current conception of mental retardation focuses attention on the capabilities of the person related to limited intelligence and adaptive skills, the environment in which people with mental retardation live, and the presence or absence of the supports needed for them to live a meaningful life.

According to the American Association on Mental Retardation (AAMR) (1992), "mental retardation":

(a) is characterized by significantly subaverage general intellectual functioning;

(b) results in, or is associated with, concurrent impairments in at least two adaptive skill areas; and
(c) is manifested before the age of 18 (during the developmental period).

A description of each of the three components of the definition is provided below.

Significant subaverage intellectual functioning. Identification of significantly subaverage intellectual functioning occurs when a person receives a score on standardized measures of intelligence quotient (IQ) that is below the score of the average person taking the test to such a degree (two standard deviations) that society has determined this person requires assistance in development beyond what is typically provided by the family and community. The average intelligence quotient has been determined to be a score of approximately 100. A score below approximately 70-75 results in a significantly subaverage intellectual functioning. Although IQ and intelligence are frequently used interchangeably, it is important to remember that these concepts are not synonymous. The IQ score is only an estimate of an individual's rate of intellectual development as compared with the average rate for same-age peers (Gottlieb, 1987).

A person's lack of performance on a particular standardized measure of IQ can be the result of many factors other than actual intelligence. Some people may not have been exposed to the items presented on the test due to cultural and environmental differences, or perhaps people may have difficulty communicating their response due to physical or neurological impairments. Other individuals may be experiencing pain and sickness, and the attitudes of the examiner and examinee can also influence test scores (Zigler & Butterfield, 1968). These situations may reduce the performance of a person on an intelligence test, and perhaps bring into question the reported scores.

Adaptive skills. "Adaptive skills" are a collection of competencies which allows for individuals' strengths, as well as limitations, to be defined. The specific adaptive skill areas identified by the AAMR (1992) include:

(a) communication;
(b) self-care;
(c) home living;
(d) social;
(e) community use;
(f) self-direction;

(g) health and safety;
(h) functional academics;
(i) leisure; and
(j) work.

To be prepared to meet the demands of the specific adaptive skill area identified as leisure, it is helpful to understand all the adaptive skills areas, because they are interrelated. However, for the purposes of this book, the adaptive skill area of **leisure** will be highlighted. The AAMR (1992) described the adaptive skill area leisure as:

> the development of a variety of leisure and recreational interests (i.e., self-entertainment and interactional) that reflect personal preferences and choices and, if the activity will be conducted in public, age and cultural norms. Skills include choosing and self-initiating interests, using and enjoying home and community leisure and recreational activities alone and with others, playing socially with others, taking turns, terminating or refusing leisure or recreational activities, extending one's duration of participation, and expanding one's repertoire of interests, awareness, and skills. Related skills include behaving appropriately in the leisure and recreation setting, communicating choices and needs, participating in social interaction, applying functional academics, and exhibiting mobility skills (p. 41).

Developmental period. According to AAMR (1992, p. 9), mental retardation begins in childhood when "limitations in intelligence coexist with related limitations in adaptive skills. In this sense, it is a more specific term than developmental disability because the level of functioning is necessarily related to an "intellectual limitation."

The "developmental period" refers to the time after conception when growth and change occur at a rapid rate. This rate of development typically begins to slow as the person enters adulthood (identified as age 18, 21, or 22). Mental retardation is one particular type of developmental disability. A developmental disability, as reported in Public Law 95-602 enacted in 1978, refers to a severe, chronic disability that:

(a) is attributable to a mental and/or physical impairment;
(b) is manifested before age 22;
(c) is likely to continue indefinitely; and
(d) results in substantial functional limitations (Grossman, 1983).

Although the age of 22 has been identified as the age for which eligibility of services under The Developmental Disabilities Act is discontinued, the oldest a person can be to receive a diagnosis of mental retardation is 18 years (AAMR, 1992).

AAMR's (1992) definition of **mental retardation** contains the following underlying assumptions:

(a) mental retardation is not a general phenomenon;
(b) intelligence, as defined by tests, has limited use;
(c) no behavior clearly defines potential;
(d) adaptive behavior can be assumed;
(e) development is lifelong;
(f) educate people and avoid testing them; and
(g) mental retardation is most meaningfully conceptualized as a phenomenon existing within the society which can only be observed through the depressed performance of some of the individuals in that society.

Therefore, although the phrase "mental retardation" is used throughout this section, the label alone means very little. The unique profile of cognitive, adaptive, educational, and recreational ability, as well as the health status associated with each person, is critical for appropriate planning and implementation of effective services (Woodrich & Joy, 1986).

More important than the definition is the classification of mental retardation established by AAMR (1992). That is to say that mental retardation refers to a level of functioning which requires from society significantly above-average training procedures. Therefore, the person with mental retardation is classified by the extent of support required for the person to learn, and not by limitations to what the person can learn. The height of a person's level of functioning is determined by the availability of training technology and the amount of resources society is willing to allocate, and not by significant limitations in biological potential.

The intensity levels of support have been defined and described by the AAMR (1992) as:

(a) intermittent supports that are provided as needed;
(b) limited supports that are limited in time, but consistent across time rather than intermittent;
(c) extensive supports that are not limited in time and are provided on a regular basis in some environments such as the home; and
(d) pervasive supports that are constant, intense, and have the potential to sustain life.

According to AAMR (1992, p. 34):

> The concept of needed supports reflects the contemporary perspective regarding the expectation for growth and potential of people; focus on personal choice, opportunity and autonomy; and the need for people to be both in and of the community. This step applies the zero reject model in which all persons are given the supports necessary to enhance their independence/interdependence, productivity, and community integration.

This classification system represents a shift toward understanding mental retardation as a multidimensional concept that requires comprehensive assessment, rather than reliance on intelligence tests as the primary indicator of mental retardation. In addition, the classification system removes the previous IQ-based levels of mild, moderate, severe, and profound mental retardation.

Considerations for Inclusion

When relating to people who have been grouped together, for whatever reason, it is important to consider these individuals as people first and then, if relevant, consider their group affiliation. It is much easier to interact with a person if we initially concentrate on the similarities we share with this person as opposed to our differences. Therefore, as much as possible, attempt to avoid the tendency to make generalizations about people who, in addition to many of the other characteristics that effect their humanness (e.g., sense of humor, reliability, honesty), happen to be identified as having mental retardation.

When recreation professionals are working with persons with mental retardation, they may examine the results of individuals' scores on standardized measure of IQ and adaptive behavior scales and determine that the person with mental retardation has significant problems as well as limited potential for growth and development. If this conclusion has been drawn, with the focus of the problem on the individual with mental retardation, the specialist's work has ended. However, if practitioners view people with mental retardation, no matter how severe the disability, as having the potential for growth and development, then professionals have before them a lifetime of challenges as they continuously attempt to determine the most effective and efficient procedures to assist these individuals in achieving their maximum potential.

Frequently, practitioners mistakenly treat a person with mental retardation as a child. A problem occurs when an adult who happens to have mental retardation is compared to a child because he or she performs some skills (e.g., reading) at a level similar to some children. Because the adult with mental retardation has many more years of experience at living and has developed a variety of skills, the comparison to a child is misleading. Recreation professionals must avoid viewing adults with mental retardation as children and instead give them the respect provided to other adults in our society. This view of people with mental retardation will encourage professionals to develop recreation programs that are appropriate for the age of the participants and do not require persons with mental retardation to compromise their dignity.

Meet Amanda, Who Enjoys Music

Amanda is a 15-year-old high-school student. Amanda does well in quiet areas with small numbers of students present, but has difficulty in public areas of the school, such as hallways or the cafeteria, because she does not like loud noises or anyone touching her. When not at school, she can usually be found in her bedroom. Amanda enjoys listening to music and, although she has many cassette tapes, Amanda listens to two songs, which she plays repeatedly. She has a book collection which is displayed in precise order. Amanda is a proficient swimmer; however, when the pool is crowded, she is too distracted to swim. Recently she indicated that she would like to learn to ride a horse.

About Autistic Disorders

An autistic disorder (also known as autism) is a complex developmental disability that is diagnosed through observation of an array of specific communication, social, and behavioral impairments. Some examples of impairments common to individuals with an autistic disorder include:

(a) lack of awareness of others;
(b) lack of social play;
(c) inability to establish friendships with peers;
(d) inability to communicate verbally or nonverbally;
(e) lack of imaginative activity;
(f) inability to initiate or sustain conversation;
(g) body movements that are stereotyped and repetitive; and
(h) the need to follow routines precisely (American Psychological Association [APA], 1994).

Although the etiology (cause) of this disorder is unknown, the behavioral manifestations usually appear during the first three years of life and is more common among males (APA, 1994).

An autistic disorder can occur in conjunction with other disabilities. Mental retardation has been demonstrated to occur in some of the population with an autistic disorder (Siegel, 1991); however, with the advent of computer-assisted assessment, the ability to more accurately assess individuals with an autistic disorder may result in a lower incidence than previously thought. Many individuals with an autistic disorder begin experiencing epileptic seizures before adolescence (Sloman, 1991).

The character Raymond in the movie *Rain Man* is a semibiographical depiction of an individual with an autistic disorder. Raymond was able to perform many self-care skills. He seemed to take pride in his room and the orderliness he maintained. Raymond had difficulty making eye contact, poor social skills, could repeat a joke but did not understand the humor, and became upset when his routines were interrupted. He had unusual body posturing, and when anxious would rock forward and back repeatedly. Raymond also exhibited characteristics of a savant: an extraordinary talent in one precise ability, such as music, art, mathematics, or amassing facts on a particular subject. It is important to note that few people with autistic disorder actually have savant characteristics.

Considerations For Inclusion

Consistency with equipment placement and routine is often helpful to develop a positive and relaxed atmosphere. People with an autistic disorder often use alternative communication techniques, such as electronic communication boards, picture boards, and sign language. Regardless of the method of communication or level of response, leisure services providers should speak to the participant with age-appropriate language about subjects of interest.

Meet Christopher, Who Finds Freedom in the Written Word

Christopher has an acute mind that has found its liberation in writing, according to Sherrid (1988). Christopher was unable to make a meaningful mark on paper until age 11, when the drug Lioresal helped his muscle spasms. He approached words much as another child might approach an overturned truck of candy, says one critic. Just four years later, he published a book of poetry, *Dam-Burst of Dreams,* which won him comparisons with such literary giants as James Joyce and the 17th-century poet John Donne. Christopher taps out letters on a typewriter with the help of a "unicorn" stick strapped to his forehead. His chin is supported by his mother who stands behind her son in his wheelchair for hours at a stretch in a study in their middle-class Dublin home.

His autobiography, *Under the Eye of the Clock,* won Britain's most prestigious literary award early this year and has zoomed to the top of the London best-seller lists. The autobiography chronicles his struggle—ultimately successful—to attend high school. While heaping praise upon his family, teachers, and friends, Christopher writes unflinchingly of society's pity, intolerance and hypocrisy.

Christopher plans to write a novel, but even some of his supporters are skeptical that his personal experience is wide enough to sustain fiction. His mother doesn't entertain any doubts. Nodding to a visiting journalist, she asks: "What do you think he is doing with all the people he meets?" Regardless of what the future brings, his work already may have changed attitudes toward people with disabilities. Says his teacher, Brendan: "Christopher experiences life so intensely, no one who reads his book could pity him."

About Cerebral Palsy

Some individuals who have difficulty with communication have **cerebral palsy.** This condition is characterized by the inability to control muscular and postural movement. It is caused by damage to the motor portions of the brain. The condition is not degenerative (it will not get worse). There are many causes of cerebral palsy, including prenatal infection, anoxia before or during birth, fetal cerebral hemorrhage, and metabolic disturbance.

People with cerebral palsy are classified by the muscular condition and degree of bodily involvement they display. People who have **spasticity** display increased muscle-tone stiffness (hypertonia) and immediate contraction when stretching affected muscles. Another type of cerebral palsy is **athetosis.** People with athetosis have difficulty controlling movement associated with affected muscles, resulting in "worm-like" movements. Individuals with **ataxia** have a more subtle form of cerebral palsy that results in balance problems. **Rigidity** is a term used to describe an individual who is rigid and appears stiff. The neck, back, or limbs may be hyperextended and mental retardation is often present. Individuals who exhibit frequent or constant involuntary shaking of body parts, especially the hands and arms, have a form of cerebral palsy identified as **tremors** (Carter, Brown, LeConey, & Nagle, 1991). Individuals with more than one type are said to have **mixed cerebral palsy**.

Individuals with cerebral palsy are also classified according to the extremities that are affected. If only one limb is affected, individuals are said to have **monoplegia.** If the person's legs are impaired, the person is said to have **paraplegia.** If one side of the person's body is affected, the person is said to have **hemiplegia.** When all four extremities are impaired as a result of cerebral palsy, the person has **quadriplegia.**

Considerations for Inclusion

Work with the individual to determine what accommodations they have already devised. When teaching activities, try to avoid excessively loud sounds and sudden, unexpected motions that may increase uncontrollable movements and trigger the startle reflex. Consider that some individuals may have balance difficulties and be prone to falling. Make necessary adaptations based on some people's limited mobility. Since gross motor coordination can often be a problem, accommodations should be made when introducing physically active activities. Fine-motor activities using hand-eye coordination or delicate finger movements can be very difficult for some people; therefore, efforts to enhance hand-eye coordination are recommended. When encouraging the grasping of an object, you may use sponges for individuals with spastic cerebral palsy and create a firm, hard surface for people with athetosis.

Meet Jennifer, Who Likes to Climb

Jennifer had her first seizure just before her 13th birthday. Because of initial difficulty in regulating her medications, she had memory problems that resulted in poor grades. Fortunately, Jennifer's school was understanding and explored options for assisting her to be a successful student. She graduated from prep school with honor grades and left home to attend college and live in a dorm. In the spring, Jennifer went rock climbing with skilled mountaineers. "I never thought the best solution was to live a limited life. I'd rather do things and take risks than do nothing at all. Going to college far from home wasn't something I felt afraid of. I felt very capable of taking care of myself" (Lovell & Lovell, 1993, p. 6).

Jennifer is careful to explain to those around her that she has epilepsy and forewarn them what to do in case she has a seizure. She states, "What to do and what not to do is something I explain to everyone I know. I try to explain what seizures look like, why I have them, what may set them off, what I'm like afterward. (I usually forget things.) Although I've felt frustrated and occasionally angry, I've never felt embarrassed by it. I have epilepsy, but epilepsy doesn't have me" (Lovell & Lovell, 1993, p. 6).

About Epilepsy

Epilepsy, affecting an estimated two million Americans, is the most common neurological disorder (Kraus & Shank, 1992). It is a condition that occurs when there is a sudden brief change in how the brain works. When brain cells are not working properly, a person's consciousness, movement, or actions may be altered for a short time. Epilepsy is therefore called a seizure disorder.

Not all seizures are classified as epilepsy. For example, many young children have convulsions from fevers. These convulsions are one type of seizure. Other types of seizures not classified as epilepsy include those caused by an imbalance of body fluids or chemicals, or by alcohol or drug withdrawal. A single seizure does not mean a person has epilepsy.

Epilepsy is classified according to three specific features:

(a) generalized or partial seizures;
(b) whether the seizures are the primary or secondary disorder; and
(c) the age of onset of recurrent seizures (Engel, 1989).

According to Engel (1989), seizures that are generalized involve cells from both hemispheres of the brain, whereas when only one hemisphere of the brain is involved, partial seizures result. One type of generalized seizure consists of a convulsion with a complete loss of consciousness, called a **grand mal** seizure. **Petit mal,** also a generalized seizure, is characterized by brief periods of fixation, called "absences," in which the individual appears to be staring into space and does not respond to external stimuli (Broglin et al., 1992). An example of a partial seizure is the **jacksonian,** in which convulsions begin in one part of a limb, such as a foot or hand, and quickly spread throughout that entire side of the body (Loiseau, 1992). Other partial seizures may cause periods of automatic behavior, such as rubbing movements with one hand or wandering, or periods of altered consciousness (Veilleux et al., 1992).

Considerations for Inclusion

Frequent occurrence of seizures by a person with epilepsy is very rare. The majority of individuals with epilepsy are able to manage their seizures with medication; therefore, there is very little adjustment to leisure services delivery. Individuals with petit mal seizures may miss part of a sentence and be unclear on instructions, requiring repetition. The most important consideration for recreation professionals is to be prepared to follow basic first-aid if a person has a grand mal seizure.

Treatment during a seizure is the same regardless of etiology, and should focus on preventing injury. The following is a list of procedures to follow when a person has a seizure:

(a) keep calm (there is nothing you can do to stop a seizure);
(b) do not try to restrain the person;
(c) clear the area so the person doesn't injure self;
(d) do not interfere with movements, unless it is to cradle the head to prevent injury;
(e) do not force anything between teeth or into mouth;
(f) if the person is choking, turn their head to the side;

(g) treat the incident in a calm, matter-of-fact manner, do not crowd around the individual; and
(h) let the person rest after the seizure.

Meet Tara, Who Helps Other People Have Fun

Tara's favorite activity is spending time on cruise ships headed for warm sandy beaches. She loves traveling with friends to remote, isolated islands. Although she enjoys her work as a supervisor of a community recreation and parks department, she is constantly planning, saving for, or going on a cruise.

Tara has always enjoyed traveling. She enjoys meeting new people and seeing new lands. After she received a traumatic brain injury as a result of a car accident when she was in college, she was determined to reacquire skills needed to continue to travel. She used thoughts of beaches and foreign sites to motivate her during rehabilitation. Although she requires adaptations in many activities, she is able to continue to travel. Tara reports that when hospitality staff are open to making accommodations for her, she almost always has a great vacation.

About Traumatic Brain Injury

A **traumatic brain injury** is a physical insult to the brain that may cause problems with physical, emotional, and social functioning. These changes influence not only the present, but the future status of a person. A traumatic brain injury frequently means that the person may never quite be the same again.

According to Vernon-Levett (1991), each year approximately 100,000 to 250,000 people with acute brain injuries are admitted to hospitals in the United States. In all age groups, the most common cause of acute neurologic injury is from a motor-vehicle accident. Males are typically affected twice as often as females. Other common sources of acute neurologic injury include falls and child neglect or abuse. Common cognitive processes influenced by traumatic brain injury are attention, memory, general intellectual performance, language, and perceptual abilities.

Closed head injury is one type of traumatic brain injury that is often caused by the brain being whipped back and forth in a quick motion. This pull-and-tug places extreme stress on the brain stem—the part that connects the larger part of the brain with the spinal cord and the remaining portion of the body. A large number of functions are packed tightly into the brain stem, such as controls of consciousness, breathing, heartbeat, eye movements, pupil reactions, swallowing and facial movements. In addition, all sensations going to the brain, as well as signals from the brain to the muscles, must pass through the brain stem. Anoxia (loss of oxygen to the brain) is another form of closed head injury. Anoxia may occur following cardiac arrest, stroke or accident, such as drowning or choking.

Open head injury is a second type of traumatic brain injury. It is a visible assault that results from an accident, gunshot wound, fall, or other trauma, such as brain surgery to remove a clot or tumor. As with closed head injuries, symptoms can vary greatly and are unique, depending on the extent and location of the brain injury. Physical disabilities, impaired learning ability and personality changes are common. Physical impairments can include disruption in speech, vision, hearing and other sensory impairments, headaches, lack of coordination, spasticity of muscles, paralysis of one or both sides and seizure disorders.

All types of head trauma may damage that part of the brain crucial to memory. Both short-term (recall of recent information) and long-term (recall of past information) memory may be impaired (Misenti, Lucas, & Thompson, 1992). **Amnesia** is a common type of memory loss, where the person can only remember bits and pieces of events that occurred in the past. Amnesia does not affect one's ability to learn new information. Seizures, another typical result of traumatic brain injury, may also affect memory. According to Misenti and colleagues, (1992), "seizures can occur immediately after the injury or may not develop until months or even years later" (p. 5). At times, the memory loss may persist because a tiny seizure, called a partial complex seizure, will originate from the injured area and continue for an indefinite period afterward. This brain damage is often not diagnosed, however, because the identifying seizure is sometimes hard to recognize: there is only a short staring spell or period of unusual behavior, and only a momentary lapse of concentration occurs. If recognized, however, the condition is often readily treatable with prescription drugs.

A person's emotions can also be influenced by a traumatic brain injury. As many as one-fourth of individuals with traumatic brain injury experience severe behavior disorders that disrupt daily life (Uomoto & Brockway, 1992). Disorders may include mood swings, denial, self-centeredness, anxiety, depression, lowered self-esteem, sexual dysfunction, restlessness, lack of motivation, inability to self-monitor, difficulty with emotional control, inability to cope, agitation, excessive laughing or crying and difficulty in making choices. Treatment for these symptoms usually includes behavior management and medication (Uomoto & Brockway, 1992).

Any or all of the symptoms of traumatic brain injury may occur in different degrees, and there may be other symptoms not mentioned. Intellectual ability may cease to improve after a period of time, but memory, social, and behavioral functions may improve over long periods of time. For many people, ongoing involvement in activities can decrease the severity of these symptoms.

Considerations for Inclusion

Individuals who have had a traumatic brain injury often have impaired planning ability and may need individualized reminders for activities of daily living, including leisure choices. Calendars, notes and telephone calls may facilitate increased attendance and participation. Abstractions or generalizations often present difficulty for a person who has experienced a traumatic brain injury. It may help to introduce novel activities by relating them to a familiar activity. It is often helpful to conduct a task analysis by breaking an activity into its components, teaching small steps, and allowing for additional practice time. To gain the person's attention, saying the person's name before giving key directions may be helpful. Consistently model, demonstrate, and provide manual assistance using physical guidance, visual cues, and verbal directions when conducting activities. One- or two-step directions are more appropriate than a series of commands. However, try to avoid using more guidance, direction, or cues than necessary to encourage the person to take more responsibility.

If having a short attention span is a problem, it may help to simplify verbal instructions. Often participants will take cues from how something sounds rather than from what is said. Consistency in voice tone, quality, and communication pattern is helpful. Directions should be brief and simple (to increase the person's attention to the most important parts of the task). Use repetitious, slow, meaningful progression. Implement rules and procedures, especially as related to health and safety, before the activity starts. Learning by example, repetition, reminders, verbal feedback and experience will foster comprehension. Vary activities, introducing new skills early in a session. Alternate active and quiet games to avoid overstimulation and to compensate for short attention spans. You can assist the participants to control high and low energy levels by structuring the pace and tempo of a session. Structure the environment so that all participants may become involved. The circle formation is an excellent leadership tool; clients are then able to take advantage of modeling, imitation, demonstration, and peer interaction.

Individuals who have experienced a traumatic brain injury may have difficulty working toward long-term goals. To maintain continued interest in a program, provide opportunities that include gratifying experiences. Preparation for participation is just as important as the activity itself. Plan activities that encourage social interaction, cooperation, challenge, and success for everyone. Measuring self-improvement in a skill is more meaningful to the person's self-concept than is competition against others, especially with people who are less skilled. Ensure full participation to promote interaction in an increasingly mature manner. Individuals may have a slower learning rate, but can still accomplish a great deal. With improvement, you can replace larger objects with smaller objects, and replace stationary objects, positions, and people with those that move. It is often helpful to keep the objective or reason for doing the activity in mind as modifications are made and maintain the intended purpose of the activity.

Meet Calvin, Who Enjoys Playing Cards

One morning in 1990, Calvin awoke early as usual and swung his legs over the side of the bed. To his surprise, he fell to the floor, unable to speak or move. When his wife, Ruby, awoke, she assumed he had gone for his ritual walk. Not until his grandson came by two hours later did they find Calvin on the floor. The doctor told his family he had experienced a stroke.

After one month in a rehabilitation hospital, Calvin returned home and began a new phase in his life. Many of his favorite pastimes still gave him pleasure: listening to gospel music, enjoying his grandchildren and attending their Little League baseball games. Other activities were no longer pleasurable. He no longer enjoyed church due to the emotional arousal which brought on tears and embarrassment. He also had difficulty talking to acquaintances due to the impaired speech caused by the stroke. One of his greatest pleasures is playing cribbage with his wife and best friend, Charlie. For a long time, Calvin did not think he would ever be able to remember the rules and hold the cards, but with Charlie's patient tutoring and the help of an adaptive card holder, Calvin is now the reigning cribbage champion of the neighborhood.

About Stroke: A Cerebrovascular Accident

A stroke, or **cerebrovascular accident,** is a form of traumatic brain injury which originates inside the brain itself. A stroke occurs when a portion of the brain is deprived of blood. The incidence is higher for men than women, and higher for African-Americans than other racial groups. Individuals 40 and younger account for less than 4 percent of the total stroke population (Adunsky, Hershkowitz, Rabbi, Asher-Sivron, & Ohry, 1992). Long-standing hypertension (high-blood pressure) is a major cause of stroke (Dorsch, 1987).

The most common form of stroke among people who are older is a **cerebral thrombosis,** which occurs when a blood clot **(thrombus)** forms in an artery that supplies blood to the brain (Kart, Metress & Metress, 1988). A **cerebral embolism** is a stroke which occurs when a blood clot travels to the brain from another part of the body, often from the heart. In both of these instances, the brain is deprived of blood due to the clot and damage ensues.

A **cerebral hemorrhage** is a stroke caused by a blood vessel bursting in the brain. Not only is the area beyond the burst deprived of blood, but the blood which spilled out puts pressure on the brain tissue in the area of the rupture. A cerebral hemorrhage is the most serious form of stroke, and frequently causes coma and death. Strokes are the third-leading cause of death among older adults in the United States (Kart et al., 1988).

There may be no warning that a stroke will occur, although some individuals may be forewarned by a series of small strokes known as **transient ischemic attacks** (brief episodes of circulatory deficiency to the cerebrum). These small strokes may cause sudden weakness or numbness on one side of the body in the face, hand, arm or leg; sudden and sharp dizziness; dimness or loss of vision, especially in one eye; or loss of the ability to speak clearly or understand speech (Staff, 1989). The individual may not realize that a stroke has actually occurred. Transient ischemic attacks are a warning sign that a major stroke may occur if medical attention is not sought and occur days, weeks, or months before the major stroke.

The amount of injury caused by a stroke depends on the type and location of the damage. A right-brain stroke affects the left side of the body and may cause **hemiplegia** (paralysis or weakness), memory loss, and impulsive behavior. Individuals who have had a right-brain stroke often experience inappropriate reflex crying, reflex laughter, or reflex anger. These reflexes occur when some emotion is triggered, and the area of the cerebral cortex that controls emotions has been damaged (Judd, 1991). A left-brain stroke causes right-side hemiplegia, memory loss, speech and language problems, and slow, cautious behavior (Kart et al., 1988). It is interesting to note that these patterns may be opposite for those who are left-handed.

The brain damage caused by stroke may suddenly alter every aspect of the person's life. In addition to paralysis, some individuals have a condition known as **hemianopsia.** This condition causes half of the visual field to disappear. The person may eat only the food on one side of the plate and may not be aware of the other food unless the plate is turned. Likewise, the person may only respond to people who approach on one side and seem to ignore those who are standing on the other side. The individual who has hemianopsia should be guided to a position in the room where he or she will be able to see the most (Kart et al., 1988). Care should also be taken not to approach the person from the affected side, since it may startle the person when you suddenly appear in the field of vision.

Aphasia is the term used to indicate difficulties in processing language. **Receptive aphasia** means that the person can no longer understand the messages received as either spoken or written language. **Expressive aphasia** describes the condition in which the person can understand what is said or written but cannot respond to it. Some people may be able to sing or count but not speak, or may be able to say only a few words such as "OK," "Amen," or "bye-bye." Families are often shocked when their relative is only able to say swear words which were never used before the stroke.

Considerations for Inclusion

Social support is very important for those who have sustained a stroke (Friedland & McColl, 1992). To this end, support groups are available throughout the country for individuals who have had strokes, their families, and friends.

It is important to treat the individual in an age-appropriate manner and not to respond as though the person is a child. The individual should be encouraged to speak and to indicate personal preferences. Families and others should be patient and allow the person sufficient time to speak, rather than finishing sentences or thoughts for the person. Likewise, the individual should be given opportunities to do as much independently as possible. Enabling independence will enhance the dignity and help the recovery of the person.

One aspect of maintaining the participant's dignity is how we respond to reflex crying. According to Judd (1991), it is important to "understand that crying doesn't necessarily reflect the person's mood" (p. 7). He suggests asking the participant what they are really feeling in order to respond appropriately. Reflex crying has a tendency to come and go suddenly and may look different than real crying. Judd (1991) advised speaking with people who are reflexively crying when they are not crying to determine how they would like to be treated when an episode occurs. Similar steps should be taken with reflex anger and laughter as well.

Meet Thomas, Who Enjoys the Outdoors

Thomas likes taking long walks in the woods nearby his home. He often brings his binoculars so that he can identify birds and more closely observe other wildlife. Although many of us may enjoy such an activity, for Thomas it brings a sense of pride in himself. It was not long ago when he had difficulty leaving his home because he experienced hallucinations as a result of his schizophrenia.

When his schizophrenia emerged during his early 30s, Thomas withdrew from his friends and family and from activities that brought him joy. He lost his job and finally sought psychiatric assistance. After actively participating in therapy sessions with mental health professionals and following a scheduled plan for taking medication, Thomas has returned to his community. He is now employed with the Postal Service and takes advantage of many recreation programs within his community.

Thomas expresses concern about the prejudice he has experienced as a result of his clinical diagnosis of schizophrenia. He hopes that in the future people will keep an open mind about people and focus on them as an individual rather than a label.

About Problems with Mental Health

Fox (1985) reported that many people believe that individuals receiving a psychiatric diagnosis are dangerous and should be locked up. As a result of certain news reports and horror movies, many people harbor the misconception that people who are receiving psychiatric care are a menace to society. While it is true that a small minority of people with psychiatric diagnoses have a history of violence, the majority of them do not engage in violent behavior. Some experts report that less than one percent of all people discharged from a psychiatric hospital can be considered dangerous, and most of them are a danger to themselves, not to others.

Unfortunately, other people believe that individuals with mental disorders do not really need help. People still have the general belief that others should be able to handle mental health problems by themselves. The view that one should pull oneself up by the bootstraps or talk oneself out of it is closely related to the belief that problems with mental health are shameful. There is a tendency to think that there is something weak or morally wrong with someone seeking help for a mental impairment. According to Michels (1985):

> The irony of this popular view is that growing evidence links cancer, heart disease and other "traditional" health problems to such personal behaviors as cigarette smoking or improper eating habits. In fact, as many as half the deaths from the 10 leading causes of death in our country can be traced to people's lifestyle. It would be fairer to attribute these diseases to "weak characters and poor decisions" than to make the same claim about the most familiar mental disorders, such as schizophrenia or depression which stem from causes that have little to do with voluntary choice.

Some mental disorders are identified as those that are associated with problems with moods, such as depression and mania. **Clinical depression** is different than the temporary experience of "everyday" depression which results from such emotions as sadness, frustration, and discouragement, but tends not to impair significantly a person's ability to function over time. Depression becomes a psychiatric diagnoses based on the frequency of the depressed mood, the intensity of the depressed feelings, and the degree to which it impairs an individual's ability to participate in daily activities.

Clinical depression is characterized by people having diminished interest and pleasure in their life, fatigue and energy loss, and a sense of worthlessness or guilt. It is also a common cause of memory loss. The loss of concentration that accompanies depression makes it difficult for the affected person to acquire new information. The slowed thinking process associated with clinical depression makes the retrieval of information more difficult and sometimes even impossible for certain periods of time. In addition, people experiencing clinical depression may reflect their feeling in changes in their weight (excessive losses or gains in weight) or in their sleeping patterns (insomnia or oversleeping). At times, severe depression can result in thoughts of, or attempts at, suicide.

Manic episodes are another type of mood disorder, and are characterized by extreme elevated, expansive, or irritable mood states (APA, 1994). According to Kinney and Sottile (1991), during a manic episode the person may exhibit several of the following behaviors: inflated self-esteem, decreased sleep need, excessive talkativeness, racing thoughts, distractibility, physical activeness and risk-taking behavior. Individuals who shift between states of depression and mania are often diagnosed as having Bipolar Disorder.

A mental disorder with which many people are familiar is schizophrenia, although in truth it affects less than one percent of the population and does *not* refer to someone who has multiple personalities. **Schizophrenia,** a psychotic disorder, is characterized by an individual who at various times departs from reality. The lack of awareness of reality can be manifested in a variety of ways. Some individuals with schizophrenia experience hallucinations which involve the perception, through any of the senses, of objects or beings which are not actually there, such as hearing voices telling one what to do. Delusions are another symptom of schizophrenia, and involve false beliefs about self, others, or objects which persist despite presentation of facts to the contrary, such as the belief that one's thoughts are not their own, but imposed by some outside force (APA, 1994). Individuals with schizophrenia may have disturbances in speech, motor activity and expression of emotion. One characteristic of schizophrenia that is strongly tied to leisure participation is disturbances associated with volition. That is, people experience difficulty making a choice or decision which often results in the absence of a sense of self-determination.

Another classification of mental disorders are those associated with **anxiety.** These disorders are associated with intense fear or panic of a situation, object or person that is not justified and should not result in fear. Many situations justify fear; however, a person experiencing an anxiety disorder will have continuous intense fears about something for no good reason, such as worrying about the welfare of a loved one. Physical symptoms include shortness of breath, accelerated heart rate, dizziness, abdominal distress, and chills or hot flashes. Anxiety disorder results in a decreased ability to function and relate to other people.

Closely linked to anxiety disorders is a category of mental disturbances identified as **phobias.** Phobias involve continuous fears that are unrealistic and dominate a person's thinking, such as agoraphobia, a fear of going out of one's house, or claustrophobia, a fear of closed spaces. Other phobias include fear of speaking in public, fear of snakes, and fear of seeing blood.

Obsessive-compulsive disorders result in people not being able to think clearly because of recurring thoughts and repetitive behaviors. Obsessions involve a persistent disturbing preoccupation with unreasonable ideas or feelings. Compulsions are irresistible impulses to perform irrational acts. The two conditions are linked in that a person may be obsessed with an idea, such as cleanliness, which may result in a compulsion, such as washing hands hundreds of times in a brief period of time.

Considerations for Inclusion

We view people who have problems related to mental health as different from us, so we are uncomfortable in interacting with them. If we view them as similar to us, we can interact with them more comfortably. With careful planning, activity inclusion can help to enhance self-esteem and provide a sense of well-being for the individual. Mental health disorders are often concealed, and leisure providers are not qualified to make formal diagnoses; however, it is important to establish rapport with all program participants. The following conversation guidelines are effective for all individuals.

To start a conversation, choose a topic you think the person may be interested in, something that has happened to them lately, or a "safe" topic like the weather or sports. If you receive no response, it may be that the person did not hear you or did not understand you. Repeat the question, point to what you are talking about, rephrase the question, make eye contact. If there is still no response, try to put them at ease by telling about something that happened to you or make light conversation. As with anyone who may have difficulty holding a conversation, the person may still very much like to listen to others and be spoken to.

If you can not understand people when they speak, you may ask them to repeat themselves or, if someone is talking about a topic you know nothing about, you may ask to change the subject or just listen politely. Even though you may feel awkward, your listening will be appreciated by the person and you may begin to understand some of their speech. It is acceptable to tell them you do not understand or ask them to repeat something.

If someone responds to you on a totally different topic, be polite and either bring the topic back, or speak to the new topic. You could say, "That's interesting, but let me ask you again about your job." Or you could respond to the new topic.

If someone asks a personal or embarrassing question, honesty is the best way to handle this. A good response is, "That is not something I want to talk about. Let's talk about something else." The person can learn from you that some things are not to be asked. If someone is extending a conversation, honesty is the best policy. "I'm sorry, but I need to move on. Could we talk more another time? Right now I don't have time to listen further." If someone is rudely interrupting your conversation, you can say something like, "I'm talking with Mary now, come talk to me some other time."

Conclusion

People who have disabilities originating in the brain are unique individuals. Some people may have difficulty communicating their needs and preferences. People who meet individuals with cognitive impairments may have incorrect perceptions about their skills and abilities. For those whose brain-related impairment is acquired later in life, there are inevitable changes that people experience as they transition back into their families and communities. With the necessary assistance and support, people with cognitive impairments can live meaningful and often enjoyable lives.

Discussion Questions

1. Which of the disabilities discussed in this chapter may be apparent at birth or within the first year?
2. Which disabilities are likely to appear in the period from childhood to young adulthood?
3. Which of the disabilities in this chapter is most likely to occur later in life?
4. List three behaviors common to traumatic brain injury?
5. What is the difference between intelligence and IQ?
6. List three factors that can affect IQ scores?
7. Describe the difficulties in adjustment that may occur following the acquisition of a brain-related disability during adulthood.
8. What is the best way to assist a person who is having a grand mal epileptic seizure?

9. How would you determine the best way to proceed with a participant who exhibits reflex crying?

10. Name at least six impairments common to persons with autistic disorder.

11. Which of the disabilities discussed in this chapter may result in the person having a normal range of intelligence despite behavioral deficits?

Kathy Sullivan, Jane Mazur, RoseBary Trammell, and Christine Eckman

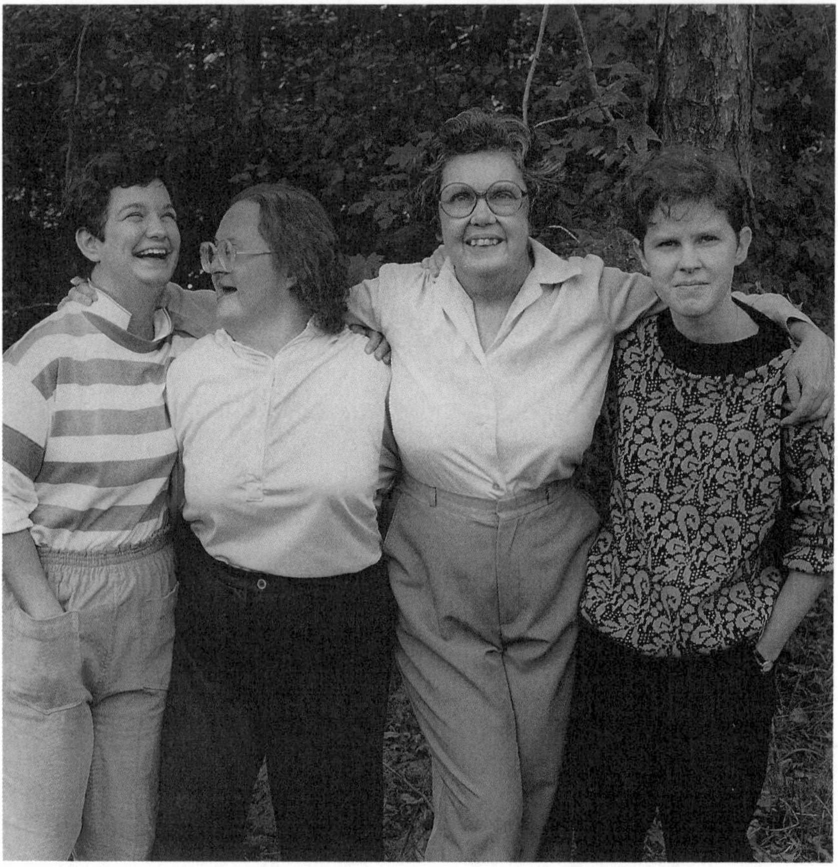

Photograph courtesy of Lynda Greer

Pictured from left to right are Kathy Sullivan, Jane Mazur, RoseBary Trammell and Christine Eckman, who were born with various types of mental retardation. All are employed and live together, with a resident manager, in a house in Roswell, Georgia.

The Stories of Kathy, Jane, RoseBary, and Christine

Kathy

My family . . . mother, stepfather, brother and sister live near in Atlanta and I live at Barrington Landing. I really love the people here. We mostly get along really well. I'm supposed to move my room into the basement soon . . . and I'll have more privacy. I work at the Haynes Bridge Kroger where I make pizzas in the deli and help Chris [Eckman] in the bakery if I can. Right now we need more people to work at Kroger. I like to ride my exercise bike, listen to music . . . mostly rock and roll. At night I do what I need to to get dinner ready and clean up. Then I relax, watch TV.

Jane

My sister and brother live in Atlanta; I see them holidays, weekends, sometimes. The rest of the time I live with my friends. I love my friends here! I work at Herman Miller, where they make furniture. Now I am gluing furniture pieces together and I like that job a lot. When I'm not working, I love to look at TV Guide. And I like listening to music and coloring.

RoseBary

Mom and Dad live on E. Wesley Rd. in Atlanta. My brother lives near Atlanta. Whenever I can, I see my family, but we're very busy at Barrington Landing. It's almost three years since I moved here. I love Jane and Kathy and Chris. And I like this house a lot. I work at RRA [Resources for Retarded Adults], helping with the cleaning. I also go to the training center and do different things. This Christmas we're helping the homeless and the needy, giving food; and I took some pennies to school today. I like to read my encyclopedias, *Reader's Digest,* things like that. I ride my exercise bike sometimes, and when the weather is nice, I like to take walks and talk to the neighbors.

Christine

My parents live in Atlanta and I have a sister in New York. For three years I have lived at Barrington Landing with Sasha, the cat; RoseBary, Jane, Kathy, and now, Tanya [resident manager at the time]. I'm happy here. I work at the Haynes Bridge Kroger. I bake cookies and some bread; I enjoy baking cookies the best. My friend, Kathy, works there, too. We eat lunch together when we can. At night I watch television, listen to music . . . many kinds of music. I like to sing, too. Every night I write in my diary about my day.

Chapter 16

People, Inclusion, and Sensory Limitations

Will and Robby Smith

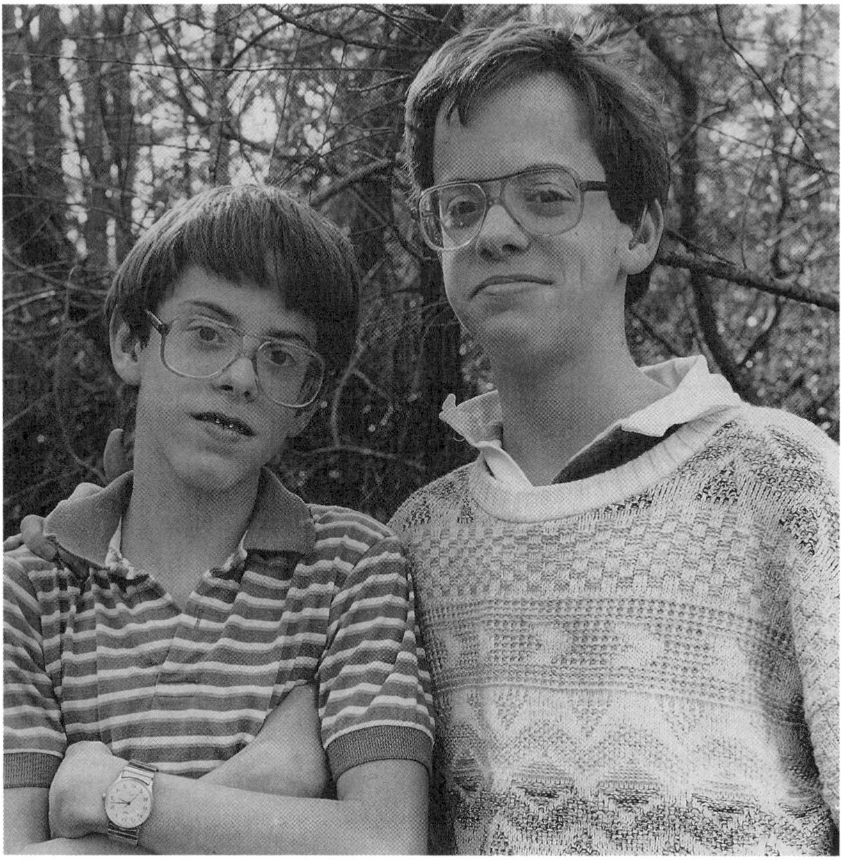

Photograph courtesy of Lynda Greer

Fraternal twins Will (left) and Robby Smith are high school students in Gainesville, Georgia. Born prematurely, they sustained severe hearing losses during neo-natal care.

The Stories of Will and Robby Smith

Will

I was born in Augusta, GA. I have a brother who is named Robby Smith. My father is a doctor and my mother deals with art. When I was three years old, the whole family moved to Gainesville, GA. Now I go to a school called Gainesville Middle School. I have some friends named Chip and Justin, and a bunch of others that I cannot remember their names.

I am an editor and a movie reviewer for the Gainesville Middle School's newspaper, "The Mirror." I hate "The Mirror" but I always wanted to be an editor and a movie reviewer so I got no choice. I always get a feeling like I am a special guest of the newspaper and I try to take a break from it whenever possible.

I have a lot of hobbies. I am not sure exactly how many, but I got comic books, rockets, stamps, books, movie reviews, articles, posters, and role-playing games.

I have told you not all, but some parts of my life.

Robby

Hey! Well, my name is Robby Smith and I have a hearing loss and eyesight problem. I'm heavily addicted to *Cheers, Night Court,* and *L.A. Law.* I love reading books, and usually stake out the local bookstore when I hear that a good book has been published.

I enjoy living life to the fullest and relaxing. I like to go to the beach, the city, and the mountains. As of 1989 I'm going to be a freshman at high school. My favorite movies are the Indiana Jones trilogy, *Who Framed Roger Rabbit?, Midnight Run,* and *Mr. North.*

My hearing/sight losses never bother me, and I really don't make a major deal out of it.

"Detachment will not do . . . . And there ought to be mutual respect, regard for each one's competence and integrity."
—M. Green

Orientation Activity

Directions: Read the following situations. On a separate sheet of paper respond to the task posed at the end of each scenario.

1. Silvia would like to use your cruise line to take a vacation with her husband. She has communicated to you that she has **diabetic retinopathy,** a disorder of the retina due to diabetes. As a member of the recreation department on the ship, identify some adaptations or considerations you may make when attempting to make this vacation one of the best Silvia has ever experienced.
2. Joseph, a teenager, would like to participate in the basketball league offered by the local parks and recreation department. Since Joseph happens to have a **sensorineural hearing loss** caused by a childhood disease, identify some ways you may assist Joseph in having a successful experience with the basketball league.

Debriefing

To permit Silvia to access your cruise line, you could provide her with an orientation to the ship and ask her for suggestions on how you could best serve her. The lighting is often a consideration: natural daylight varies from extremely bright sun that creates glare, to overcast skies that provide insufficient light. These conditions may make it difficult for individuals to see demonstrations, environmental obstructions, or signage. Leisure services providers can assist passengers by checking the signs on the ship for compliance with the Americans with Disabilities Act regarding positioning, color and use of raised letters or Braille. When making visual demonstrations, attempt to use an increased number of verbal instructions and directions. Providing large-print playing cards may assist Silvia if card games are a desired activity. During the evening entertainment, reserve a place at one of the front tables for Silvia and her party so that she can enjoy the show. If Silvia is on a reduced sugar diet, then the leisure services provider will want to have a selection of refreshments that includes sugar-free options.

To promote Joseph's ability to play in the basketball league, you should determine the level of his residual hearing and learn how to maximize his hearing abilities on the basketball court. Many athletes with hearing impairments play successfully by using signs to represent verbal instructions. Work with your local basketball officials to educate them on accommodations required for compliance with the ADA. For example, it may help to have a light flash to signal Joseph each time the whistle is blown. Joseph's teammates will also be an important component in his successful participation. Identify a player to be an informer to ensure Joseph understands verbal discussions that may occur. If desired, this person could go to Joseph each time there was a break in the action and be available to clarify any situation. If Joseph uses sign language, he may choose to teach you and his teammates a couple of signs a day to help with communication. Once you have learned the signs, it will help to always use the sign and the spoken word together. The American Athletic Association for the Deaf, headquartered at Gallaudet University in Washington, DC, will provide additional information on sports for individuals with hearing impairments. Consider the following questions when thinking about the orientation activity:

1. Why is lighting an important consideration when working with individuals with visual impairments?
2. Why is it important to include Sylvia's entire party at a front table if only she is visually impaired?
3. What is the purpose of using an informant during activities?
4. Why is it important to use sign language and the spoken word together when addressing individuals with deafness?

Introduction

Visual and hearing impairments can be congenital, or acquired at any point across one's life span. These impairments can affect a person's ability to perform daily tasks at home and in their communities. Sensory impairments can also have an effect on the individual's leisure lifestyle. Without leisure options, the individual may eventually become isolated from other people. This chapter will present information on the causes and treatments for visual and hearing impairments and offer suggestions for inclusion into leisure services.

Meet Donna, Who Enjoys Nature with an Imagination

The following description is based on the testimony given in 1986 by Donna before the President's Commission on Americans Outdoors. Excerpts have been used and adaptations made to reflect sensitive terminology.

> . . . I still hear professionals in the recreation field tell me that they do not know why they should make their parks or programs accessible to blind people. "No blind people ever come here," they explain, while, to me, their attitude screams "Keep Out!" How little they know about blind people and our ability to see beauty around us. These professionals ask me why someone with no sight would be interested in seeing mountains, or watching the sun as it rises over the ocean. It is sad that they clearly believe life's beauty can only be experienced through the eyes.

One day I boarded a ski lift and went to the summit of Mount Wild Cat. On the way I leaned as far as I could out of my window (which, of course, is against the rules), and listened intently to the trees passing by me. This ride actually ascends the face of the mountain. That enabled me to sense the rock formations, smell the pines, hear the wind blowing through the trees, and listen to a stream descending the mountain, twisting and curving beneath me.

Then I arrived at the summit. As I moved about, I saw some areas thick with vegetation. The flowers felt beautiful and soft as I looked at them. How can I describe to professionals the joy I felt standing on the top of the mountain, listening to its silence and seeing it not with my eyes, but with every part of me!

Descending the mountain provided me with the opportunity to drop heavy stones from the ski lift's window and listen to them roll down, down, down. The trees rose up to greet me; the air became warmer, and soon I was at the base. I kept a stone from my mountain; it now sits in a dried arrangement I made for my living room. The stone and the cassette tape I made of the mountain's sounds are my photograph!

Those with sight admire the sun as it rises above the horizon; I listen to the sounds created by daybreak, feel the increase of light and warmth, and become part of the total experience. True, I do not see the beautiful colors; but what is color when you have a world of sounds, smells and feelings around you to absorb?

According to Donna Veno, a free lance writer who happens to be blind, people with visual impairments will be best served when service providers stop viewing blindness through their eyes. "Most of us do not feel restricted or disadvantaged; we lead normal, healthy and active lives. We work hard and want to play hard as well. While you who see stand at a distance and view the beauty of the mountain, I go to the top and become one with it."

Meet Alex, Who Likes to Plan His Strategy

Alex is faced with some tough decisions these days. The 17-year-old high-school senior has to decide where to go to college next year—University of Pennsylvania, University of Michigan, or the University of California at Berkeley—whether to attend a conference, accept a scholarship he has been awarded, start guide dog training, or take a computer training class—all of which start at about the same time.

Not an easy set of decisions for any 17-year-old, but certainly not any less difficult for a teenager who is blind and about to start a new life away from home for the first time. Home for Alex is Staten Island. A borough miles outside of Manhattan, Staten Island is far enough away to require his daily commute of a bus, a ferry, and a subway to Hunter College High School, one of Manhattan's public schools for children who are academically gifted.

But commutes do not seem to bother Alex. When he is not running uptown to complete his senior year internship, he is dashing downtown to meet with his chess teacher. Alex has won accolades in both areas. This year, he won a Class-C national chess championship and has garnered top scores in the New York state exams in Spanish.

Alex, who returned from a solo two-week trip to Spain in April, says he has always been interested in Spanish culture and language. "I plan to major in Spanish and other foreign languages, and then go on to law school where I will specialize in international law." Ambitions aside, Alex is not all that different from any other 17-year-old testing new waters as a young adult. Alex's mother would prefer a college closer to home and family, while Alex thinks otherwise. But mother and son are willing to compromise. Says his mother: "After all, this is the beginning of a new life."

About Visual Impairments

The American Foundation for the Blind (Cockerham, 1987) suggests that the terms **blind** and **blindness** be reserved for persons who have no usable sight at all. The terms **visually impaired, partially sighted,** or **low vision** describe "a serious loss of vision that cannot be corrected by medical or surgical procedures, or with conventional eyeglasses" (Cockerham, 1987).

In the early 1930s, the federal government developed a "legal" definition for blindness to determine whether individuals are eligible for special benefits. Because of this definition, there is often confusion between the terms blindness and visual impairment. The government adopted the same terms used by medical specialists to describe low vision—acuity and visual field.

Acuity describes the amount of detail an individual sees compared to what a person with normal vision sees. It is the measurement taken of the best eye with the best correction to determine what the individual can see at 20 feet, compared to what a person with unimpaired vision sees. For example, if a person has to be 20 feet away from an object that a person with normal vision can view from at least 70 feet away, the person would be said to have low vision. The larger the second number, the less vision a person has (20/100, 20/200, etc.). The common phrase "20/20 vision" means the individual's sight is normal and needs no correction for distance.

Your **visual field** includes the entire area that can be seen at one time with the fixed eye. The normal visual field is 180 degrees. According to the American Foundation for the Blind (Cockerham, 1987):

> visual field refers to how great an area a person can see and is measured, in degrees, as an angle. If a person with normal vision looks straight ahead, he should be able to see nearly all of the objects in a half-circle (180 degrees), with an equal area perceived on each side of the nose. The central one-third of the visual field is seen by both eyes. A visual deficit may be a central field loss, or may occur elsewhere in the visual field . . . The particular definition of field used for legal blindness is 20 degrees. In either case, a loss of visual field restricts either central vision (what is seen in the center of either eye) or peripheral (side) vision (p. 3).

A person is said to have low vision if he or she can only see a 20- to 40-degree field, or less, in their best eye (Cockerham, 1987).

Legal blindness occurs when a person's visual acuity is 20/200 or less in the better eye (with the best possible correction) and/or the visual field is 20 degrees or less at the widest point. It is interesting to note that 72 percent of people identified as legally blind are 65 or older. Eighty percent of people who are legally blind have some degree of usable vision, such as perception of light and dark.

Having **low vision** or a severe visual impairment means that a person's vision can range between 20/70 and 20/200 acuity or 30 degrees or less visual field. There are five times as many individuals with low vision as people who are legally blind. People with low vision often encounter reading and mobility problems; however, with the aid of special devices, they are able to read and perform tasks requiring vision.

Visual impairments can be **congenital** (present at birth) or acquired. **Rubella** (German measles) is an infectious disease that can cause multiple disabilities, including blindness, in the fetus if contracted during the first trimester of pregnancy. Although once common, rubella can now be prevented by immunizations that are mandatory in the U.S. and many industrialized nations. **Trachoma** is an infectious disease caused when a bacterium-like microorganism spread by flies enters the eye, producing infection and scarring the cornea or eyelid (Hollins, 1989). Although rare in the U.S., trachoma is the major cause of blindness in the world, found most often in areas with poor hygienic conditions (Hollins, 1989).

Accidents are another common cause of visual impairments. Pieces of flying metal (from construction, home workshops, etc.) cause more eye wounds than any other type of object (Hollins, 1989), which is why safety glasses are strongly recommended. School-aged children (5-14) sustain sports-related eye injuries which could be prevented with proper head gear and eyewear. For children of preschool age, cigarettes, cigars and pipes that dangle at eye level are the most hazardous type of item (Hollins, 1989).

In addition to these accidents that puncture, rupture, or burn the eye, two additional accidents are **retinopathy of prematurity (ROP)** and **detached retina.** ROP is blindness that occurs when premature infants are exposed to 100-percent oxygen for prolonged periods of time (Hollins, 1989). There is often accompanying brain damage. Detached retina occurs when the retina (the sensory tissue upon which the lens image is formed) detaches and rips a hole in the outer wall (Cockerham, 1987). This creates a blind spot as the blood supply decreases. Detached retina can be surgically repaired, often using laser technology. The condition is often associated with trauma and is most common with young males (Treavor-Roper & Curran, 1984).

Diabetic retinopathy is a vascular disease that is the leading cause of blindness in U.S. for people aged 20 to 74 (Hollins, 1989). Retinal blood vessels degenerate due to an imbalance of insulin, the hormone that the pancreas does not secrete in diabetes (Hollins, 1989). There is no cure for this disorder; however, it is possible to slow the loss of sight through laser technology to coagulate and seal off leaking blood vessels (Hollins, 1989).

Glaucoma is a blinding disease caused by increased pressure in the eye. The intraocular pressure is usually due to a malfunction in the system that controls the amount of fluid in the eye (Hollins, 1989). If the pressure rises high enough, it may damage structures in the back of the eye, particularly the optic nerve. Glaucoma may be acute, but is usually progressive (gradual peripheral sight loss) and unnoticed until peripheral vision is lost, causing a condition known as **tunnel vision** (Hollins, 1989). Glaucoma is most often treated with eyedrops or, if ineffective, with surgery to drain the excess fluid in the eye to relieve pressure on the optic nerve.

Cataracts describe opacity (fogging) of the lens, and are found at the two extremes of the life span: infancy and advanced age. Cataracts are usually caused by a breakdown of the metabolic process that keeps the lens transparent (Hollins, 1989). For older adults, vision decreases very gradually as the developing cataract blocks more and more of the light needed for vision. Cataracts can also be caused by external factors, such as electrical shock, wounds, or X-rays. Treatment ranges from the use of prescription eyeglasses and contact lenses to surgically implanted lenses to replace the opaque natural lens. For infants born with cataracts, removal must occur prior to 8 weeks of age for the greatest likelihood of normal vision (Hollins, 1989).

The macula is the region of the retina that is the most important for such activities as reading or sewing (Hollins, 1989). **Macular degeneration,** a leading cause of new cases of legal blindness, is a malfunction of the pigment epithelium which removes waste from the inner fluid of the eye. This condition tends to run in families and is most common in people who have blue, gray, or green eyes. There is little treatment for macular degeneration; however, it usually does not result in total blindness (Hollins, 1989).

Retinitis pigmentosa, another inherited disease, often leads to blindness in adolescence or young adulthood. The cause of the disease has not been fully established. However, the result is the failure of normal process in which the rods and cones (receptor cells) of the eye rejuvenate. Over time, the receptor cells grow shorter, resulting in night blindness, tunnel vision, and loss of central vision (Cockerham, 1987). There is no cure or treatment at this time.

Considerations for Inclusion

Ask participants. As always, it is best to ask program participants to determine how best to meet their needs. The individual may disclose information regarding residual vision which will help you to maximize their participation and enjoyment.

Communicate with participants. When first meeting individuals with visual impairments, introduce yourself and let them know you are speaking to them. Speak directly to the individual rather than through a companion, parent, or sibling. Speak in a normal tone of voice. Someone who has loss of vision probably does not also have a hearing impairment. Do not hesitate to use "sighted" terminology such as "look," "see," etc. People who are blind usually use such words themselves to help their social interaction with those who are sighted. When others enter or leave the room, use their names when greeting them or saying good-bye to help the person who is visually impaired keep track of who is in the room. When you leave people with visual impairments, tell them so and do not leave them guessing about your presence.

Provide an orientation. People with visual impairments often depend on familiar landmarks, sounds and smells for successful mobility. It may be helpful to provide an orientation to the environment by touring the facility and describing the location of distinctive landmarks to help them locate restrooms, water fountains, and emergency exits. Environmental barriers such as posts, changes in floor level and other obstructions should be located and described. For the safety of all participants, doors and cupboards should be kept either completely closed or open (Torres & Corn, 1990).

Consider balance. Some individuals with visual impairment may also have impaired balance and may benefit by knowing the location of hand railings, counters, and other features that can provide support. The goal at all times is to facilitate independence for the participant. Loud, monotonous noises of prolonged duration are discouraged because they interfere with the participants' ability to utilize auditory cues.

Act as a sighted guide. For ease in moving through the environment, people with visual impairments often use a **sighted guide.** When assuming the role of a sighted guide, allow an individual with a visual impairment to grasp your bicep. The person with the visual impairment walks beside you about a half-step behind. In addition, communication occurs through subtle movements in the sighted guide's arm. The advantage of sighted guiding is that it includes and promotes social interaction. As a sighted guide, you should concentrate on orienting the person with a visual impairment to the surroundings and inherent dangers. Let the person know if you must leave them and make sure they are oriented to their current location.

Understand methods of mobility. Canes provide the most independent means of mobility for people with visual impairments. However, some people resist using a cane because of the stigma associated with it. Some parents may be embarrassed if their child were to use a cane, and may not allow children to learn the procedure. Some current technological developments in the area of mobility are sonic guides and laser canes. **Dog guides** assist some individuals with visual impairments to move about their communities and, by law, are permitted to enter most facilities within the community, with hospitals as one exception.

Use teaching methods. When special teaching methods must be used, the techniques should be geared to the individual. Lighting, colors, textures, size of objects and print, space and boundaries may all be modified for successful participation. If glare is a concern, recommend that the individual wear sunglasses or a hat. Consider the speed of the activity and, if appropriate, slow the action down. Provide auditory and tactile cues and be consistent with material placement. If the person is partially sighted, the teaching techniques should be adapted to make use of residual vision. You would not teach dancing, for example, to a person who has been blind since birth in the same way as to a person who was previously sighted and has danced or has seen dancing performed.

Use techniques to assist. Touch may be helpful when instructing a person with a visual impairment, but *always ask* before doing so. In teaching golf, for example, you might position the person's fingers and hands around the golf club. Verbal instruction may have to be more detailed and consistent to compensate for lack of vision. It is helpful to conduct a task analysis (break down skills into components) and teach one skill at a time.

Purchase adaptive equipment. Consider equipment requirements to determine if adaptive equipment would be helpful. Beep baseballs and dart boards, raised checkerboards, and Braille sheet music are examples of adaptive equipment that is commercially available. A complete catalog of aids and appliances is available free in Braille and printed editions from the American Foundation for the Blind, 15 West 16th St., New York, N.Y. 10011.

Modify activities. Skating requires no more equipment for the person who is blind than for the person who is sighted, but a sighted skating partner might accompany the person who is blind. Music coming from a central speaker may be helpful in giving the person who is blind a sense of direction while moving around the rink. Likewise, no special equipment is needed for swimming, but the person who is blind must be warned about any hazards in the area. Activities such as wrestling can be successful when competitors who are blind compensate with their senses of touch and balance. In all active sports, athletes should be warned of potential danger.

Facilitate integration. Many of our parks provide special trails with Braille signs guiding the blind along their way. Make a general trail usable by visitors with visual impairments rather than designing off-the-beaten-track trails with big signs indicating only people who are blind may use them. Most people with visual impairments are not asking for specialized services; rather, they are demanding an equal opportunity to use the existing services and facilities.

Advertise. Taped information is often less costly than Braille, and is accessible to at least as many, if not more, people with visual impairments. Local radio services can assist in advertising to people with visual impairments.

Include people in planning. Including people with visual impairments in the planning process makes sense—and it saves dollars. Therefore, involve people with disabilities at all levels of recreation, from planning of services to participation in programs. In addition, professionals should discourage separate services, like segregated trails in parks, or specially designed tactual rooms in museums.

Though the opportunities to enjoy services at parks and recreation areas have increased, there are still barriers which must be eliminated. A barrier may be physical, such as a lack of materials in Braille or on tape, or it may be attitudinal. Attitudinal barriers are by far the worst to encounter, and the most difficult to break down. For both types of barriers, solid planning is essential, and planning bodies must not only include recreational professionals and providers, but participants with visual impairments, as well.

Veno (1986) encouraged recreation professionals to:

> Look at who we are and what we have, not at what you think we lack. Accept the reality that people with visual impairments are like others, except we do not see with our eyes. Be assured, however, we see with our hands, feet, ears and minds. Blindness allows me to use the gift of imagination. I create my own beauty in the space around me. You see your world as it is; I see the same world as I want it to be in my own mind's eye. Who can tell, then, whose appreciation is greater? (p. 14)

Meet Reba, Who Advocates for Rights

Nelson (1987) reported that like most pageant winners, Reba is talented, attractive, and articulate. She has used her status as a pageant winner to advocate for the rights of people with disabilities, especially those with hearing impairments. Reba has asked people she meets to help remove the communication and attitudinal barriers between people who hear and those who do not. "I want people to learn that people with hearing impairments should not be looked upon as having a handicap that can not be overcome. We must reciprocate the best way we can and overcome communication difficulties."

Reba was raised in a family with parents who are deaf and several brothers and sisters, some of whom hear and others who do not. In response to the varying hearing abilities of her family members, Reba is fluent in oral and manual communication. Reba herself has had a severe hearing impairment since birth.

Since her days as pageant winner, Reba has completed her degree in recreation and leisure studies and is a practicing Certified Therapeutic Recreation Specialist. She enjoys helping others, as she recognizes that others have helped her along the way. Not only is Reba able to help people with disabilities develop meaningful leisure lifestyles, but she also acts as a role model to them. In addition, Reba continues to be a strong advocate for people with disabilities, trying to educate all citizens regarding the ability of people with disabilities to be successful members of their communities.

Meet John, Who Has Signed His Way to the Top

John founded a high-tech computer company and turned it into a multimillion-dollar enterprise. What is interesting about his company is that more than 12 percent of the 375 employees have some form of hearing impairment and at least half of the employees without visual impairments use sign language (Andersen, 1988). They do so because it is the most effective way to communicate with their boss, John, who is deaf.

John remembers when he was 10 and had just moved to new community. The neighborhood children decided to test the newcomer by setting a firecracker off behind his back. Of course, the small boy never heard the explosion. The humiliation drew tears. How did John cope with the cruelty? Did he fight back? "No, I made friends with them."

John continues to make friends wherever he goes. He enjoys the social contact and values his relationships. For relaxation, he spends time with this wife and their three children. John also feels it is important to advocate for the rights of people with disabilities. "I want the business world to understand that any person has capabilities. They can work and perform well if given the opportunity."

About Hearing Impairments

A **hearing impairment** is an invisible condition that affects 21 million people in the United States, making it one of the most prevalent disabilities (Turkington & Sussman, 1992). Hearing loss can range from total congenital deafness to mild partial deafness, causing the person to strain to hear. Hearing losses are experienced by about 12 million Americans as they age, resulting in 50 percent of those 75 years or older having some hearing loss (Turkington & Sussman, 1992). Although hearing impairments are common, many persons who are affected do not fully understand the problem and may be unaware of the need for, or unwilling to seek, treatment. Those who have adjusted to a gradual loss of hearing through the years often do not realize that the sounds reaching them are greatly diminished.

Hearing impairments include all losses of hearing, regardless of type or degree. Total or partial impairment of hearing may result from a variety of causes, the onset being either insidious (having a gradual and cumulative effect) or acute (having a sudden onset, sharp rise and a short course). **Deafness** is defined as the state occurring when a person is unable to understand speech through the ear alone, either with or without a hearing aid (Turkington & Sussman, 1992).

People are said to be hard-of-hearing if they have mild to moderate hearing loss resulting in decreased perception of conversational speech, but sufficient hearing to permit understanding under optimal circumstances. These people have losses that can result in sound distortions or trouble interpreting sounds. Depending on the causes of the hearing loss, some people who are hard-of-hearing can benefit from the use of a hearing aid. According to Turkington and Sussman (1992), the term **hard-of-hearing** is preferred by members of the deaf community rather than the term "hearing impaired;" however, **hearing impairment** is the term of choice by the general public.

Hearing impairment is categorized by the degree of hearing loss in one or both ears. **Mild hearing loss** is a loss of some sounds while **moderate hearing loss** indicates "a loss of enough sounds so that a person's ability to understand his surrounding environment is affected, including some speech sounds" (Turkington & Sussman, 1992, p. 59). When both ears have some hearing loss and the better ear has some difficulty hearing and understanding speech, the individual is said to have significant **bilateral loss. Severe loss** indicates that many sounds are not heard including most speech. Finally, **profound loss** indicates the inability to hear almost all sounds.

Hearing is measured by units of sound intensity called **decibels (dB).** "Zero decibel is the softest intensity of sound or speech that can be heard" (Turkington & Sussman, 1992, p. 59) by a person with normal hearing. People who can hear sounds from 0-25 dB and up are considered to have normal hearing. As a point of comparison, 20 dB is at a level of a whisper. People who can only hear sounds starting at 25-40 dB are considered to have a mild hearing loss, whereas those who begin to hear at 40-55 dB are said to have a moderate loss: 50-60 dB is at typical conversational speech volume. Moderately severe loss occurs when the individual cannot hear at volumes lower than 55-70 decibels. Severe loss refers to the inability to hear sounds and speech under 70-90 decibels: 80 dB is the volume of an alarm clock from two feet away. Not being able to hear until a sound is at least 90 decibels or above is termed a profound hearing loss. Beyond 90 decibels, many people would be called deaf, but with modern hearing devices some people can obtain usable sound. People with hearing in the normal range begin to experience discomfort at volume levels of 90-100 dB, such as when using a lawn mower (90 dB) or a chain saw (100 dB). Stereo headphones (100 dB) and rock band concerts in front of speakers (120 dB) pose danger to one's hearing that increases with exposure (Turkington & Sussman, 1992).

Hertz (Hz), the unit of measurement of the frequency of sound waves, describes pitch. Persons who have difficulty understanding speech generally have losses of high or low pitch. Some people may find it easier to understand deeper voices than high voices, or vice versa.

There are three basic types of hearing impairments. With a **conductive loss,** sound waves are blocked as they travel through the auditory canal or middle ear and cannot reach the inner ear. Sounds seem muffled and an earache may be present. Both children and adults are often affected by conductive hearing loss caused by wax blocking the ear canal, infection, or a punctured eardrum. Another cause of conductive-type loss is otosclerosis. In this disorder, the bones of the middle ear soften, do not vibrate well, and then calcify. This, and other conductive hearing problems, can often be treated successfully with surgery or other procedures.

A **sensorineural hearing loss,** commonly termed "nerve deafness," involves the inner ear and is the result of damage to the hair cells, nerve fibers, or both. Sounds are distorted, high tones are usually inaudible, and ringing or buzzing sounds (tinnitus) may be present. Speech can be heard, but is not easily understood. This type of loss is permanent and irreversible. "Every year, about 5,000 infants are born with sensorineural hearing loss caused by genetics, birth injury (Rh incompatibility or loss of oxygen during labor) or damage to the developing fetus because of maternal infection (rubella, herpes or other viral diseases) (Turkington & Sussman, 1992, p. 96). Other causes include high fevers, excessive noise, heredity, adverse reaction to drugs, diseases such as meningitis, head injuries, and the aging process.

A third, although rare, form of hearing loss is **central hearing loss.** With this type of impairment, because the pathways to the brain or the brain itself are damaged, sound levels are not affected, but understanding of language becomes difficult (Turkington & Sussman, 1992). Central hearing loss results from excess exposure to loud noise, head injuries, high fever, or tumors.

Many people try to "pass" without a hearing impairment being detected, preferring lost sound to the perceived stigma of using a hearing aid. Some people do not respond to suggestions that encourage the use of a hearing aid or medical advice. Despite wishful thinking, a hearing loss can never be successfully concealed. In the attempt, the significant benefits available through medical and scientific technology are missed, friendships may be severed, and the person may gradually retreat to a life of isolation.

Considerations for Inclusion

Use meaningful communication. When speaking to a person with a hearing impairment, use a normal tone of voice and speak in complete sentences. Speak slowly and distinctly. Enunciate clearly, but do not "mouth" the words. Overarticulation does not make it easier to read lips. Look at the person when speaking and be sure the person is looking at you. "V-" or "U-" shaped and semicircles are the best seating formations. It is necessary to maintain face-to-face contact while communicating.

Ensure that adequate lighting on the face of the speaker is available to facilitate reading the person's lips. When interacting with the person, watch their gestures and face to gain additional cues to understand them. Use demonstration when teaching skills or explaining activities, because demonstrations are often more meaningful to the person who is hearing impaired than lengthy explanations.

Consider technology. It is often helpful for leisure services providers to be aware of the technology that is available to assist individuals with hearing impairments to hear as effectively as possible. The most common and best-known assistive hearing device is the hearing aid. **Hearing aids** are assistive devices that improve hearing in many instances, but the aids do not correct hearing or necessarily restore it to normal levels. A hearing aid will, however, lessen the degree of severity of hearing loss and enable the user to hear many sounds that previously were inaudible. If a hearing aid is recommended, there are many types from which to choose. These range from tiny, all-in-the-ear models for mild to moderate losses to large body aids for profound impairments. Hearing aids may also be worn in eyeglasses or behind the ear. Some people require only one aid **(monaural),** while others receive the most benefit from **binaural** aids—one aid for each ear. Many hearing aids are equipped with a telephone switch, which enables the sound from the telephone to go directly into the hearing aid, greatly increasing clarity.

The **earmold,** or **ear insert,** is a vital component of any hearing aid. Some earmolds are made from a solid plastic material, others from a more pliable substance. Some are simple tubular inserts, while other molds fill the entire cavity of the outer ear. They are made in a manner similar to taking an impression for dentures. Like hearing aids, earmolds eventually need replacement. Danger signs are whistling noises (feedback), indicating the earmold no longer fits snugly in the ear.

In various situations, and especially with a severe to profound loss, a hearing aid may not be enough. Modern technology has provided a variety of assistive listening devices and systems for telephones, one-to-one and small groups, conferences, classrooms, theaters, and places of worship. They include both portable and permanent telephone amplifiers, direct audio input devices, personal infrared systems, alarm systems and telecaptioning devices (Kasper, 1990). For additional information on assistive technology, refer to Chapter 17.

Understand methods of assistance. Speech reading and sign language are other modalities available to persons with severe hearing loss. Speech reading is a virtual necessity in cases of severe or profound loss and can be self-taught to some extent. However, professional training may be indicated for many persons. Depending upon the degree of impairment and individual needs, each person must decide what options offer the most advantages.

Understand classification of hearing impairments. It may be helpful for leisure services providers to consider when the onset of the hearing impairment occurred, if the individual chooses to disclose the information. People with hearing impairments can be placed into two distinct classes based on when their impairment occurred. People are identified as having **prelingual** deafness if deafness occurs before language skills have been acquired (Turkington & Sussman, 1992). The deafness can be congenital or acquired in infancy. The second category is termed **postlingual.** This term is used if the deafness occurs after language has been acquired. Although nearly half of all adventitious hearing problems are of unknown etiology, the most common known causes of postlingual hearing impairments are certain childhood diseases (e.g., meningitis, encephalitis, measles, mumps, influenza) and high fevers during childhood.

Meet Lisa, Who Tends the Garden

One look at the flower garden in Lisa's front yard tells you how much she enjoys beauty. Lisa has been blind since birth. She lost her hearing at the age of 5 from complications of meningitis. She tells all of the people she meets how fortunate she was to have learned to speak.

> I remember the sound of the piano—my mother was a music teacher when I was a girl. The fragrance of the flowers, the subtle ways they move with the breeze, the delicate, velvety texture of their petals, all remind me of the music that came from my mother's piano. One doesn't need to be able to see or hear to find beauty in the world. My flower garden gives me so much pleasure. I grow different flowers every season. Every type is unique in fragrance, shape, and texture. Of course, the gardenias are my favorite: simple, pungent, yet delicate. Unlike me, they don't like to be touched.

Another source of pleasure for Lisa is her imagination. She knows Braille and reads at least one new book a week that she receives from her public library's Talking Book program.

> The books I enjoy reading the most are the stories with rich descriptions about people and their environment, you know, like Charles Dickens or John Steinbeck. I also love poetry, especially Maya Angelou. The written word can so eloquently convey beauty.

About Deaf-Blindness

Most people who are deaf-blind are over 65 years of age, and most are women. This is due to the longer life span for women in the U.S. According to Turkington and Sussman (1992), only 1.7 percent of people who are deaf-blind "are institutionalized, which means that for every person institutionalized, more than 50 are living in the general population (p. 57)."

Between 250 and 300 children who are deaf-blind are born each year due to accidents, diseases, and genetic problems. Prior to the advent of rubella vaccine, incidence of deaf-blindness was much higher. During the rubella epidemic of 1964, 30,000 infants were born with visual or auditory deficits, 1,500 of whom were born with deaf-blindness. This epidemic brought deaf-blindness to the attention of the U.S. Congress and lead to special funds appropriations in 1968. The Education for All Handicapped Children Act of 1975 and, later, the Individuals with Disabilities Education Act (IDEA) of 1990, guarantees the right to education for all children who are deaf-blind.

The condition that caused the deaf-blindness may cause other impairments. However, the majority of children with deaf-blindness are just as intelligent as children without disabilities (Turkington & Sussman, 1992). Infants require immediate and intense stimulation to the remaining senses to increase their awareness of the world around them. Without outside stimulation, infants with deaf-blindness withdraw and develop behaviors such as rocking, finger waving, and eye rubbing (Turkington & Sussman, 1992). Even though toddlers with deaf-blindness may have balance difficulties, it is important for them to walk frequently, rather than being carried, because they develop space perception through mobility (Harrell, 1984). Children who are born deaf-blind can learn, but in different ways and at a different pace. Providing educational and leisure services often requires perseverance of the family and professionals.

Considerations for Inclusion

The family is the greatest resource for information on how to provide meaningful recreational opportunities for the person with deaf-blindness. Learn from them how you can best communicate with the individual to discover their leisure preferences. The recommendations given for providing services to individuals with visual impairments, such as assuring a barrier-free environment, and those for individuals with hearing impairments, such as teaching through demonstration, will be helpful when providing services for participants with deaf-blindness.

Conclusion

One goal of leisure services providers is to facilitate meaningful recreation opportunities for all participants. People who have sensory impairments can successfully participate in recreation programs when provided with appropriate support. When first meeting individuals with sensory impairments, avoid the often incorrect assumption that they have limited skills and cognitive abilities. In fact, they may only have difficulty communicating their preferences and needs. It is the leisure services provider's responsibility to discover the best way to communicate with each individual who happens to have a sensory impairment.

All participants with sensory impairments have the right to be served with dignity and respect. The National Federation of the Blind has published the following narrative to communicate courtesies to follow when interacting with people with visual impairments. Many of these recommendations are equally applicable to people with hearing impairments.

> I am an ordinary person, just blind. You don't need to raise your voice or address me as if I were a child. Don't ask my spouse if I want "cream in the coffee"—ask me. I may use a long white cane or dog guide to walk independently, or I may ask to take your arm. Let me decide. And please don't grab my arm. Let me take yours. I'll keep a half-step behind to anticipate curbs and steps. I want to know who's in the room with me. Speak to me when you enter. And please introduce me to the others. Include the children and tell me if there's a cat or dog. A partially opened door to a room, cabinet or car can be a hazard to me. Please be considerate.
>
> I have no trouble with ordinary table skills and can manage with no help. Don't avoid words like "see." I use them, too. I'm always glad to see you. Please don't talk about the "wonderful compensations" of blindness. My sense of smell, touch and hearing didn't improve when I became blind. I rely on them more and therefore may get more information through those senses, but that's all. If I'm your house guest, show me the bathroom, closet, dresser, window and the light switch. I like to know whether the lights are on, so please tell me. I'll discuss blindness with you and answer all your questions if you're curious, but it's an old story to me. I have as many other interests as you do.

Don't think of me as just "a blind person." I'm just a person who happens to be blind. In all 50 states the law requires drivers to yield the right-of-way when they see my white cane. Only the blind may carry white canes. You see more blind persons today walking alone, not because there are more of us, but because more of us have learned to make our own way.

Discussion Questions

1. What is the difference between blindness and low vision?

2. What is legal blindness?

3. What is tunnel vision and the two conditions that can cause it?

4. What are two hereditary causes of a visual impairment?

5. What is acuity?

6. What is the visual field?

7. What are five functional disorders that result in visual impairment as discussed in this chapter?

8. What are two infectious disease processes that cause visual impairments?

9. What are the accidental causes of visual impairment discussed in this chapter?

10. What are the techniques for using the three mobility aids described in this chapter? What are the advantages and disadvantages of each?

11. What are at least eight considerations for inclusion of individuals with visual impairments?

12. What is a cause of visual impairment that is associated with infancy, adolescents, as well as middle and later adulthood?

13. What is the difference between the terms deaf, hearing impairment and hard-of-hearing?

14. What are prelingual and postlingual deafness?

15. How are hearing impairments categorized? List and describe the five categories discussed in this chapter.

16. What are decibels? How are they related to each of the categories of hearing loss? Provide four examples.

17. What are the three basic types of hearing impairments?

18. What are four causes for each of the basic types of hearing impairments as discussed in this chapter?

19. What is a hertz? How does it affect hearing?

20. What are at least five considerations for inclusion of individuals with hearing impairments?

Mary Jane Owen

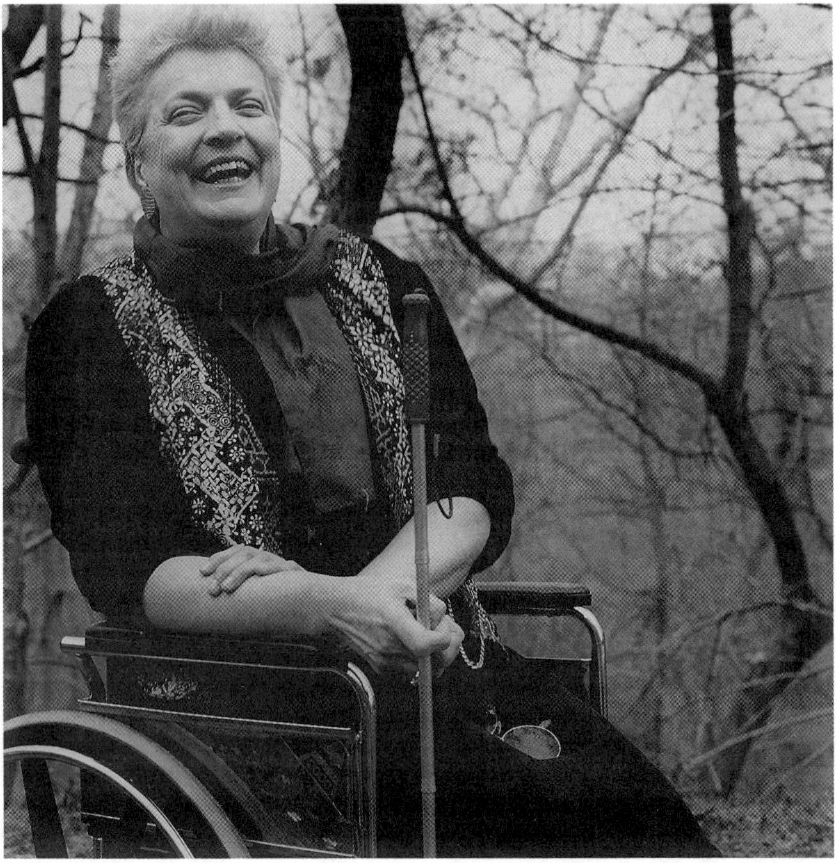

Photograph courtesy of Lynda Greer

Mary Jane Owen lives in Washington, DC, where she is Executive Director of Disability Focus, Inc., as well as Executive Director of National Catholic Office for Persons with Disabilities. She also works as a freelance writer and public speaker. Mary Jane's loss of sight in 1972 was the result of a hereditary ophthalmic disorder. An inner ear dysfunction caused hearing impairment and severe loss of balance which requires her to use a wheelchair.

Mary Jane's Story

I'm a lot of things rolled into one package: laughter and tears; triumphs and defeats; dreams and disappointments; foolishness and wit; self-concern and willingness to sacrifice for others. Sometimes I wonder how I manage to balance so many differing abilities and disabilities. I'm proud of my American heritage and humble before those who have prevailed without my advantages.

I'm strong, intelligent, principled, articulate and very stubborn woman (who happens to be blind, partially hearing, and a wheelchair user) who will probably continue to fill roles I consider essential in the struggle to create opportunities and allow my species to fulfill its potential.

I started out with all the obvious gifts life had to offer. I was born to young parents who cared about racism and a religious life and lived in small northern Illinois towns where my father published a small newspaper and both shared responsibilities for ministering to small congregations within the Rock River Conference of the Methodist Church. I gained my sense of women's roles when my mother assumed total responsibilities following the death of my father when I was six. From my family I gained an inquiring mind, a strong attractive body, a sense of moral obligation to others, an orientation toward art and literature and a life-long interest in ideas and education.

With such unlimited possibilities I learned to be complacent. The miracles which life holds became apparent only as I personally began to explore the all-too-common experience of evolving flaws. The mysteries of human vulnerability and the strength of the human spirit to survive and thrive has been a fascinating puzzle for the last few decades of my life.

Several years ago it became evident to me that the risks and stresses of the living process itself bring assorted impairments but also awaken one of the evolving joys of life. Therefore, I recognize the power of experiences I would never have selected for myself. Through them I have gained a firm knowledge of the power of the human spirit and its drive toward self-determination. The weakest among us is empowered by a dream of possibilities and the gift of "being."

Chapter 17

People, Inclusion, and Assistive Technology

C. Anthony Cunningham

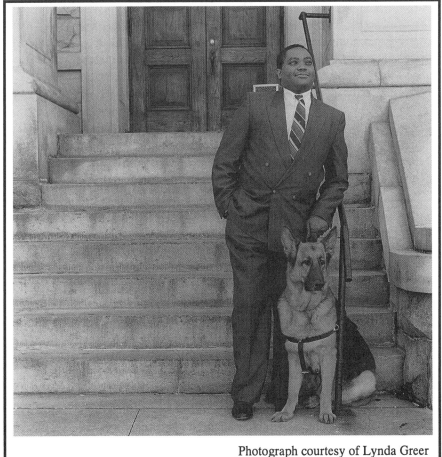

Photograph courtesy of Lynda Greer

C. Anthony Cunningham is an attorney in Decatur, Georgia. Born with a detached retina and glaucoma, he was totally blind by the age of 23.

C. Anthony's Story

My eyesight was never any good, but nobody really knew for a long time. My mother worked in domestic and restaurant service; my father was a heavy equipment operator. They stayed busy, working and raising ten kids. Of course when I started to school, I had to deal with it. I developed certain "tricks of the trade" to compensate and conceal my poor vision. They worked pretty well most of the time. I went through school as a sighted person and graduated a quarter early. But by the time I was seventeen I was legally blind in my left eye and had no vision in my right.

Between 1973 and 1978 my sight deteriorated rapidly, but after working for three years I was finally able to start college . . . while still working, in 1976.

In 1978 I began to come to grips with the fact of my blindness. I quit working and took time off from school to do rehabilitation training. During this time I came to the realization that I'm me, blind or not blind, and that was fine. After the time in rehab training I had the confidence to go back to college full time.

Since I was young I've wanted to be in a helping profession, to do something socially responsible. I grew up hearing the cries of the sixties and seventies, aware of the need to create social change. So while in college I decided to become a criminal lawyer . . . to help those accused of crimes. I'm not talking about corporate types, rich people who hire big names for big money. I mean the little guy, usually not much money, no real understanding of the system, who is in trouble and scared. For five years after law school I worked on the civil side of poverty law practice for the Atlanta, Georgia, Legal Aid Society; and now I'm practicing on my own. I just opened my office in early 1990. It's a big step. There are no guarantees it will work out. But it's a step I had to take.

"Ability is of little account without opportunity."
—Napoleon Bonaparte

Orientation Activity

Directions: Read the following situation. On a separate sheet of paper, identify the technological advances in this scenario which were not available to people just fifty years ago.

> Carmen leaned back in her chair, took off her glasses, and rubbed her eyes. It had been a productive afternoon at the computer and time had slipped away. Gazing out the window, she was surprised to see that it was dusk and the street lights were on. A glance at the digital clock confirmed the time—6:06 p.m. and she had not started dinner. Carmen saved her document, then hurried to the kitchen. This would be a good night for the frozen gourmet dinners she had put away for just such an evening. Placing them in the microwave, she turned her attention to the remaining portion of the meal. By the time the aroma of chicken and rice filled the kitchen, Carmen had whipped an instant chocolate mousse in the blender, started the coffeemaker, and put a loaf of brown-and-serve French bread in the convection oven. Place mats and tablewear were put into place just as she heard the automatic garage door begin to open. Carmen rolled her wheelchair into the living room to turn on the CD player and ignite the gas log. At 6:30 p.m., Juan walked in the house to find his smiling wife, a fire, his favorite music, and wonderful smells. It was good to be home!

Debriefing

Innovations appear so rapidly in modern society that we quickly forget the way things "used to be." Many people cannot remember televisions without remote control, kitchens without a microwave oven, and music systems that played only records or eight-track tapes. Eyeglasses, electric lights, processed foods, central heating and air conditioning—the list of technological wonders that we take for granted goes on and on. The scenario above has many examples of inventions not available 50 years ago—how many did you find? The inventions include: computer, automatic streetlights, digital clock, frozen dinners, microwave oven, instant chocolate mousse, blender, automatic coffeemaker, brown-and-serve French bread, convection oven, automatic garage door opener, CD player, and gas log. Consider the following questions when reflecting on the orientation activity:

1. What are some technological advances that may increase the leisure opportunities for people with disabilities?
2. Why is technology important to consider relative to leisure participation of people with disabilities?
3. What is meant by the phrase "assistive technology?"

Introduction

While technological advances and conveniences are often viewed as modern necessities, many of these advances have transformed the quality of life for people who have disabilities. Some technological developments have made it possible for people with disabilities to participate in previously inaccessible leisure opportunities (Bedini, 1993). According to Chandler, Czerlinsky, and Wehman (1993), "**assistive technology** involves the use of new or modified devices, materials, or equipment, which enables people with disabilities to be more effective and competent in daily life activity" (p. 117). Today there are many assistive devices available to help people with disabilities learn more efficiently, communicate more effectively, live more independently, and experience leisure more easily. Mann and Lane (1991, p. 7) offered the following description:

> Technological tools that restore or extend human functions are called assistive devices, and the field concerned with research, development, and service on assistive devices is called **assistive technology.** New assistive devices for persons with disabilities are based on technologies from many fields. Computer-based devices (hard technology) come from the electronics industry, while applications (soft technology) come from health and education. Controls, switches, and robotics are based on advances in the industrial and aerospace programs. Commercial and military developments generate new composite materials useful for mobility devices. Advances in biotechnology will generate unimaginable devices and functions for persons with disabilities.

According to Crouse and Deavours (1993), there are many arguments for incorporation of technology in inclusive leisure services. The authors identified some of the following benefits associated with technological assistance:

(a) increases independence;
(b) promotes expression and creativity;
(c) affords choice-making opportunities;

(d) facilitates inclusion; and
(e) enhances self-esteem.

This chapter will consider four general categories of technology and assistive aids which enhance independence. In the first section, devices that are implanted in, or attached to, the body to simulate more typical functioning are described. Examples of assistive technology that substitutes for impaired functions such as speech, hearing, or walking are contained in the second section. The third section of this chapter contains information on technology that helps individuals to control their environment. Assistive animals that are simultaneously the oldest and newest of resources are presented in the final section.

Meet the Six-Million-Dollar Family

A popular television program during the 1970s, "The Six-Million Dollar Man," portrayed a futuristic Air Force test pilot whose shattered body had been rebuilt with artificial parts, giving him powers of speed, strength, and vision to rival a comic book hero. Bill likes to tell friends that his family is making the fantasy come true. When his rheumatoid arthritis finally became too painful, Bill had two artificial hip replacements. One year later, he is able to take his grandchildren fishing again. Bill's wife, Edna, is able to go with them now that she has been implanted with a heart pacemaker. Their oldest son, Rodney, is also enjoying better health since being fitted with an insulin pump to automatically monitor and treat his diabetes. Finally, Bill is happy that granddaughter Celeste has received permanent dental implants to replace the teeth she lost in a fall from her bicycle.

About Biotechnology

Devices that are implanted in, or attached to, the body to simulate more typical functioning may sound like science fiction, but they are very real and are making differences in the lives of individuals with disabilities. Since there are too many innovations to discuss them all (and more are being developed rapidly), this section of the chapter only provides an overview of biotechnology.

Hearing. Several instruments have been created to assist hearing processes. **Cochlear implants** are electrode devices that are surgically implanted in the mastoid bone behind the ear to stimulate the hearing nerve (Turkington & Sussman, 1992). Although they do not restore total hearing, they have helped people to gain some understanding of spoken words. In addition, technology has been helpful for those who have hearing impairments but are not candidates for implants. While **hearing aids** are helpful for some individuals, others find the background noise that is picked up to be very distracting. Amplification systems consist of a wireless microphone worn by the speaker, and a headset or insert earmold worn by the listener. This may be the ideal solution in an instructional situation allowing the instructor to move about freely, all the while "broadcasting" to an audience of one. Another hearing-related instrument is an electronic metronome device worn outside the ear, which has been successful in reducing stuttering for some individuals. Finally, a hearing-aid type device is available to mask the ringing of the ear caused by tinnitus. The device produces a soothing "white noise," a soft whooshing sound, that makes the ringing less distracting for many individuals.

Manage health problems. **Neuroimplantation** is a procedure that implants electrodes on the spinal cord, in limbs, or directly in the brain (Fox, 1993). The electrical impulses that are generated help to alleviate dysfunctions such as seizures and spasticity found in individuals who have cerebral palsy, closed head injuries, spinal cord injury, and multiple sclerosis. To benefit people with heart problems, the **artificial pacemaker** is a small device that is permanently implanted under the skin of the chest wall. A pacemaker regulates the heart rate by sending out electrical impulses at a set rate to force the heart to contract rhythmically (Dorsch, 1987). Pacemakers are powered by batteries that last about four years before replacement.

Control one's body. Technology has enabled people with disabilities to have more control over their bodies. Personal cooling systems help individuals with spinal cord injuries to regulate the temperature of their bodies. Custom-made gloves assist those who use wheelchairs to experience less strain on their hands and wrists. People with disabilities may need assistance with personal care, and welcome products that enable more privacy and independence. An instrument is available that uses completely external ultrasound to inform individuals who have no lower body sensation when it is appropriate to mechanically empty their bladder. Technological advances have made it possible for men with paralysis due to spinal cord injury to father children and for women with disabilities to conceive and carry pregnancies satisfactorily (Maddox, 1988).

Improve muscle tone. Research continues on ways people with paralyzing disabilities might be able to walk. **Neurorehabilitation** is an experimental system of stimulating muscles to contract by sending electrical impulses to them through surface electrodes. In addition to enabling a few people with partial paraplegia to walk again, the technology has greater potential for the improvement of muscle tone and circulation in many people with paralysis.

The alternate contracting and relaxing of the muscle via electrical impulse helps to build muscle mass, which improves the health of the skin, helps to build bone, and increases cardiovascular health (Maddox, 1988).

Considerations for Inclusion

It is helpful for leisure services providers to be aware of the potential that biotechnology holds for increasing leisure experiences for people with disabilities. Often, professionals will be unaware that participants are using biotechnological aids. However, if information about biotechnology is provided by participants, it is important to be aware of participation consideration and actions that should be followed if problems should arise. The key ingredient is a willingness to work with individuals and facilitate their leisure involvement.

Meet Stephen, Who Enjoys a Joke and an Occasional Dance

Berger (1992) wrote about Stephen, who may be the world's most brilliant physicist and is best-known as the developer of the black hole theory. Stephen, who has amyotrophic lateral sclerosis (Lou Gehrig's Disease), rolled noiselessly into the darkened conference room, accompanied by two nurses. Fingering a control panel with the partial motion remaining in his left hand, he positioned himself at the back of the center aisle, quietly attended the lectures of his fellow physicists, and took in their illustrative slides. When he had a comment to interject, he fingered the same panel, triggering an artificial voice that emanated from somewhere beneath him.

Midway through the conference, Stephen rolled to the front of the room to give his own talk, "My Biggest Mistake." It was not clear how much of the voice from under the chair had been preprogrammed and how much he was improvising with the panel in his hand. His admitted "mistake" was that he formally assumed time would flow the opposite way when the expanding universe reached its outer limits and began to collapse; now, after years of reconsideration, he thought that time would continue in the same direction.

After the presentation, over lunch, a friendly discussion ensued about why Americans often groan rather than laugh at puns. Was it backhanded appreciation or were they seriously offended? As the debate proceeded, Stephen began fingering his panel and gazed around the table, eyes sparkling mischievously, and a voice beneath him said, in elevated tones, "I am trying to get my synthesizer to groan."

During the last night of the conference, participants were bused to a flamenco club for dinner and entertainment. Guitarists, singers, and dancers took to the stage, gave an accomplished performance, then invited the physicists to dance with them. When one of the dancers made her way through the tables to dance in front of Stephen, I thought it might cross that nebulous boundary into bad taste. Here was a young woman stomping her feet in front of a man who could barely move. Other physicists stood aside to make room. Grinning asymmetrically, Stephen programmed his chair to move back and forth in synchronicity with the dancer. As correctly as his fellow physicists, Stephen ended the conference by dancing flamenco.

About Technology that Improves Functioning

Stephen is able to continue his work because he has a combination of human and technological assistance. For a person with severe disabilities, no amount of computerized, robotic, or biomechanical equipment can completely substitute for human assistance with activities of daily living. The computer is a tool, and thoughtful human beings are the critical ingredient (Moore, 1991). People, not machines, make technological adaptations work for people with disabilities. The application of technology is especially meaningful for people with severe disabilities. Assistive technology can help people to learn or relearn materials and to perform tasks that lead to increased self-sufficiency (Chandler, Czerlinsky, & Wehman, 1993). Equipment can provide new ways to:

(a) write;
(b) work;
(c) hear;
(d) communicate;
(e) speak;
(f) see;
(g) move;
(h) maneuver;
(i) transport; and
(j) recreate.

Write better. Computer technology is a great equalizer. Consider the last time you spoke to a telephone operator—you have no way of knowing whether the person wore glasses, used a wheelchair, or was visually impaired. All you know is that you needed assistance and the operator was able to provide it. Computers are tools that can enable the person to write more rapidly and legibly than by hand. Individuals who have difficulty manipulating the letters on a keyboard can benefit from adaptive hardware. With one such device installed, the computer displays the alphabet, numbers, and important symbols on the bottom of the screen and slowly moves the cursor across the display.

The person hits the switch when the desired letter is highlighted and it is then pasted on the screen. By selecting one letter at a time, the user can type an entire document by pressing one switch (Dutton & Dutton, 1990). The switch could be placed under the hand, foot, chin, elbow, or against the cheek. The switch could also be triggered by blowing air through a **sip-and-puff** control.

Work better. People with quadriplegia are often eager to work, but some find it difficult to be without an attendant in the workplace to assist work-related tasks such as turning on the computer, answering the phone, and tearing off printer sheets, as well as activities of daily living such as providing water, dispensing medication, and adjusting the wheelchair. A case study in California (Hammel, Van der Loos, & Perkash, 1992) profiled a man who was furnished with a desktop robot to assist him in his work as a database programmer for a major utility company. The man was asked to compare the robot with a human attendant in a controlled study. The man declared afterwards that he preferred the robot over a human attendant for all tasks except feeding. According to the researchers, training attendants for assistance incurs an additional period of reduced productivity for the person. Given the economic implications of an attendant, an alternative is highly desirable (Hammel, Van der Loos, & Perkash, 1992, p. 683). Furthermore, the increased self-sufficiency resulting from the use of assistive technology is physically and psychologically empowering for an individual both at work and in other aspects of the individual's life (Chandler, Czerlinsky & Wehman, 1993).

Hear better. Human beings communicate in a variety of ways: vocalizations, hand gestures, body movements, and facial expressions. If one means of communication is removed, most people usually compensate with another—so, too, can people with disabilities. Individuals who have natural speech but are not able to produce volume may be assisted with a personal amplifier, a small, lightweight, battery-powered device that is fully portable and has adjustable volume. The amplifier enables the person to carry on conversations, speak up in class, or make public presentations. If the larynx (voicebox) is removed, speech is still possible with an electronic device held against the throat that converts vibrations into sound.

Another innovation features a highly sophisticated miniature computer that converts spoken language to print and displays it at the bottom of the lens of special eyeglasses. People with hearing impairments are then able to read the words said to them and carry on more typical conversations. This technology is most useful for individuals whose hearing loss occurred after their spoken language had developed.

Communicate better. An **augmentative and alternative communication (AAC)** system describes the symbols, aids, strategies, and techniques that are used by individuals whose disabilities prevent typical communication (Beukelman & Mirenda, 1992). Systems can be simple paper charts or elaborate computers with keyboards. Systems can utilize pictures in the form of simple line drawings, full-color photographs (Mirenda, 1985), or picture symbols. One such symbol set is Blissymbolics, a complex vocabulary of nearly 2,000 symbols developed in the early 1970s and used in countries around the world (Beukelman & Mirenda, 1992).

AAC systems are typically about the size and shape of a large computer keyboard and are usually mounted on a wheelchair, desk, or table in front of the individual at an angle to insure maximum comfort and ease of operation (Prentke Romich, 1992). Some units even come in a choice of colors. Once the device is selected, the communication options are customized to the needs of the person.

Some AAC systems operate as a simple display format: the user activates the system and the desired message appears on the screen. The advantage of such a system is that it is silent and can be used anywhere; among the many disadvantages is the tendency of the listener to focus on the system, rather than the face of the person who is communicating. Another disadvantage is that the person cannot communicate with anyone who is not able to read the screen, such as a young child, someone in another room, a person who has a visual impairment, or one who is not literate.

Speak better. Other AAC systems have **auditory output** in the form of **synthetic** or **digitized speech** that convert the written message to sound (Beukelman & Mirenda, 1992). The manufacturer of one AAC system offers a choice of ten different voices—four male, four female, one boy, and one girl. Synthetic speech can enable people to participate in discussions, to call across the room, and above all, to have a voice and speak for themselves. For active people, a device about the size of a Walkman™ is available that can be used for both receptive and expressive communication.

See better. Computers hold great promise for people who have visual impairments. Characters can be displayed on the computer screen in very large type and with varying degrees of color and contrast to assist readers who have reduced vision. Printers are also available that produce the message in Braille or raised standard print.

Move better. For people who cannot see, there are technological advances such as laser canes and other electronic travel aids to help lead the way. These instruments can provide information about objects in the vicinity, including the distance, direction, and surface characteristics (Jacobson & Smith, 1983). The electronic travel aids are most useful in unfamiliar areas but are not preferred in rainy, snowy, or noisy conditions.

Maneuver better. Power wheelchairs have undergone major improvements since the first motor was attached to a manual chair. Lightweight materials, improved shock-absorbing features, better batteries, and other advances have created more reliable, customized chairs. Power chairs are generally used by individuals who have cervical (high) spinal cord injuries, severe developmental disabilities, post-polio weakness syndrome, or other degenerative disease processes. Manual chairs are recommended for individuals who are able to self-propel and will benefit from the aerobic demands of such exercise. (See Chapter 14 for information on manual wheelchairs.)

Specialized battery-operated cushions are available that automatically shift the pressure points of the cushion at regular intervals in order to prevent skin ulcers (Maddox, 1988). Power chairs have been developed that raise the individual to a standing position and roll forward and back. According to Maddox (1988), periods of standing can have great psychological importance for some individuals and can help simulate a more typical life. An individual with such a chair could stand to work at a drawing board, or stand face-to-face with others at a party.

Manual and power chairs are not the only option for moving about the community. Individuals with arthritis or multiple sclerosis often use electric scooters. These compact, battery-powered scooters are often collapsible to fit into the trunk of a car.

Transport better. To transport a power chair requires a van with specialized lifts and other equipment (Maddox, 1988). Under the requirements of the ADA, most metropolitan areas are now purchasing power wheelchair accessible buses and vans as the buses currently in use need replacement. Individuals with disabilities are also able to operate their cars and vans with adaptations. Hand controls installed on the steering column can brake and accelerate the vehicle. For those who do not have the range of motion to turn a standard steering wheel, there are miniature wheels and joysticks as substitutes. There is a joystick-type invention that replaces the steering wheel, throttle, and brakes of a converted van. A person who can move a joystick only three inches is able to drive independently (Maddox, 1988).

Recreate better. Fitness is a goal shared by many people, including those with disabilities. For people with physical disabilities who would like to body-build, weight-lift, or simply work out at home, exercise equipment is available with stations for biceps curl, bench press, rowing and more that are accessible for people using wheelchairs (Axelson, 1993). For those who want to participate in rigorous outdoor activities, all-terrain vehicles can be adapted (Colston, 1991). There is an all-terrain vehicle that is amphibious and can travel 25 mph on land and 4 mph in the water, allowing a person to hike and fish.

Sailors with disabilities are assisted by specialized systems to adapt racing boats. Those who prefer to spend their time on the water fishing, rather than racing, can do so with a push-button drive system to operate a fishing reel. Chesapeake Region Accessible Boating has developed a weatherproof, salt-water resistant portable lift device to transfer sailors from their wheelchairs on and off watercraft (Brady, 1993). Mono-skis, sit-skis, and bi-skis enable both water and snow enthusiasts who have physical limitations to enjoy skiing.

Wheeled sports are enjoyed by people of all ages. Bicycles have been adapted to allow individuals to pedal with the hands instead of the feet, and are available in three-wheel and tandem models. Carbon fiber spoked wheelchair wheels, first used by the French team in the 1992 Paralympics in Barcelona, Spain, offer less resistance and facilitate faster acceleration than conventional wheels (Paciorek, 1993). Throwing events such as discus, shotput, and javelin are benefitting from an anchor system that utilizes four strong suction pads to hold wheelchairs in place instead of the traditional ropes and rigging systems (Paciorek, 1993). Golf, scuba diving, fencing, archery . . . the list of activities being transformed by technology goes on and on.

Considerations for Inclusion

When incorporating technology in leisure participation, it can be helpful to ask questions about the person's social and emotional responses to the technology. For example:

(a) What is the impact of the use of technology on the environment and peers?
(b) What are the positive or negative psychological impacts of the use of technology with certain participants?
(c) How will the person deal with the use of technology?

Technological systems have been used with clear results by people at all levels of cognitive ability. For example, Dattilo & Camarata (1991) demonstrated the ability of an AAC system to enable both a college student and a man with mental retardation to have synthetic speech that greatly enhanced their quality of life. However, simply providing an individual with an AAC system, a mobility aid, or a sophisticated piece of sports equipment does not enable them to have a better quality of life if they have not learned how to use the device. Skills training and on-going consultation must be available to the prospective person. Sharing conversation, for example, is a technique which can be taught to individuals with disabilities (Dattilo & O'Keefe, 1992) and service providers (Dattilo & Light, 1993) to set the stage for leisure. In addition, Bedini (1993) encouraged community recreation professionals to consider acquiring and maintaining selected assistive devices that could be available for use to enhance leisure of people with disabilities.

Meet J. D., Who Makes His World Move

Hallem (1991) reported on J. D., who has quadriplegia and is unable to move his arms or legs, yet can walk his dachshunds, escape a house fire, answer the phone and set his burglar alarm — all without any assistance. These tasks are completed with the assistance of an electronic box the size of a clock-radio. The high-tech device rests on his bedroom dresser, lighting up in red. This environmental control unit is a sophisticated, centralized system that is connected to his wheelchair and almost every electronic device in his home— from his TV, VCR and personal computer to the back door that swings open for his dogs. Using either a mouthstick or a sip-and-puff mechanical straw attached to his wheelchair, he can activate these systems and function without someone constantly at his side. That independence is important to J. D.

About Technology to Control the Environment

Environmental control units can increase independence and personal safety. The manufacturer of one advertises the following capabilities: "control lights, electric beds, electric doors, appliances and TVs; make phone calls and detect intruders; lights can turn on and off when you are away; an alarm will waken you in the morning; if you fall out of bed, the system will awaken an attendant; you can make phone calls and answer phone calls." These services are controlled by the owner's voice (in English or any other language), from a distance up to 20 feet away (Mastervoice, 1992). Another manufacturer sums the advantages of their system with the words, "If you can move your head . . . you can move your world" (Prentke Romich, 1992).

Technology can help people to find their way around public buildings. One such system consists of small transmitters placed throughout public buildings such as shopping malls and museums. Individuals with visual or cognitive impairments obtain a pocket-size receiver when they enter the building. As the person moves through the environment, the transmitter provides information (in multiple languages, as needed) on the location of the nearest exit, public phone, elevator, restroom, or office. According to the manufacturer, a typical message might be, "Welcome to the City Hall Second

Street entrance—nine steps up to double door entry—Verbal Landmark Directory to your right." The person may replay the message as often as desired and at the desired volume.

Technological advances have greatly improved the opportunities for individuals with disabilities to enjoy a wide range of typically passive recreational and leisure choices. For the youngest participants, toys and games have been adapted to utilize switches and computers. Levin and Enselein (1990) give clear, illustrated instructions on adapting toys for children as young as 2 or 3 years. Interactive computer programs allow children to touch the computer screen and have immediate results.

Popular children's books are available in interactive computer versions, complete with voice narration and sound effects. When the child touches the portion of the screen that shows a bird in the tree, for example, the bird chirps and flies away. Touching the mailbox causes it to open, allowing a frog to jump out one time, an ocean wave to roll out the next. The random display of these many interactive choices—and finding unexpected things in unexpected places—entertains and teaches young children for long periods of time. Older children enjoy making popcorn (Levin & Enselein, 1990), using a blender to make a milkshake, watching slides (Dattilo & Mirenda, 1987), and playing video games using electronic adaptations. Adult hobbies can be made more accessible by use of such devices as a battery-powered card shuffler for card enthusiasts who have some use of their hands (Levin & Enselein, 1990). Poker, blackjack, bridge, and chess are also available in computer versions for one or more players to enjoy. For those who like to sew, electric scissors and chin-controlled sewing machine power units are a couple of the adaptations available.

Considerations for Inclusion

The leisure services provider may inquire about the skills and interests of the participant who uses assistive technology. It may be helpful to contribute to the customization of various technological systems to reflect aspects of the recreation environment. For example, if a participant enjoys soft drinks, an AAC might be programmed to say, "I want to buy a Coke.™" Other words to include in an AAC system might be the names of the leisure services providers, activities the participant enjoys, rooms or spaces in recreation centers (the pool room, the baseball diamond), and personal needs (restroom).

Computers may also be used by leisure services providers to assess the preferences of program participants. Dattilo (1988) utilized a computer and switches to discover the music preferences of children with severe disabilities. Such information will be useful in both the recreation setting and in the home to provide the individual with satisfying choices.

Meet Kim, and Her Best Friend Sophie

Kim and Sophie are a familiar sight around the university campus. Like other best friends, they share a dorm room, rely on each other, enjoy ice cream, and spend time together outdoors whenever possible. Sophie walks to class with Kim and waits quietly during the lecture. She always seems to know when Kim is feeling sad and does her best to let her know that she is there for her. Kim is proud to be seen with Sophie, who always attracts admirers with her golden hair and big brown eyes. Kim likes to tease her boyfriend, Lee, by telling him that he only hangs around her because he has a crush on Sophie. Lee laughs and responds that he is not interested in younger females, especially the four-legged type who get fleas. You see, Kim's best friend, Sophie, is a 5-year-old golden retriever trained as a dog guide for Kim, who is blind.

About Animal Assistants

Assist people with visual limitations. Although dogs have aided humans for thousands of years as watchdogs and farm helpers, they have only recently been trained to guide owners who are blind. The German army first trained dogs to carry messages during World War I. Following the war, a program was started to adapt the original training and teach the messenger dogs to assist war veterans who had been blinded. The first American dog guide school was opened in 1929. Since that time, **dog guides** for people with visual impairments have enabled thousands of individuals to move about their communities in confidence and safety.

According to Murphy (1987), to qualify for a dog, an applicant must be between the ages of 16 and 55, be in good health, have good hearing and at least average intelligence, possess the temperament and emotional stability to maintain a working relationship with the dog and be responsible for it. The applicant must be totally blind or without any useful vision that might interfere with reliance on the dog (Murphy, 1987), and must also like dogs. Dog guides require daily airing, exercise, grooming, and use as a guide. Generally, dogs are not suitable for children, who may lack the necessary maturity. The applicant and the dog must train together for four weeks at a dog guide school. For all of these reasons, only one percent of people who are blind actually use a dog (Murphy, 1987).

Assist people with hearing limitations. **Hearing-ear dogs** are trained to assist people who have hearing impairments. Such dogs are often obtained from animal shelters and may be almost any breed. During a six-month training program, hearing-ear dogs are taught to alert the owner to such sounds as the doorbell ringing, a pot boiling over on the stove, a baby crying, or a smoke detector alarm. The dogs respond to these noises by going to the owners and leading them to the cause of the sound. Hearing-ear dogs can be recognized by a blaze orange collar and leash (Turkington & Sussman, 1992).

Assisting people with physical limitations. **Assistive dogs** (also called ***helper dogs*** or *service dogs*) are trained to accompany individuals who have disabilities which affect their strength and balance, such as multiple sclerosis or spinal cord injury. Each dog is trained to help with the specific needs of its owner. The dogs are often fitted with backpacks to help carry objects, are trained to pick up dropped objects such as pencils and keys, to turn light switches on and off, and to provide a stable support for the person to lean on when transferring from wheelchair to bed or car. Some dogs can answer the phone and bring it to the owner, change the television channel, push elevator buttons, and pull wheelchairs up the curb (Maddox, 1988). Canine Companions for Independence of Santa Rosa, Calif., breeds dogs and trains them to respond to approximately 100 instructions before they are placed with the new owner (Maddox, 1988).

Lesser-known animal helpers are **simian aides**—capuchin monkeys that are trained to perform activities of daily living for owners with disabilities (Maddox, 1988). The owner must be able to operate a motorized wheelchair and to operate the equipment needed to signal the monkey. Three-year-old female monkeys receive extensive training in the activities of daily living that are difficult for the owner. The five-pound, 18-inch-tall capuchins can retrieve a snack from the refrigerator, open it, feed it to the owner, wipe the owner's mouth, and put the dirty container in the sink. They can brush the owner's hair, hold up a mirror, and return the brush and mirror to the bathroom. The owner controls the monkey through verbal commands or by pointing with a light beam attached to a mouth stick. Fruit-flavored pellets are dispensed from a device attached to the owner's wheelchair to reward the monkey for tasks completed. The possibilities for simian help are limited only by the imagination and patience of the owner and trainer. As an added bonus, the little monkeys are affectionate, playful, and fun to watch.

Provide companionship. Recently, dogs have been trained as companion animals **(therapy dogs)** for some people with depression and mental illness. The affection that an animal gives the person helps to enhance the self-esteem of the owner. Knowing that the dog depends on the owner for food, water, and care can be therapeutic and can encourage the owner to develop relationships (Maddox, 1988).

Considerations for Inclusion

The use of animal assistants in public is guaranteed by ADA. Leisure services providers are responsible to educate all participants about proper etiquette with animal aides. The owners can help everyone understand how their animals have been trained to respond in public. Most animal aides are very protective of their owners, but will enjoy a kind word and pat when they are not working—but only after the owner has given you permission to approach the animal.

Conclusion

Most people have a limited awareness of assistive technology rehabilitation engineering. A fundamental problem is the lack of awareness that individuals with disabilities can be productive and capable citizens. As a society, we need to increase our awareness that people with disabilities have widely ranging skills and capabilities. The term **"reasonable accommodation"** helps to suggest that there is an expanding array of options and resources available to integrate people with disabilities in our society. The role that assistive technology can play in inclusion of people into leisure opportunities needs to be more widely known and understood. The delivery of assistive technology services is directly impacted by the awareness of what is available.

Technological advances do not solve all problems for people with disabilities and are only as helpful as the people who design them for the user. Anyone who has used a computer knows that systems must be programmed, debugged, and updated. Some products just do not perform as advertised or break down before they are broken in. Even the best advances are often a bit temperamental and will not always work the first time they are used.

Advanced technology can be costly. A device that looks as if it should cost hundreds of dollars usually costs thousands. One system, which recognizes the voice of the speaker, converts it to print on the screen and then transmits it via a modem, costs up to $20,000 (Smith, 1990). For that reason, the U.S. Congress passed the Technology-Related Assistance for Individuals with Disabilities Act (PL 100-407) in 1988. While this law does not directly provide technological systems to individuals, it does enable states to set up information and referral centers. In some states, for example, individuals have the opportunity to borrow a system for a four-week trial period before making a decision to purchase it. Unsatisfactory systems can be returned and another tried until the best possible match is determined (Enstrom, 1992).

Technology can greatly enhance the person's abilities and may open new ways to explore the world around them. However, using these new technologies can be frustrating and difficult for some people with disabilities. For example, there are word processing systems that can be activated by merely sipping and puffing on a straw connected to a special switch. Such devices make it possible for people who are immobile and lack speech to communicate in ways that were not previously possible. Yet, sipping and puffing through the 2,000 characters of a short one-page letter is laborious and mentally demanding. And for every other similar technological solution, there is a corresponding challenge. Technology enables many people with disabilities to exercise control over their lives and to become more fully integrated into society. Assistive technology extends the same options commonly available for people without disabilities by offering tools necessary for access. Unfortunately, persistent misconceptions about assistive technology services and devices limit their use as a solution for people with disabilities. As a result, this "great equalizer" is underutilized despite the growing number of technology-related options currently available.

Technology can provide a means for people with disabilities to experience enjoyment facilitated through the leisure experience. Construction of a supportive environment that is responsive to people using assistive technology and aids is needed in the area of leisure services delivery (Dattilo, 1993). Parette and Van Biervliet (1991), stated that the use of technology for people with disabilities must be guided by values and philosophy that, according to Bedini (1993), focuses on choice and dignity.

So what can leisure service providers do to promote technology for people with disabilities? It may be helpful to encourage agencies to develop a position paper on assistive technology devices and services. Being proactive and initiating forums and discussions of assistive technology issues as they relate to recreation participation can be helpful. Professionals can develop a public awareness campaign on assistive technology and describe its benefits to leisure involvement. It may be helpful to conduct surveys on present levels of technology knowledge and availability of resources in homes, agencies, communities, and local businesses. Another suggestion is to establish a peer support network for the sharing of ideas and resources. Some leisure services professionals have begun to document existing technology resources as they relate to enhancing recreation participation. It is useful to identify needs of your participants and develop a list of priorities for incorporating assistive technology, secure appropriate technology devices to meet priority needs, and make a "wish list" for additional devices and target potential funding groups. All leisure services professionals are encouraged to take responsibility for supporting technology recommendations by becoming familiar with funding sources and the needs of participants.

Discussion Questions

1. What is meant by biotechnology?

2. What are some examples of biotechnology?

3. What are some ways that assistive technology can improve people's abilities to write, work, hear, communicate, speak, see, move, maneuver, and participate in recreation activities?

4. What do the initials "AAC" represent?

5. What are two mobility aids for individuals who are visually impaired or blind.

6. Name four recreation activities that are available to people with disabilities through the use of assistive technology.

7. How could environmental control devices influence leisure participation for some people with disabilities?

8. How can animals be used to assist people with disabilities in participation in recreation activities?

9. What are some advantages and disadvantages for people with disabilities using assistive technology?

10. What can be done to encourage the use of technology that increases leisure participation for people with disabilities?

Paul Guest

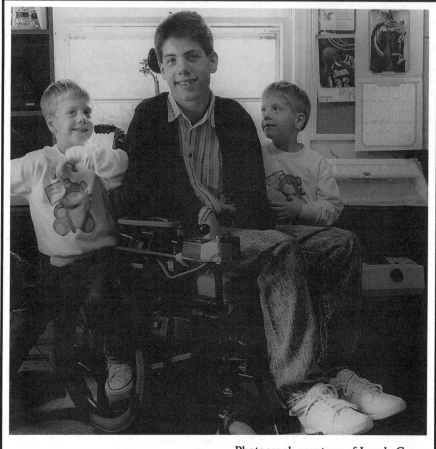

Photograph courtesy of Lynda Greer

Paul Guest lives in Fort Oglethorpe, Georgia, with his parents and younger brothers Chan, and Bo and Clay (pictured here). He is currently a sophomore in high school. When he was 11 he sustained a spinal cord injury in a bike accident.

Paul's Story

Several years ago, when I was hurt, the other kids didn't make a big deal of it when I went back to school. They still don't. I have some really great friends and we have great times together. But there are a number of things that I like about being in high school . . . this year I'm a sophomore. So . . . I'm on the editorial staff of our yearbook, THE WARRIOR. I'm one of the people responsible for the design of the yearbook; I also design motifs, do a little editing . . . whatever is needed.

The yearbook work is really good, but I especially like being on the Toss-Up Team . . . that's our academic competition team. We meet twice a week to practice, but mostly you just have to read a lot and keep up with current events to prepare for matches with other teams. We have to try out every year for Toss-Up. I hope I can make it every year until I graduate, and then I'd like to continue in college on a college bowl team. I guess I have to say that the competition is what I really love about it.

Another thing I really like is basketball . . . professional basketball. My teams are the Detroit Pistons and the Atlanta Hawks. I guess home state loyalty gives the Hawks an edge on the Pistons for me, but they're both great teams . . . very different teams.

When it comes to academics, the areas that interest me most are biological science and computer science. In the 7th and 8th grades my enrichment teacher turned me on to an IBM computer . . . I loved it! Working with computers seems to come easily to me most of the time; when it doesn't, I enjoy the challenge. Computer science is definitely a career choice I consider for the future. BUT my first love is writing . . . science fiction, fantasy. Right now I keep my stories to myself, but someday I want to be a published writer . . . I wouldn't mind a career like Stephen King's! Of course, I could do something in the field of computer science AND be a writer. Well, I've got a little while to think about it!

Conclusion

"The end is where we start from."
—T.S. Eliot

After reading this book you may still be concerned about the importance of including people with disabilities in community leisure services. Perhaps to better understand the need for inclusion consider that even at the lowest estimate, people with disabilities could be the nation's largest minority. Disability, however, is the one minority that anyone can join at any time, as a result of a sudden automobile accident, a fall down a flight of stairs, cancer, or disease—less than fifteen percent of Americans with disabilities were born with their disabilities (Shapiro, 1993).

Although many suggestions have been presented in this text on how to relate to people, I have found one idea that helps guide my interactions with all people, including those who happen to have a disability. When I encounter a man older than me, I think to myself, if that were my father, how would I want others to behave toward him? When I encounter a woman older than me, I think to myself, if that were my mother, how would I want others to behave toward her? When I encounter a child, I think to myself, if that were my child, how would I want others to behave toward him or her? When I encounter a woman about my age, I think to myself, if that were my wife, how would I want others to behave toward her? When I encounter a man my age, I think to myself, if that were me, how would I want others to behave toward me? I use my answers to these questions to help determine my actions toward all individuals. When I do this, I am then more likely to act toward people with kindness, dignity and respect.

Although various disabling conditions have been described in this text, you are encouraged to focus on the principles that facilitate individuals' inclusion into community leisure services. Hutchison and McGill (1992) provided the following similar sentiments:

> People working in the field of leisure must resist the temptation to view a diagnosis as the only important truth and begin to looking for other ways to determine people's interests and abilities. They can begin by building relationships with people and providing supports based on people's assessment of their own situation. (p. 20)

Inherent in leisure service delivery, at any level, is the need to communicate to potential consumers the availability of services. Therefore, as attempts at marketing are made, it may be helpful to consider that, although people with disabilities are a minority, they are many in number. People with disabilities have clearly emerged as a consumer group with money to spend on leisure pursuits. Shapiro (1993) described an incident that identified people with disabilities as a market to be targeted:

> The Minneapolis-based Target department store chain put its first model with mental retardation, a young girl with Down syndrome, in a Sunday newspaper advertising insert in 1990. "That ad hit doorsteps at six A.M. Sunday and a half hour later my phone was ringing," recalls George Hite, the company's vice-president for marketing. "It was the mother of a girl with Down syndrome thanking me for having a kid with Down syndrome in our ad. 'It's so important to my daughter's self-image,' she said. That ad, one small picture among dozens in the circular, generated over two thousand letters of thanks to stunned Target executives. (p. 36)

Since I have spent some of my life interacting with, befriending and providing services to people with some very severe disabilities, I have been asked: "How do you know if a person will respond to you or even knows you are there?" My response to this question is always the same. I tell people that sometimes, I am not sure whether a person is aware I am there; however, I always assume that the person is aware of me and benefits from my contact. I would much prefer to assume that a person is benefiting by my actions and be wrong, than to assume that they could not, and not give them the chance. As I explain this concept I often share the quote by Baer (1981) when he responded to the question "Why should we proceed as if all people are capable of learning under instruction?"

> If I proceed in this way, sometimes—perhaps often—I will be right, and that will be good. What will be good is not that I will have been right (much as I enjoy that), but rather that some children who we otherwise might have thought could not learn will learn at least something useful to them. (p. 93)

As you read the text you may have noticed that the chapter titles and the various headings used throughout the book began with action verbs. I intentionally included these words to encourage readers to take action and implement what they have learned. Now that you possess the knowledge presented in this book you have a responsibility . . . a responsibility to advocate for people with disabilities, to promote their inclusion into community in general, and, more specifically, promote inclusion into recreation and leisure opportunities within their communities. To help emphasize this point, Fulghum (1989) stated:

> I do not want to talk about what you understand about this world. I want to know what you will do about it. I do not want to know what you *hope.* I want to know what you will *work for.* I do not want your sympathy for the needs of humanity. I want your muscle. As the wagon driver said when they came to a long, hard hill, "Them that's going on with us, get out and push. Them that ain't, get out of the way." (p. 107).

Glossary

Access — the freedom and ability to enter, approach, communicate with, or pass to and from a facility, agency, or individual.

Accessibility — the degree to which a person with limitations can get to, enter and use a building or area surrounding the facility.

Acuity — the amount of detail a given individual sees compared to what a person with normal vision sees.

Adaptive behavior — individual's ability to meet standards of personal independence and social responsibility expected of their age and cultural group. Includes maturation, learning, and social adjustment.

Advocate — to recommend, to be in favor of, to plead for a cause. A person who pleads the cause of another or gives support to a particular policy, or proposal.

Affective predispositions — feelings or emotions that are fairly consistent and that set the stage for a pattern of behaviors.

Americans with Disabilities Act (ADA) — passed by Congress in 1990, required that the federal mandate for access to public accommodations and programs be extended to the private sector.

Amnesia — a common type of memory loss whereby the person can only remember bits and pieces of events that occurred in the past.

Amputation — the removal of all or a portion of a limb as the result of a trauma or infection.

Antecedent to beliefs — condition that "sets the stage" for beliefs to develop.

Anxiety — intense fear or panic resulting from a situation, object or person.

Aphasia — the loss of the ability to express oneself by speech or writing or to comprehend spoken or written language due to injury or disease of the brain centers.

Architectural barrier — any feature of the physical environment constructed by humans which impedes or restricts the mobility of people to the full use of a facility.

Architectural Barriers Act — passed by Congress in 1968, states that all facilities receiving direct or indirect federal funds must provide access to all people.

Arthritis — a group of conditions that involve an inflammation of the joints, tissues, or bones.

Artificial pacemaker — a small device that is permanently implanted under the skin of the chest wall and regulates the heart rate by sending electrical impulses at a set rate to force the heart to contract rhymically.

Assistive device — technological tool that restores or extends human functions.

Assistive dog — a dog trained to accompany a person who has a disability which affects their strength and balance, such as multiple sclerosis or spinal cord injury.

Assistive listening device and system (ALDS) — equipment that includes portable and permanent telephone amplifiers, direct audio input devices, personal infrared systems, alarm systems and telecaptioning devices designed to help people with disabilities.

Assistive technology — the field concerned with research, development, and service on assistive devices.

Ataxia — a subtle form of cerebral palsy that results in balance problems.

Athetosis — a form of cerebral palsy in which individuals have "worm-like" movements because of difficulty controlling affected muscles.

Attitude — a learned predisposition to respond in a consistently favorable or unfavorable manner with respect to a given object.

Attitudinal barrier — a way of thinking about or perceiving a disability in a restrictive, condescending or negative manner.

Auditory output — the product of the conversation of written messages to synthetic or digitized speech.

Augmentative and alternative communication (AAC) system — the symbols, aids, strategies, and techniques that are used by individuals whose disabilities prevent typical communication

Autism — a complex developmental disability of unknown etiology that typically effects communication, social, developmental, and behavioral functions.

Autonomy — the freedom and independence to manage one's life.

Barrier — any obstacle or obstruction, natural or man-made, that impedes progress but is not necessarily impassable.

Behavioral predisposition — a consistent desire to act in a particular way.

Behavior(s) — any observable and measurable act, response, or movement by an individual.

Belief(s) — what a person perceives to be true that is composed of an individual's perception of information that has been available in the form of antecedent conditions.

Bilateral hearing loss — hearing loss in both ears.

Binaural aid — a hearing aid for each ear.

Blind(ness) — a condition which causes a person to have no usable sight.

Boredom — a mental state which may result from the perception that activities are worthless, meaningless, frustrating or monotonous.

Cataract(s) — opacity of the lens that is found at the two extremes of the lifespan: infancy and advanced age. Cataracts are usually caused by a breakdown of the metabolic process that keeps the lens transparent.

Central hearing loss — reduced ability to hear because the brain or pathways to the brain are damaged; although sound levels are not affected, the understanding of language becomes difficult. Central hearing loss results from excess exposure to loud noise, head injuries, high fever, or tumors.

Cerebral embolism — a cause of stroke due to a blood clot traveling to the brain from another part of the body, often from the heart.

Cerebral hemorrhage — caused by a blood vessel bursting in the brain, frequently resulting in coma and death. It is the most serious form of stroke.

Cerebral palsy — a developmental disability caused by damage to the motor portions of the brain resulting in an inability to control muscular and postural movements.

Cerebral thrombosis — a cause of stroke due to a blood clot (thrombus) that has formed in an artery that supplies blood to the brain.

Cerebrovascular accident — commonly called a stroke; it is a form of traumatic brain injury that originates inside the brain when a portion of the brain is deprived of blood.

Childhood muscular dystrophy — the most common type of muscular dystrophy that occurs prior to age six and affects the pelvic musculature.

Choice — refers to the act of selecting one option, ideally a preferred one, from among others that are simultaneously available.

Clinical depression — an extended period where individuals experience diminished interest and pleasure in life, fatigue and energy loss, and a sense of worthlessness or guilt.

Closed head injury — one type of traumatic brain injury that is often caused by the brain being whipped back and fourth in a quick motion.

Cochlear implant— electrode device that is surgically implanted in the mastoid bone behind the ear to stimulate the hearing nerve.

Cognitive predisposition — the consistent way that people think or develop ideas.

Conductive loss — a type of hearing loss in which sound waves are blocked and cannot travel through the auditory canal or middle ear to reach the inner ear.

Congenital anomaly — a problem that has occured at birth.

Congenital disability — a problem that exists at birth that results in reduced ability.

Deaf(ness) — hearing loss which prevents understanding of conversational speech, even with a hearing aid.

Decibel (db) — a unit of measurement used to assess the volume of sound.

Detached retina — the retina detaches and rips a hole in the outer wall of the eye, creating a blind spot as the blood supply decreases.

Developmental disability — a severe, chronic mental and/or physical impairment, manifested before the age 22, will likely continue indefinitely, and results in substantial functional limitations.

Deviancy — implies that an individual has strayed away from the majority of society, an established standard, or a highly regarded principle.

Diabetic retinopathy — a vascular disease and disorder of the retina due to diabetes that is the leading cause of blindness in United States.

Direct competition — competition which involves pitting oneself against another.

Disability — a condition resulting from a physical or mental impairment that substantially limits one or more major life activities, a record of such impairment, or being regarded as having such an impairment.

Discrimination — judgments made about people based on their affiliation with a group rather than on who they are as individuals.

Dog guide — dog trained to guide a person with a visual impairment.

Earmold (or **ear insert**) — a vital component of any hearing aid. Some earmolds are made from a solid plastic material, others from a more pliable substance.

Empower(ment) — to give power or authority to a person.

Enjoyment — the experience derived from investing one's attention in action patterns that are intrinsically motivating. Often assumed to be synonymous with fun, enjoyment requires psychological involvement such as concentration, effort, and a sense of control and competence.

Epilepsy — a seizure disorder in which a temporary chemical imbalance of the brain causes a disturbance of brain functioning.

Exacerbation — a new outbreak of lesions with an increase in the severity of symptoms in multiple sclerosis.

Exclusion — the barring of another person from oneself, resulting in the disregard of that person as a human presence in a face-to-face situation.

Expressive aphasia — the condition in which a person can understand what is said or written but is unable to respond.

Facio-scapulohumeral muscular dystrophy — form of muscular dystrophy that causes facial paralysis that spreads to the shoulders and upper arms.

Freedom — the state of having personal independence and full rights of citizenship, including access to, and unrestricted use of, public and private facilities.

Free time — unobligated time not occupied by work or activities of daily living.

Glaucoma — a blinding disease caused by increased pressure in the eye; increases in intraocular tension may be acute or progressive.

Grand mal seizure — one type of generalized epileptic seizure which consists of a convulsion accompanied by complete loss of consciousness.

Handicap — a disadvantage caused by an interaction between environmental conditions and an individual, and not simply inherent in the person.

Hard of hearing — a mild to moderate hearing loss resulting in decreased perception of conversational speech, but sufficient hearing to permit understanding under optimal circumstances. Preferred term of the deaf community.

Head injury — a traumatic insult to the brain that may cause physical, intellectual, emotional, and social changes.

Hearing aid — assistive device that improves hearing in many instances, but does not correct hearing or necessarily restore it to normal levels.

Hearing ear dogs — dogs trained to assist people who have hearing impairments.

Hearing impairment — a range of conditions that includes all losses of hearing, regardless of type or degree. Term preferred by the general public.

Hemianopsia — defective vision or blindness in half of the visual field.

Hemiplegia — paralysis of one side of the body.

Hertz (Hz) — the unit of measurement of the frequency of sound waves, describing pitch.

Impairment — an identifiable organic or functional condition that may be permanent (e.g., amputation) or temporary (sprain).

Indirect competition — competition against one's own internal standards.

Integration — making the use of activities, community resources, and facilities available to all people, including those with disabilities.

Intentions — behavioral plan an individual makes with respect to the presence of an individual.

Internalized oppression — the tendency to accept negative stereotyping about oneself.

Intrinsic motivation — doing an activity out of one's own volition and free from expected results or external rewards.

Jacksonian seizure — a partial epileptic seizure in which convulsions begin in one part of a limb, such as a foot or hand, and quickly spread throughout that entire side of the body.

Legal blindness — a condition which occurs when a person has visual acuity of 20/200 or less in the better eye (with the best possible correction) and/or a visual field of 20 or less at widest point.

Leisure — an experience that transcends time, environments, and situations, integrating elements of activity, time, and the perception of freedom to choose to participate in meaningful, enjoyable, and satisfying experiences.

Limb girdle muscular dystrophy — a form of muscular dystrophy resulting in paralysis of the shoulder and pelvic musculature.

Low vision — a severe visual impairment that results in a visual acuity range between 20/70 - 20/200, or 30 degrees or less visual field.

Macular degeneration — a malfunction of the pigment epithelium which removes waste from the inner fluid of the eye.

Mania — an extreme elevated mood state.

Manic episode — a type of mood disorder which is characterized by extreme elevated, expansive, or irritable mood states.

Mental retardation — a developmental disability characterized by significantly subaverage general intellectual functioning resulting in, or associated with, concurrent impairments in at least two adaptive skill areas, and manifested before the age of 18.

Mild hearing loss — a loss of the ability to hear some sounds.

Mixed hearing loss — a reduced ability to hear as a result of both conductive and sensorineural losses.

Mixed cerebral palsy — a condition that occurs when an individual has more than one type of cerebral palsy.

Moderate hearing loss — indicates a reduction in the ability to hear sounds which limits one's ability to understand the surrounding environment as well as some speech sounds.

Monaural aid — hearing aid device for one only ear.

Monoplegia — paralysis of only one limb.

Multiple sclerosis — a disease of the central nervous system in which spontaneously appearing lesions at the nerve endings of the central nervous system, and the disappearance of the protective nerve coverings, impair nervous impulses to the brain.

Muscular dystrophy — a group of chronic, hereditary diseases characterized by the progressive degeneration and weakness of voluntary muscles.

Networking — establishing and maintaining connections with professionals and paraprofessionals from various disciplines and organizations.

Neuroimplantation — a procedure that inserts implant electrodes on the spinal cord, in limbs, or directly in the brain.

Neurorehabilitation — an experimental system of stimulating muscles to contract by sending electrical impulses to them through surface electrodes.

Obsessive-compulsive disorder — a mental impairment resulting from the inability to think clearly because of recurring thoughts and/or repetitive behaviors.

Open head injury — a visible type of traumatic brain injury that results from an accident, gunshot wound, fall, or other trauma, such as brain surgery to remove a clot or tumor.

Orthopedic impairment — a group of limitations involving the locomotor components of the body including the bones, joints, and muscles.

Osteoarthritis — a degenerative form of arthritis that creates stiffness, swelling and pain in the joints.

Overjustification effect — occurs when intrinsic motivation is undermined by extrinsic rewards. Extrinsic rewards, while offered, increase interest in participation, but once they are withdrawn, interest in participation is lower than before the rewards were offered.

Paraplegia — paralysis and/or loss of sensation of the lower body resulting from a variety of conditions including injury to the sacral, lumbar, or thoracic area of the spine, and polio.

Partially sighted — a severe visual impairment that results in a visual acuity range between 20/70, 20/200, or 30 degrees or less visual field.

Partial participation — adaptations and assistance provided so that one may participate in the leisure activity of choice, without regard to degree of assistance required.

Peer tutoring — linking individuals without disabilities with individuals of a similar age who have disabilities to promote positive interactions and attitudes.

Perceived freedom — self-determined behavior or having the feeling of being the origin of the activity.

Petit mal seizure — a generalized epileptic seizure resulting in brief periods of fixation (absences) in which the individual appears to be staring into space and does not respond to external stimuli.

Phobia — an unrealistic fear which dominates a person's thinking.

Postlingual hearing impairment — a reduction in the ability to hear that is acquired after language development.

Preference — a desire for an option following a comparison of that option against a continuum of other options.

Prejudice — the development of a judgment in disregard of a person's rights that results in that individual being injured or damaged in some way.

Prelingual hearing impairment — a limitation to hearing that is acquired before language acquistion, typically congential or occuring in infancy.

Profound hearing loss — the inability to hear almost all sounds.

Prosthesis — an artificial body part.

Quadriplegia — paralysis and loss of sensation of the body below the neck resulting from a variety of conditions including spinal cord injury, stroke, and multiple sclerosis.

Reasonable accommodation — action taken to include people with disabilities into programs based on the premise that there is an expanding array of options and resources available to promote integration.

Receptive aphasia — inability to understand messages received as either spoken or written language.

Recreation — an activity developed and accepted by a society that is designed for the primary reasons of fun, enjoyment and satisfaction.

Rehabilitation Act — legislation passed by Congress in 1973 that focused on the rights of all people to have equal access to jobs, education, housing, transportation, and all programs which directly, or indirectly, received federal funds.

Remission — the healing of lesions and the relief of some symptoms in various medical conditions, including multiple sclerosis.

Retinitis pigmentosa — a disease in which the rods and cones (receptor cells) fail to rejuvenate, resulting in night blindness, tunnel vision, and loss of central vision.

Retinopathy of prematurity (ROP) — blindness that occurs when premature infants are exposed to 100% oxygen for prolonged periods of time.

Rheumatoid arthritis — progressive, profound form of arthritis typically resulting in severe inflammation that primarily attacks the joints, but can also affect other body tissues and organs and is characterized by unpredictable changes in pain and stiffness.

Rigidity — a form of cerebral palsy causing individuals to be physically rigid and appear stiff. The neck, back, or limbs may be hyperextended.

Rubella — German measles which, when passed from mother to child during the first trimester of pregnancy, can cause a variety of disabiling conditions such as visual, hearing, and cognitive impairments.

Schizophrenia — a psychotic mental disorder which is characterized by departures from reality.

Segregation — the separation or isolation of a group or individual in a restricted area by discriminatory means that results in members of the group, or an individual, receiving treatment that is different from other people.

Self-advocacy — individuals and groups who have traditionally been powerless and largely voiceless, who speak up on their own behalf to try to change their social status and situation.

Self-determination — the feeling of being the origin of the activity, sometimes regarded as the basis of intrinsic motivation.

Sensorineural hearing loss — commonly termed "nerve deafness," involves the inner ear and is the result of damage to the hair cells, nerve fibers, or both.

Severe hearing loss — indicates that many sounds are not heard including most speech.

Sighted guide — an individual who guides a person with a visual impairment through subtle arm movements, and verbal communications.

Simian aide — a capuchin monkey trained to perform activities of daily living and safety for owners who typically have quadriplegia.

Similarity — the perception of a general likeness, of having common characteristics.

Sip and puff — assistive device which allows individuals with quadriplegia to control their wheelchair and other electronic devices through a straw which, when air is forced in or out, signals the device to operate.

Social role valorization — a critical aspect of integration occuring when a person who holds a valued social role is given the respect typically given to people fulfilling that valued social role and, therefore, becomes less vulnerable to devaluation.

Spasticity — increased muscle tone stiffness (hypertonia) and immediate contraction when stretching the affected muscles.

Spina bifida — a congenital disability of the spinal column that occurs early in prenatal development and results in incomplete formation of the vertebrae.

Spina bifida meningocele — a moderate form of spina bifida in which the meninges, the protective covering around the spinal cord, protrudes through the vertebrae.

Spina bifida mylomeningocele — the most serious form of spina bifida, in which a portion of the spinal cord itself protrudes through the back, sometimes exposing tissue and nerves.

Spina bifida occulta — the most mild variety of spina bifida in which no neural damage occurs.

Spinal cord injury — damage to the spinal cord resulting in the loss of function below the level of injury because of impaired transmission of neural impulses. Severity is a result of the extent and location of the injury to the spinal column.

Spread phenomenon — the association of additional imperfections to a person on the basis of an actual disabling condition.

Stereotype — a standardized mental picture held in common by members of a group that represents an oversimplified opinion, attitude, or judgment.

Stigma — an undesired differentness which separates a person from the rest of society.

Synthetic or **digitized speech** — auditory output by an augmentative and alternative communication device that converts the written message to sound.

Therapy dog — dog trained as a companion for people experiencing problems with their mental health.

Thrombus — a blood clot which forms in and obstructs a blood vessel.

Trachoma — an infectious disease that is the major cause of blindness in the world, but rare in the United States, caused when a bacterium-like microorganism enters the eye producing infection and scarring the cornea or eyelid.

Transient ischemic attack (TIA) — brief episode of circulatory deficiency to the cerebrum.

Traumatic brain injury — a physical insult to the brain resulting in changes to cognitive, physical, emotional, and social functioning.

Tremors — a form of cerebral palsy where individuals exhibit frequent or constant involuntary shaking of body parts, especially the hands and arms.

Tunnel vision — loss of peripheral vision.

Visual field — the area a person can see; it is measured, in degrees, as an angle and includes the entire area that can be seen at one time with the fixed eye. Normal visual field is 180 degrees.

Visual impairment — a condition in which a person experiences a loss of vision that cannot be corrected, but in which they retain some usable vision.

References

Abery, B. (1994). A conceptual framework for enhancing self-determination. In M. Hayden, & B, Abery (Eds.), *Challenges for a service system in transition: Ensuring quality community experience for persons with developmental disabilities.* Baltimore, MD: Paul H. Brookes.

Abramson, L., Seligman, M., & Teasdale, J. (1978). Learned helplessness in humans: Critique and resolution. *Journal of Abnormal Psychology, 87*, 49-74.

Adunsky, A., Hershkowitz, M., Rabbi, R., Asher-Sivron, L., & Ohry, A. (1992). Functional recovery in young stroke patients. *Archives of Physical Medicine and Rehabilitation, 73*, 859-862.

AFB News. (1991). The politics of access for blind and visually impaired persons. *American Foundation for the Blind (AFB) News, 26*(1), 3-4.

Agosta, J., Jennings, D., & Bradley, V. (1985). Statewide family support programs: National survey results. In J. M. Agosta, & V. J. Bradley (Eds.), *Family care for persons with developmental disabilities: A growing commitment* (pp. 94-112). Boston, MA: Human Services Research Institute.

Ajzen, I., & Driver, B. L. (1991). Prediction of leisure participation from behavioral, normative, and control beliefs: An application of the theory of planned behavior. *Leisure Sciences, 13*, 185-204.

Alderson, G. (1985). *Tips for tabs: Temporarily able bodied.* Altoona, PA: GHA Publications.

Algozzine, B., Mercer, C. D., & Countermine, T. (1977). The effects of labels and behavior on teacher expectations. *Exceptional Children*, 131-132.

Allport, G. W. (1954). *The nature of prejudice.* New York, NY: Addison-Wesley.

American Association on Mental Retardation. (1992). *Mental retardation: Definition, classification, and systems of supports (9th ed.).* Washington, DC: American Association on Mental Retardation.

American Psychiatric Association. (1994). *Diagnostic and statistical manual of mental disorders: DSM-IV-R.* Washington, DC: Author.

Americans with Disabilities Act, PL 101-336, (July 26, 1990). 42 U. S. C. 12101, et seq: *Federal Registrar, 56*(44), 35544-35756.

Amir, Y. (1969). Contact hypothesis in ethnic relations. *Psychological Bulletin, 71*, 319-342.

Anderson, A. (1981). Exclusion: A study of depersonalization in health care. *Journal of Humanistic Psychology, 21*(3), 67-68.

Anderson, J. (1988, January). Success in a world of silence. *Parade Magazine,* 31.

Anderson, S. C., & Allen, L. R. (1985). Effects of a leisure education program on activity involvement and social interaction of mentally retarded persons. *Adapted Physical Activity Quarterly, 2*(2), 107-116.

Anthony, P. (1985). The recreation practitioner as change agent and advocate for special populations. *Journal of Leisurability, 12*(1), 19-23.

Anthony, W. A. (1969). The effects of contact on an individual's attitude toward disabled persons. *Rehabilitation Counseling Bulletin, 12*, 168-170.

Antia, S. D., & Kreimeyer, K. (1992). Project Interest: Interventions for social integration of young hearing-impaired children. *OSERS: News in Print, 4*(4), 14-20.

Arthritis Foundation. (1986). *Basic facts: Answers to your questions.* Atlanta, GA: Author.

Ashton-Shaeffer, C., & Kleiber, D. A. (1990). The relationship between recreation participation and functional skill development in young people with mental retardation. *Annual in Therapeutic Recreation, 1*, 75-81.

Austin, D. R., Powell, L. G., & Martin, D. W. (1981). Modifying attitudes toward handicapped individuals in a classroom setting. *The Journal for Special Educators, 17*(2), 135-141.

Axelson, P. (1993). Choices, choices, choices. *Sports 'N Spokes, 18*(6) 33-70.

Axelson, P. (1994). Chairs, chairs, everywhere. *Sports 'N Spokes, 19*(6), 15-67.

Baer, D. (1981). A hung jury and a Scottish verdict not proven. *Analysis and Intervention in Developmental Disabilities, 1*, 91-97.

Ballard, M., Corman, L., Gottlieb, J., & Kaufman, J. (1977). Improving the social status of mainstreaming retarded children. *Journal of Educational Psychology,* 605-611.

Bambara, L. M., & Ager, C. (1992). Using self-scheduling to promote self-directed leisure activity in home and community settings. *Journal of the Association for Persons with Severe Handicaps, 17*(2), 67-76.

Barber, E. H., & Magafas, A. (1992). Therapeutic recreation majors' work preference. *Journal of Therapeutic Recreation, 26*(4), 43-54.

Barber, T., Calverley, D., Forgione, A., McPeake, J., Chaves, J., & Bowen, B. (1969). Five attempts to replicate the experimenter bias effect. *Journal of Consulting and Clinical Psychology, 33*, 1-6.

Baroff, G. S. (1986). Mental retardation: *Nature, cause, and management. (2nd ed.).* Washington, DC: Hemisphere.

Barton, L., Johnson, H., & Brulle, A. (1984). *An evaluation of the effectiveness of extended year programming for individuals with severe handicaps.* Unpublished manuscript, Kent State University, OH.

Baumgart, D., Brown, L., Pumpian, I., Nisbet, J., Ford, A., Sweet, M., Messina, R., & Schroeder, J. (1982). The principle of partial participation and individualized adaptations in educational programs for severely handicapped students. *Journal of the Association for the Developmentally Handicapped, 7*, 17-27.

Beaver, D. (1993). A reflection on person-first usage. *Palaestra, 9*(3), 4-5.

Bedini, L. A. (1990). Separate but equal? Segregated programming for people with disabilities. *Journal of Physical Education, Recreation, & Dance, 10,* 40-44.

Bedini, L. A. (1993). Technology and people with disabilities: Ethical considerations. *Palaestra, 9*(4), 25-30.

Bedini, L. A., Bullock, C. C., & Driscoll, L. B. (1993). The effects of leisure education to the successful transition of students with mental retardation from school to adult life. *Therapeutic Recreation Journal, 26*(2), 70-82.

Beland, R. M. (1993). Outdoor recreation for everyone. *Parks and Recreation Magazine, 28*(8), 62-63.

Belgrave, F. Z., & Mills, J. (1981). Effect upon desire for social interaction with a physically disabled person of mentioning the disability in different contexts. *Journal of Applied Social Psychology, 11*, 44-57.

Berger, A. (1994). Inclusion: Not an ideology, but a way of life. *Newsletter: The Association for Persons with Severe Handicaps, 20*(1), 4-7.

Berger, B. (1992). Dancing with time. *American Way*, February 15th, 40, 44, 89.

Berkowitz, L. (1962). *Aggression: A social psychological analysis.* New York, NY: McGraw-Hill.

Beukelman, D., & Mirenda, P. (1992). *Augmentative and alternative communication: Management of severe communication disorders in children and adults.* Baltimore, MD: Paul H. Brookes.

Black holes figured back in time. (1988, June 6). *Insight*, p. 54.

Blatt, B. (1982). *The conquest of mental retardation.* Austin, TX: Pro-ed.

Blaxter, M. (1976). *The meaning of disability.* New York, NY: Neale Watson Academic Publications, Inc.

Block, M. E., & Krebs, P. L. (1992). An alternative to least restrictive environments: A continuum of support to regular physical education. *Adapted Physical Activity Quarterly, 9*(2), 97-113.

Bogdan, R., & Taylor, S. J. (1982). *Inside out: The social meaning of mental retardation.* Toronto, ON: University of Toronto Press.

Bogdan, R., & Taylor, S. J. (1992). The social construction of humanness. In P. M. Ferguson, D. L. Ferguson, & S. J. Taylor (Eds.), *Interpreting disability,* (pp. 169-171). New York, NY: Teachers College Press.

Braddock, D., Hemp, R., & Fujiura, G. (1987). National study of public spending for mental retardation and developmental disabilities. *American Journal on Mental Deficiency, 92,* 121-133.

Brady, M. (1993, July 23). Governor William Donald Schaefer announces recreation grants for Marylanders with disabilities. *Press Release.* Annapolis, MD: Governor's Press Office.

Bray, A. (1989, September). "Attitude change:" Another instance of the readiness myth? *TASH Newsletter,* p. 7.

Brazelton, T. B. (1983). *Infants and mothers. Differences in development (rev. ed.).* New York, NY: Dell.

Bregha, F. J. (1985). Leisure and freedom re-examined. In T. A. Goodale & P. A. Witt (Eds.), *Recreation and leisure: Issues in an era of change (2nd ed.)* (pp. 35-43). State College, PA: Venture Publishing, Inc.

Brehm, J. (1977). *A theory of psychological reactance.* New York, NY: Academic Press.

Breslin, M. L. (1994). Is the ADA living up to its promise? *Mainstream, 18*(6), 31-42.

Brickman, P., & Bulman, R. J. (1977). Pleasure and pain in social comparison. In J. M. Suls & R. L. Miller (Eds.), *Social comparison processes: Theoretical and empirical perspectives.* Washington, DC: Hemisphere.

Brickman, P., Coates, D., & Janoff-Bulman, R. (1978). Lottery winners and accident victims: Is happiness relative? *Journal of Personality and Social Psychology, 36*(8), 917-927.

Broglin, D., Delgado-Escueta, A. V., Walsh, G. O., Bancaud, J., & Chauvel, P. (1992). Clinical approach to the patient with seizures and epilepsies of frontal origin. In P. Chauvel, A. Delgado-Escueta, E. Halgren, & J. Bancaud (Eds.), *Advances in neurology: Vol. 57. Frontal lobe seizures and epilepsies.* New York, NY: Raven Press.

Brolley, D. Y., & Anderson, S. C. (1988). Advertising and attitudes. *Journal of Leisurability, 15*(3), 23-26.

Brooks, N. A., & Matson, R. R. (1987). Managing multiple sclerosis. In J. A. Roth & P. Conrad (Eds.), *Research in the sociology of health care* (pp. 73-106). London, UK: JAI Press, Inc.

Brown, D. S. (1992). Empowerment through peer counseling. *OSERS: News in Print, 5*(2), 27-29.

Brown, L., Branston, M. B., Hamre-Nietupske, S., Pumpian, I., Certo, N., & Gruenewald, L. (1979a). A strategy for developing chronological age-appropriate and functional curricular content for severely handicapped adolescents and young adults. *Journal of Special Education, 13*, 81-90.

Brown, L., Branston-McClean, M. B., Baumgart, D., Vincent, L., Falvey, M., & Schroeder, J. (1979b). Using the characteristics of current and subsequent least restrictive environments in the development of curricular content for severely handicapped students. *AAESPH Review, 4*, 407-424.

Brown, L., Long, E., Udvari-Solner, A., Davis, L., Van Deventer, P., Ahlgren, C., Johnson, F., Gruenewald, L., & Jorgensen, J. (1989). The home school: Why students with severe intellectual disabilities must attend the schools of their brothers, sisters, friends, and neighbors. *Journal of the Association for Persons with Severe Handicaps, 14*(1), 1-7.

Brown, L., Shiraga, B., York, J., Zanella, K., & Rogan, P. (1984). The life space analysis: Strategy for students with severe intellectual disabilities. In L. Brown, M. Sweet, B. Shiraga, J. York, K. Zanella, P. Rogan, & R. Loomis (Eds.) *Educational programs for students with severe handicaps Vol. XIV*, 23-31. Madison, WI: Metropolitan School District.

Brown, W. H., Fox, J. J., & Brady, M. P. (1987). Effects of spatial density on three- and four-year-old children's socially directed behavior during freeplay: An investigation of setting factor. *Education and Treatment of Children, 10*, 247-258.

Bullock, C. (1993). Forward: Avoiding common problems. In L. A. Heyne, S. J. Schleien, and L. H. McEvoy (Eds.), *Making friends: Using recreation activities to promote friendship between children with and without disabilities*, p. 2. Minneapolis, MN: Institute on Community Integration (UAP).

Byrd, K., Crews, B., & Ebener, D. (1991). A study of appropriate use of language when making reference to persons with disabilities. *Journal of Applied Rehabilitation Counseling, 22*(2), 40-41.

Caldwell, L. L., Smith, E. A., & Weissinger, E. (1992). Development of a leisure experience battery for adolescents: Parsimony, stability, and validity. *Journal of Leisure Research, 24*(4), 361-376.

Calhoun, M. L., & Calhoun, L. G. (1993). Age-appropriate activities: Effects on the social perception of adults with mental retardation. *Education and Training in Mental Retardation, 28*(2), 143-148.

Cangemi, P. (1992). Accessibility and recreation trails. *Recreation Access in the 90s, 2*(2), 7-9.

Cangemi, P., Williams, W., & Gaskell, P. (1992). Going to the source for accessibility assessment. *Parks and Recreation, 27*(10), 66-69.

Carter, M. J., Browne, B., LeConey, S. P., & Nagle, C. J. (1991). *Designing therapeutic recreation programs in the community*. Reston, VA: American Alliance for Health, Physical Education, Recreation, & Dance.

Carter, M. J., & Foret, C. M. (1994). Building transitional bridges for the disabled. *Parks and Recreation, 29*(4), 79-83.

Carter, M. J., Van Andel, G. E., & Robb, G. M. (1985). *Therapeutic recreation: A practical approach*. Prospect Heights, IL: Waveland Press, Inc.

Certo, N. J., Schleien, S. J., & Hunter, D. (1983). An ecological assessment inventory to facilitate community recreation participation by severely disabled individuals. *Therapeutic Recreation Journal, 17*(3), 29-38.

Chandler, L. K., Fowler, S. A., & Lubeck, R. C. (1992). An analysis of the effects of multiple setting events on the social behavior of preschool children with special needs. *Journal of Applied Behavior Analysis, 25*(2), 249-263.

Chandler, S. K., Czerlinsky, T., & Wehman, P. (1993). Provisions of assistive technology: Bridging the gap to accessibility. In P. Wehman, *The ADA mandate for social change.* Baltimore, MD: Brookes.

Chinn, K. A., & Joswiak, K. F. (1981). Leisure education and leisure counseling. *Therapeutic Recreation Journal, 15*(4), 4-7.

Cobb, S. (1976). Social support as moderator of life stress. *Psychosomatic Medicine, 38*, 300-314.

Cockerham, P. (1987). *Low vision questions and answers: Definitions, devices, services.* New York, NY: American Foundation for the Blind.

Cole, M., & Meyer, L. H. (1991). Social integration and severe disabilities: A longitudinal analysis of child outcomes. *Journal of Special Education, 25*, 340-351.

Coleman, D., & Iso-Ahola, S. E. (1993). Leisure and health: The role of social support and self-determination. *Journal of Leisure Research, 25*(2), 11-128.

Collard, K. (1981). Leisure education in the schools: Why, who, and the need for advocacy. *Therapeutic Recreation Journal, 15*(4), 8-16.

Colston, L. G. (1991). The expanding role of assistive technology in therapeutic recreation. *The Journal of Physical Education, Recreation & Dance, 62*(4), 39-41.

Cook, S., & Makas, E. (1979). Why, some of my best friends are disabled! A study of the interaction between disabled people and nondisabled rehabilitation professionals. Unpublished manuscript, George Washington University, VA.

Cornwall, K. M., & Winn-Orr, B. (1991). Neurological and neuromuscular disorders. In D. R. Austin & M. E. Crawford (Eds.), *Therapeutic recreation: An introduction* (pp. 240-263). Englewood Cliff, NJ: Prentice Hall.

Coulter, D. L. (1992). An ecology of prevention for the future. *Mental Retardation, 30*(6), 363-369.

Crabtree, J. (1994). Overcoming adversity: Judy Clouston has turned her loss into poetry. *Independent Living, 9*(3), 34-36.

Crouse, J., & Deavours, M. (1993). Switch technology in therapeutic recreation programming: An idea whose time has come. *Palaestra, 9*(4), 41-44.

Csikszentmihalyi, M. (1975). *Beyond boredom and anxiety: The experience of play in work and games.* San Francisco, CA: Jossey Bass.

Csikszentmihalyi, M. (1982). Toward a psychology of optimal experience. *Review of Personality and Social Psychology, 3*, 13-36.

Csikszentmihalyi, M. (1985a). Emergent motivation. In D. Kleiber & M. Maehr (Eds.). *Motivation and adulthood.* Greenwich, CT: JAI Press.

Csikszentmihalyi, M. (1985b). Reflections on enjoyment. *Perspectives on Biology and Medicine, 28*, 489-497.

Csikszentmihalyi, M. (1990). *Flow: The psychology of optimal experience.* New York, NY: Harper & Row.

Csikszentmihalyi, M., & Csikszentmihalyi, I. (1988). *Optimal experience.* Cambridge, UK: Cambridge University Press

Csikszentimihalyi, M., & Larson, R. (1984). *Being adolescent.* New York, NY: Basic.

Curtis, C. K., & Shaver, J. P. (1987). Modifying attitudes toward persons with disabilities: A review of reviews. *International Journal of Special Education, 2*, 103-129.

Darley, J. M., & Fazio, R. H. (1980). Expectancy confirmation processes arising in the social interaction sequence. *American Psychologist, 35*, 867-881.

Dattilo, J. (1985). Incorporating choice into therapeutic recreation programming for individuals with severe handicaps. In G. Hitzhusen (Ed.), *Expanding horizons in therapeutic recreation, XII* (pp. 62-83). Columbia, MO: Curators University of Missouri.

Dattilo, J. (1986). Computerized assessment of preferences for persons with severe handicaps. *Journal of Applied Behavior Analysis, 19*(4), 445-448.

Dattilo, J. (1988). Assessing music preferences of persons with severe disabilities. *Therapeutic Recreation Journal, 22*(2), 12-23.

Dattilo, J. (1991). Recreation and leisure: A review of the literature and recommendations for future directions. In L. M. Meyer, C. A. Peck, & L. Brown (Eds.), *Critical issues in the lives of people with severe disabilities* (pp. 171-193). Baltimore, MD: Paul H. Brookes.

Dattilo, J. (1993). Facilitating reciprocal communication for individuals with severe communication disorders: Implications to leisure participation. *Palaestra, 10*(1), 39-48.

Dattilo, J., & Barnett, L. (1985). Therapeutic recreation for individuals with severe handicaps: Implications of chosen participation. *Therapeutic Recreation Journal, 19*, 79-91.

Dattilo, J., & Camarata, S. (1991). Facilitating conversation through self-initiated augmentative communication treatment. *Journal of Applied Behavior Analysis, 24*(2), 369-378.

Dattilo, J., & Kleiber, D. A. (1993). Psychological perspectives for therapeutic recreation research. In M. Malkin, & C. Z. Howe (Eds.), *Research in Therapeutic Recreation: Concepts and Methods.* State College, PA: Venture Publishing, Inc.

Dattilo, J., & Light, J. (1993). Setting the stage for leisure: Encouraging reciprocal communication for people using augmentative and alternative communication systems through facilitator instruction. *Therapeutic Recreation Journal, 27*(3), 156-171.

Dattilo, J., & Mirenda, P. (1987). The application of a leisure preference assessment protocol for persons with severe handicaps. *Journal of the Association for Persons with Severe Handicaps, 12*(4), 306-311.

Dattilo, J., & Murphy, W. D. (1987a). *Behavior modification in therapeutic recreation.* State College, PA: Venture Publishing, Inc.

Dattilo, J., & Murphy, W. D. (1987b). The challenge of adventure recreation for individual with disabilities. *Therapeutic Recreation Journal, 21*(3), 14-21.

Dattilo, J., & Murphy, W. D. (1991). *Leisure education program planning: A systematic approach.* State College, PA: Venture Publishing, Inc.

Dattilo, J. & O'Keefe, B. M. (1992). Setting the stage for leisure: Encouraging adults with mental retardation who use augmentative and alternative communication systems to share conversations. *Therapeutic Recreation Journal, 26*(1), 27-37.

Dattilo, J., & Rusch, F. (1985). Effects of choice on behavior: Leisure participation for persons with severe handicaps. *The Journal of the Association for Persons with Developmental Handicaps, 11*, 194-199.

Dattilo, J., & Schleien, S. J. (1991). *Consensus conference on the benefits of therapeutic recreation: A perspective on developmental disabilities. Working paper.* Philadelphia, PA: Temple University.

Dattilo, J., & Schleien, S. J. (1994). Understanding the provision of leisure services for persons with mental retardation. *Mental Retardation, 32*(1), 53-59.

Dattilo, J., & Smith, R. (1990). Communicating positive attitudes toward people with disabilities through sensitive terminology. *Therapeutic Recreation Journal, 24*(1), 8-17.

Dattilo, J., & St. Peter, S. (1991). A model for including leisure education in transition services for young adults with mental retardation. *Education and Training in Mental Retardation, 26*(4), 420-432.

Dattilo, J., & Weltner, L. (1991). Developing positive attitudes toward people with mental retardation. *Research Into Action: Applications for Therapeutic Recreation Programming, 8*, 2-8.

de Charms, R. (1968). *Enhancing motivation: Change in the classroom*. New York, NY: Irvington.

Deci, E. L. (1971). Effects of externally mediated rewards on intrinsic motivation. *Journal of Personality and Social Psychology, 18*, 105-115.

Deci, E. L. (1980). *The psychology of self-determination*. Lexington, MA: Lexington Books.

Deci, E. L., Betley, G., Kahle, J., Abrams, L., & Porac, J. (1981). When trying to win: Competition and intrinsic motivation. *Personality and Social Psychology Bulletin, 7*, 79-83.

Deci, E. L., & Chandler, C. L. (1986). The importance of motivation for the future of the LD field. *Journal of Learning Disabilities, 19*, 587-594.

Deci, E. L., & Olsen, B. C. (1989). Motivation and competition: Their role in sports. In J. Goldstein (Ed.), *Sports, games, and play: Social and psychological viewpoints* (pp. 83-110). Hillsdale, NJ: Lawrence Erlbaum Associates Publishers.

Deci, E. L., & Ryan, W. (1985). *Intrinsic motivation and self-determination in human behavior*. New York, NY: Plenum Press.

Decker, J. A. (1987). Social integration: The hard part. *Journal of Expanding Horizons in Therapeutic Recreation, 2*, 47-50.

Deutsch, M. (1969). Socially relevant science: Reflections on some studies of interpersonal conflict. *American Psychologist, 24*, 1076-1092.

de Villiers, P. (1987). Choice in concurrent schedules and a quantitative formulation of the law of effect. In W. K. Honig, & J. E. R. Staddon (Eds.), *Handbook of operant behavior* (pp. 233-287). Englewood Cliffs, NJ: Prentice-Hall.

Dietl, D. (1988). They won the roles with talent. *Worklife, 1*, 4-5.

Dolnick, E. (1993). Deafness as Culture. *The Atlantic Monthly, 272*(3), 37-53.

Donaldson, J. (1980). Changing attitudes toward handicapped persons: A review and analysis of research. *Exceptional Children, 46*, 504-515.

Donnellan, A., Mirenda, P., Mesaros, R., & Fassbender, L. (1984). Analyzing the communicative functions of aberrant behavior. *Journal of the Association for Persons with Severe Handicaps, 9*, 201-212.

Dorsch, E. (1987). Hypertension, heart attack, and stroke. In P. B. Doress & D. L. Siegal (Eds.), *Ourselves, growing older* (pp. 313-326). New York, NY: Simon & Schuster.

Dreimanus, M., Sobsey, D., Gray, S., Hamaha, B., Uditsky, B., & Wells, D. (1992). Annotated bibliography reveals strategies for education integration. *Edmonton Autism Society Update, 8*(1), 25-26. (Reprinted from Edmonton, AB: University of Alberta Severe Disabilities Program, 1990.)

Dunn, I. (1968). Special education for the mildly retarded: Is much of it justifiable? *Exceptional Children, 35*, 5-22.

Dutton, D. H. , & Dutton, D. L. (1990). Technology to support diverse needs in regular classes. In S. Stainback (Eds.), *Support networks for inclusive schooling: Interdependent integrated education* (167-183), Baltimore, MD: Brookes.

Dweck, C. S., & Light, B. A. (1980). In J. Garber, & M. Seligman (Eds.). *Human Helplessness* (pp. 197-221). New York, NY: Academic Press.

Edgar, E. (1992). Secondary options for students with mild intellectual disabilities: Facing the issues of tracking. *Education and Training in Mental Retardation, 27*(2), 101-111.

Eichmiller, S. (1990). Wheelchairs: Simulating is believing. *Penn State Journalist, 1*(1).

Eisenberg, M. G. (1982). Disability as stigma. In M. B. Eisenberg, C. Griggins, & R. J. Duval, (Eds.), *Disabled people as second-class citizens* (pp. 3-12). New York, NY: Springer.

Ellis, G. D., Maughan-Pritchett, M., & Ruddell, E. (1993). Effects of attribution based verbal persuasion and imagery on self-efficacy of adolescents diagnosed with major depression. *Therapeutic Recreation Journal, 26*(2), 83-97.

Engel, J. (1989). *Seizures and epilepsy.* Philadelphia, PA: F. A. Davis Co.

Enstrom, D. H. (1992). The Communication Resource Center: A New Jersey AAC service delivery model. *Augmentative and Alternative Communication, 8*, 234-242.

Evans, J. H. (1976). Changing attitudes toward disabled persons: An experimental study. *Rehabilitation Counseling Bulletin, 19*, 572-579.

Fabbri, P. (1991). You just can't keep Chuck down. *Sports Illustrated.*

Fenrick, N., & Petersen, T. (1984). Developing positive changes in attitudes toward moderately/severely handicapped students through peer tutoring program. *Education and Training of the Mentally Retarded, 19*, 83-90.

Ferguson, D. L., & Baumgart, D. (1991). Partial participation revisited. *Journal of the Association for Persons with Severe Handicaps, 16*(4), 218-227.

Ferguson, D. L., Meyer, G., Jeanchild, L., Juniper, L., & Zingo, J. (1992). Figuring out what to do with the grownups: How teachers make inclusion "work" for students with disabilities. *Journal of the Association for Persons with Severe Handicaps, 17*(4), 218-226.

Ferguson, P. M., Ferguson, D. L., & Taylor, S. J. (1992). Conclusion: The future of interpretivism in disability studies. In P. M. Ferguson, D. L., Ferguson, & S. J. Taylor (Eds.), *Interpreting disability*, (pp. 169-171). New York, NY: Teachers College Press.

Ficker-Terrill, C., & Rowitz, L. (1991). Choices. *Mental Retardation, 29*(2), 63-65.

Fico, L. (1992). The interface between community and therapeutic recreation: Implications for the 21st century. *NTRS Report, 17*(3), 5-7

Fink, D. (1988). *School-age children with special needs. What do they do when school is out?* Boston, MA: Exceptional Parent Press.

Fishbein, M., & Ajzen, I. (1975). *Belief, attitude, intention and behavior: An introduction to theory and research.* Reading, MA: Addison-Wesley.

Flynn, R., & Nitsch, K. (Eds.). (1980). *Normalization, social integration and community services.* Baltimore, MD: University Park Press.

Flynt, S. W., Wood, T. A., & Scott, R. L. (1992). Social support of mothers of children with mental retardation. *Mental Retardation, 30*(4), 233-236.

Ford, A., Brown, L., Pumpian, I., Baumgart, D., Nisbet, J., Schroeder, J., & Loomis, R. (1984). Strategies for developing individual recreation/ leisure plans for adolescent and young adult severely handicapped students. In N. Certo, N. Haring, and R. York (Eds.), *Public school integration of severely handicapped students: Rational issues and progressive alternatives* (pp. 245-275). Baltimore, MD: Paul H. Brookes.

Foster, G. G., Schmidt, C., & Sabatino, D. (1976). Teacher expectations and the label "learning disabilities." *Journal of Learning Disabilities, 9*, 58-61.

Foster, G. G., Ysseldyke, J. E., & Reese, J. H. (1975). I wouldn't have seen it if I hadn't believed it. *Exceptional Children, 41*, 469-473.

Fox, J. (1985, May 31). Image of mentally ill distorted by society: Point of view. *Lincoln Journal Star.*

Fox, S. (1993, August 16). Rehab is important aspect of neuroimplantation program. *Advance: For speech-Language Pathologists & Audiologists, 3*(17), 10, 40.

Fredricks, B. (1987). Tim becomes an Eagle Scout. *The Exceptional Parent, 17*, 22-27.

Friedland, J. F., & McColl, M. (1992). Social support intervention after stroke: Results of a randomized trial. *Archives of Physical Medicine and Rehabilitation, 73*, 573- 581.

Friedrich, W., Wilturner, L., & Cohen, D. (1985). Coping resources and parenting mentally retarded children. *American Journal of Mental Deficiency, 90*(2), 130-139.

Fulghum, R. (1989). *It was on fire when I lay down on it.* New York, NY: Ivy Books.

Funk, R. (1987). Disability rights: From caste to class in the context of civil rights. In A. Gartner & T. Joe (Eds.), *Images of the disabled, disabling images*. New York, NY: Praegel Publisher.

Galambos, L., Lee, R., Rahn, P., & Williams, B. (1994). The ADA: Getting beyond the door. *Parks and Recreation, 29*(4), 67-71.

Gall, E. (1992). What can be done when arthritis starts in the hands causing lumps in the joints? *Arizona Alumnus, 1*, 15.

Gallagher, J., Beckman, P., & Cross, A. (1983). Families of handicapped children: Sources of stress and its amelioration. *Exceptional Children, 50*(1), 10-19.

Garber, J., & Seligman, M. (1980). *Human Helplessness*. New York, NY: Academic Press.

Georgia Advocacy Office. (1992). *Promoting inclusion*. Atlanta, GA.

Gething, L. (1992). *Person to person*. Baltimore, MD: Paul H. Brookes.

Gibbons, D. & Jones, J. (1975). *The study of deviance: Perspectives and problems*. Englewood Cliffs, NJ: Prentice-Hall.

Gill, C. (1994). Disability and the family. *Mainstream, 18*(5), 30-35.

Girdano, D. A., Everly, G. S., & Dusek, D. E. (1990). *Controlling stress and tension: A holistic approach (3rd ed.)*. Englewood Cliffs, NJ: Prentice Hall.

Goffman, E. (1963). *Stigma: Notes on the management of spoiled identity*. Englewood Cliffs, NJ: Prentice Hall.

Goffman, E. (1974). *Stigma*. New York, NY: Jason Aronson.

Gold, D., & Crawford, C. (1989). *Leisure connections: Helping people with a disability lead richer lives in the community*. Toronto, ON: G. Allan Roeher Institute.

Goldenson, R. M. (1978). Muscular dystrophy. In R. M. Goldenson, J. R. Dunham, & C. S. Dunham (Eds.), *Disability and rehabilitation handbook* (480-485). New York, NY: McGraw-Hill, Inc.

Goldfard, L., Brotherson, J. J., Summers, J. A., & Turnbull, A. P. (1987). *Meeting the challenge of disability or chronic illness: A family guide.* Baltimore, MD: Paul H. Brookes.

Goldstein, H., Kaczmarek, L., Pennington, R., & Schafer, K. (1992). Peer-mediated interventions: Attending to, commenting on, and acknowledging the behavior of preschoolers with autism. *Journal of Applied Behavior Analysis, 25*(2), 289-305.

Goodale, T. (1992). Roger Mannell, social psychology of leisure researcher, receives 1991 Roosevelt Award. *Parks and Recreation, 27*(4), 18-21, 82.

Gordon, J. (1977). *Parent effectiveness training.* New York, NY: Wyden Books.

Gottlieb, M. (1987). Major variation in intelligence. In M. Gottlieb & J. Williams (Eds.), *Textbook of developmental pediatrics,* (pp. 127-150). New York, NY: Plenum Medical.

Green, F. P., & DeCoux, V. (1994). A procedure for evaluating the effectiveness of a community recreation integration program. *Therapeutic Recreation Journal, 28*(1), 41-47.

Grossman, H. J. (Ed.). (1983). *Classification in mental retardation.* Washington, DC: American Association on Mental Deficiency.

Gunn, S. L. (1975). *Basic terminology for therapeutic recreation and other action therapies.* Champaign, IL: Stipes.

Guralnick, M. J., & Groom, J. M. (1988). Peer interactions in mainstreamed and specialized classrooms: A comparative analysis. *Specialized Children, 54,* 415-426.

Guskin, S. (1981). Directions for research on attitudes related to mental retardation. In P. Mittler (Ed.), *Frontiers of knowledge in mental retardation, Vol. 1,* (pp. 397-405). Baltimore, MD: University Park Press.

Hale, G. (1979). *The source book for the disabled.* New York, NY: Bantam Books.

Hallem, J. J. D. controls his environment. *Spinal Column, 49.*

Halliwell, W. (1978). The effects of cognitive development on children's perceptions of intrinsically and extrinsically motivated behavior. In D. Landers & R. Christina (Eds.), *Psychology of motor behavior and sport - 1977* (pp. 403-419). Champaign, IL: Human Kinetics Publishers.

Hamilton, E. J., & Anderson, S. (1991). Effects of leisure activities on attitudes toward people with disabilities. *Therapeutic Recreation Journal, 17*(3), 50-57.

Hamilton, J. A. (1983). Development of interest and enjoyment in adolescence. Part II. Boredom and psychopathology. *Journal of Youth and Adolescence, 12*, 363-372.

Hammel, J. M., Van der Loos, H. F. M., & Perkash, I. (1992). Evaluation of a vocational robot with a quadriplegic employee. *Archives of Physical Medicine and Rehabilitation, 73*(7), 683-693.

Hamre-Nietupski, S., Hendrickson, J., Nietupski, J., & Sasso, G. (1993). Perceptions of teachers of students with moderate, severe, or profound disabilities on facilitating friendships with nondisabled peers. *Education and Training in Mental Retardation, 28*(2), 111-127.

Hamre-Nietupski, S., Krajewski, L., Nietupski, J., Ostercamp, D., Sensor, K., & Opheim, B. (1988). Parent/Professional partnerships in advocacy: Developing integrated options within resistive systems. *Journal of the Association for Persons with Severe Handicaps, 13*, 251-259.

Handleman, J. S., & Harris, S. L. (1986). *Educating the developmentally disabled: Meeting the needs of children and families*. Boston, MA: Little, Brown, and Company.

Hanline, M. F. (1993). Inclusion of preschoolers with profound disabilities: An analysis of children's interactions. *Journal of the Association for Persons with Severe Handicaps, 18*(1), 28-35.

Hanline, M. F., & Fox, L. (1993). Learning within the context of play: Providing typical early childhood experiences for children with severe disabilities. *The Journal of the Association for Persons with Severe Handicaps, 18*(2), 121-129.

Harackiewicz, J. (1979). The effects of reward contingency and performance feedback on intrinsic motivation. *Journal of Personality and Social Psychology, 37*, 1352-1363.

Harrell, L. (1984). *Touch the baby—Blind and visually impaired children as patients: Helping them respond to care.* New York, NY: American Foundation for the Blind.

Hastorf, A. H., Wildfogel, J., & Cassman, T. (1979). Acknowledgment of handicap as a tactic in social interaction. *Journal of Personality and Social Psychology, 37*, 1790-1797.

Hawkins, B. A. (1993). A exploratory analysis of leisure and life satisfaction of aging adults with mental retardation. *Therapeutic Recreation Journal, 26*, 98-109.

Hayes, G. A. (1977). Professional preparation and leisure counseling. *Journal of Physical Education and Recreation, 48*(4), 36-38.

Herman, S., & Hazel, K. L. (1991). Evaluation of family support services: Changes in availability and accessibility. *Mental Retardation, 29*(6), 351-357.

Hersch, H. (1991). Ace of the Angels. *Sports Illustrated*, 22-29.

Heyne, L. A., Schleien, S. J., & McEvoy, L. H. (Eds.). (1993). *Making friends: Using recreation activities to promote friendship between children with and without disabilities.* Minneapolis, MN: Institute on Community Integration (UAP).

Hoenk, A. H., & Mobily, K. E. (1987). Mainstreaming the play environment: Effects of previous exposure and salience of disability. *Therapeutic Recreation Journal, 21*(4), 23-31.

Hollins, M. (1989). *Understanding blindness: An integrative approach.* Hillsdale, NJ: Lawrence Erlbaum Assoc., Inc.

Howe-Murphy, R., & Charboneau, B. G. (1987). *Therapeutic recreation intervention: An ecological perspective.* Englewood Cliffs, NJ: Prentice-Hall.

Howell, L. (1978). Brain damage. In R. M. Goldenson, J. R. Dunham, & C. S. Dunham (Eds.), *Disability and rehabilitation handbook* (pp.284-295), NJ: McGraw-Hill, Inc.

Hultsman, W. Z. (1993). The influence of others as a barrier to recreation participation among early adolescents. *Journal of Leisure Research, 25*, 150-164.

Hutchison, P. (1990). *Making friends: Developing relationships between people with a disability and other members of the community.* Toronto, ON: G. Allan Roeher Institute.

Hutchison, P., & Lord, J. (1979). Recreation integration: Issues and alternatives in leisure services and community involvement. Ottawa, ON: Leisurability Publications, Inc.

Hutchison, P., & McGill, J. (1992). *Leisure, integration and community.* Concord, ON: Leisurability Publications, Inc.

Hyser, C. L., & Mendell, J. R. (1988). Recent advances in duchenne and becker muscular dystrophy. In J. E. Riggs (Ed.), *Neurologic Clinics, 6*(3), 429-453.

Iso-Ahola, S. E. (1980). *The social psychology of leisure and recreation.* Dubuque, IA: William C. Brown.

Iso-Ahola, S. E., & Crowley, E. D. (1991). Adolescent substance abuse and leisure boredom. *Journal of Leisure Research, 23*, 260-271.

Iso-Ahola, S. E., & Weissinger, E. (1987). Leisure and boredom. *Journal of Social and Clinical Psychology, 5*(3), 356-364.

Iso-Ahola, S. E., & Weissinger, E. (1990). Perceptions of boredom in leisure: Conceptualization, reliability, and validity of the leisure boredom scale. *Journal of Leisure Research, 22*, 1-17.

Jacobson, W. H., & Smith, T. E. C. (1983). Use of the Sonicguide™ and laser cane in obtaining or keeping employment. *Journal of Visual Impairment & Blindness, 77*, 12-15.

Jansma, P., & Shultz, B. (1982). Validation and use of a mainstreaming attitude inventory with physical educators. *American Corrective Therapy Journal, 36*, 150-158.

Jesiolowski, J. (1988). Attitudes toward disabilities discussed. *The Daily Collegian*, p. 2.

Johnson, D. W., & Johnson, R. T. (1984). *Cooperation in the classroom.* Edina, MN: Interaction Book Company.

Jolly, A. C., Test, D. W., & Spooner, F. (1993). Using badges to increase initiations of children with severe disabilities in a play setting. *Journal of the Association for Persons with Severe Handicaps, 18*(1), 46-51.

Jones, E. E., Farina, A., Hastorf, A. H., Markus, H., Miller, D. T., & Scott, R. A. (1984). *Social stigma: The psychology of marked relationships.* New York, NY: Freeman.

Jones, R. (1972). Labels and stigma in special education. *Exceptional Children, 38*, 553-564.

Jones, W. J., Sowell, V. M., Jones, J. K., & Butler, L. G. (1981). Changing children's perceptions of handicapped people. *Exceptional Children, 47*, 365-368.

Joswiak, K. F. (1979). *Leisure counseling program materials for the developmentally disabled.* Washington, DC: Hawkins & Associates.

Judd, T. (1991). Reflex crying. *Evergreen Stroke Association, 13*(10), 6-7, 10.

Kart, C. S., Metress, E. K., & Metress, S. P. (1988). *Aging, health and society.* Boston, MA: Jones & Bartlett.

Kasper, R. (1990). About technology and hearing. *Independent Living*, 59-60.

Kelly, J. R. (1983). *Leisure identities and interactions.* Boston, MA: George Allen & Unwin, Ltd.

Kelly, J. R. (1987). *Freedom to be: A new sociology of leisure.* New York, NY: Macmillan.

Kelley, H. H., Hastorf, A. H., Jones, E. E., Thibaut, J. W., & Usdane, W. M. (1960). Some implications of social psychological theory for research on the handicapped. In L. H. Lofquist (Ed.), *Psychological research and rehabilitation* (Miami Conference Report, pp. 172-204). Washington, DC: American Psychological Association.

Kelley, H. H., & Thibaut, J. W. (1969). Group problem solving. In G. Lindzey, & E. Aronson (Eds.), *The handbook of social psychology* (pp. 1-101). Reading, MA: Addison-Wesley.

Kennedy, D. W., Austin, D. R., & Smith, R. W. (1987). *Special recreation: Opportunities for persons with disabilities*. Philadelphia, PA: Saunders College Publishing.

Kennedy, T., Jr. (1986, November 23). Our right to independence. *Parade Magazine*, pp. 4-6.

Keogh, D. A., Faw, G. D., Whitman, T. L., & Reid, D. H. (1984). Enhancing leisure skills in severely retarded adolescents through a self-instructional treatment package. *Analysis and Intervention in Developmental Disabilities, 4*, 333-351.

Kinney, W. B., & Sottile, J. (1991). Psychiatry and mental health. In D. R. Austin & M. E. Crawford (Eds.), *Therapeutic recreation: An introduction* (pp. 240-263). Englewood Cliff, NJ: Prentice Hall.

Kisabeth, K. L., & Richardson, D. B. (1985). Changing attitudes toward disabled individuals: The effect of one disabled person. *Therapeutic Recreation Journal, 19*(2), 24-33.

Kishi, G., Teelucksingh, B., Zollers, N., Park-Lee, S., & Meyer, L. (1988). Daily decision-making in community residences: A social comparison of adults with and without mental retardation. *American Journal on Mental Retardation, 92*, 430-435.

Kleck, R. (1966). Emotional arousal in interactions with stigmatized persons. *Psychological Reports, 19*, 1226.

Kleck, R. (1968). Physical stigma and nonverbal cues emitted in face-to-face interaction. *Human Relations, 21*, 19-28.

Kleck, R., Ono, H., & Hastorf, A. H. (1966). The effects of physical deviance upon face-to-face interaction. *Human Relations, 19*, 425-436.

Kleiber, D. A., & Dirkin, G. (1985). Intrapersonal constraints to leisure. In M. Wade (Ed.), *Constraints on leisure* (pp. 17-42). Springfield, IL: C. C. Thomas.

Kleiber, D. A., & Kelly, J. R. (1980). Leisure, socialization, and the life cycle. In S. Iso-Ahola (Ed.), *Social psychological perspectives on leisure and recreation.* Springfield, IL: C. C. Thomas.

Kleiber, D. A., & Rickards, M. (1985). Leisure and recreation in adolescence: Limitations and potential. In M. G. Wade (Ed.), *Constraints on leisure* (pp. 289-317). Springfield, IL: C.C. Thomas.

Klein, E. (1992). *Lap pillow holder. Sharing innovations: A self-help guide for people with rheumatoid arthritis*, p. 7. Summit, NJ: Lederle Laboratories.

Knox, V., Gekoski, W., & Johnson, E. (1986). Contact with and perceptions of the elderly. *The Gerontologist, 26*(3), 309-313.

Kohl, F. L., & Beckman, P. J. (1990). The effects of directed play on the frequency and length of reciprocal interactions with preschoolers having moderate handicaps. *Education and Training in Mental Retardation, 25*(3), 258-266.

Kraat, A. (1985). Developing intervention goals. In S. Blackstone (Ed.), *Augmentative and alternative communication* (pp. 197-266). Rockville, MD: American Speech-Language-Hearing Association.

Kraus, R. & Shank, J. (1992). *Therapeutic recreation services.* Dubuque, IA: Wm. C. Brown Publishers.

Krauss, M. W. (1986). Patterns and trends in public services to families with a mentally retarded member. In J. J. Gallagher & P. M. Vietze (Eds.), Families of handicapped persons: Research, programs, and policy issues (pp. 237-248). Baltimore, MD: Paul H. Brookes.

Krebs, P. L., & Block, M. E. (1992). Transition of students with disabilities into community recreation: The role of the adapted physical educator. *Adapted Physical Activity Quarterly, 9*(4), 305-315.

Laird, R. (1992, Winter). Access—It's a matter of attitude. *Integrare*, 7-8.

Lanagan, D., & Dattilo, J. (1989). The effects of a leisure education program on individuals with severe disabilities. *Therapeutic Recreation Journal, 23*(4), 8-17.

Langer, E. J. (1983). *The psychology of control.* Beverly Hills, CA: Sage Publications.

Langlois, M. (1990, Summer). Recreation choices. *Integrare*, 1-2.

Larson, R., Mannell, R., & Zuzanek, J. (1986). Daily well-being of older adults with friends and family. *Journal of Psychology and Aging, 1*, 117-126.

Larson, R., Zuzanek, J., & Mannell, R. (1985). Being alone versus being with people: Disengagement in the daily experience of older adults. *Journal of Gerontology, 40*, 375-381.

Lazar, A., Gensley, J., & Orpet, R. E. (1971). Changing attitudes of young mentally gifted children toward handicapped persons. *Exceptional Children, 37*, 600-602.

Leary, M. R., & Miller, R. S. (1986). *Social psychology and dysfunctional behavior: Origins, diagnosis, and treatment.* New York, NY: Springer-Verlag.

Ledman, S. M., Thompson, B., & Hill, J. W. (1992). The every buddy program: An integrated after-school program. *Children Today, 20*(2), 17-20.

Lepper, M. R., & Greene, D. (1978). *The hidden costs of rewards.* Hillsdale, NJ: Lawrence Erlbaum Associates.

Lepper, M. R., Greene, D., & Nisbett, R. E. (1973). Undermining children's intrinsic interest with extrinsic rewards: A test of "overjustification" hypothesis. *Journal of Personality and Social Psychology, 28*, 129-137.

Levin, J., & Enselein, K. (1990). *Fun for everyone: A guide to adapted leisure activities for children with disabilities.* Minneapolis, MN: Able Net.

Levy, J. M., Jessop, D. J., Rimmerman, A., & Levy, P. H. (1992). Attitudes of Fortune 500 corporate executives toward the employability of persons with severe disabilities: A national study. *Mental Retardation, 30*(2), 67-75.

Light, J. (1988). Interaction involving individuals using augmentative and alternative communication systems: State of the art and future directions. *Augmentative and Alternative Communication, 4*(2), 66-82.

Loiseau, P. (1992). The Jacksonian model of partial motor seizures. In P. Chauvel, A. Delgado-Escueta, E. Halgren, & J. Bancaud (Eds.), *Advances in neurology: Vol. 57. Frontal lobe seizures and epilepsies*. New York, NY: Raven Press.

Lord, J. (1981). Opening doors, opening minds! *Recreation Canada*, Special Issue, 4-5.

Lovell, J., & Lovell, J. (1993, August 15). I am not defined by my disorder. *Parade Magazine*, p. 6.

Luken, K. (April, 1993). Reintegration through recreation. *Parks and Recreation*, 54-57.

Mace, R. L. (1977). Architectural accessibility. *White House Conference on Handicapped Individuals. Vol. 1: Awareness Papers*. Washington, DC: U. S. Government Printing Office.

Maddox, S. (Ed.). (1988). *Spinal Network*. Boulder, CO: Spinal Network.

Mahon, M. J., & Bullock, C. C. (1992). Teaching adolescents with mild mental retardation to make decisions in leisure through use of self-control techniques. *Therapeutic Recreation Journal, 26*(1), 9-26.

Makas, E. (1988). Positive attitudes toward disabled people: Disabled and nondisabled person's perspectives. *Journal of Social Sciences, 44*(1), 49-61.

Mann, W., & Lane, J. (1991). *Assistive technology for persons with disabilities: The role of occupational therapy*. Rockville, MD: The American Occupational Therapy Association.

Marlowe, M. (1979). The game analysis intervention: A procedure to increase the peer acceptance and social adjustment of a retarded child. *Education and Training of the Mentally Retarded, 14*, 262-268.

Martens, R., Vealey, R. S., & Burton, D. (1990). *Competitive anxiety in sport.* Champaign, IL: Human Kinetics Press.

Martin, R. (1986a). *Is your child entitled to a summer program?* Austin, TX: Advocacy Inc.

Martin, R. (1986b). *The end of take it or leave it IEPs.* Austin, TX: Advocacy Inc.

Mastervoice. (1992). *Advertising brochure.* Los Alamitos, CA.

Matson, J., Sevin, J., Box, M., Francis, K., & Sevin, B. (1993). An evaluation of two methods for increasing self-initiated verbalizations in autistic children. *Journal of Applied Behavior Analysis, 26*, 389-398

Maughan, M., & Ellis, G. D. (1991). Effect of efficacy information during recreation participation on efficacy judgements of depressed adolescents. *Therapeutic Recreation Journal, 25*(1), 50-59.

McCarty, K. S. (1991). *Complying with the ADA.* Washington, DC: National League of Cities.

McDonald, R. G., & Howe, C. Z. (1989). Challenge/initiative recreation programs as a treatment for low self-concept children. *Journal of Leisure Research, 21*(3), 242-253.

McDowell, C. F. (1976). *Leisure counseling: Selected lifestyle processes.* Eugene, OR: Center for Leisure Studies.

McEvoy, M., Nordquist, V., Twardosz, S., Heckaman, K. A., Wehby, J., & Denny, K. (1988). Promoting autistic children's peer interaction in an integrated early childhood setting using affection activities. *Journal of Applied Behavior Analysis, 21*, 193-200.

McFadden, D. L., & Burke, E. P. (1991). Developmental disabilities and the new paradigm: Directions for the 1990s. *Mental Retardation, 29*(1), iii-vi.

McGill, J. (1984). Training for integration: Are blindfolds really enough? *Journal of Leisurability, 11*(2), 12-15.

McGill, J. (1987). *We are people first—A book on self-advocacy.* Lincoln, NE: Nebraska Advocacy Services.

McGovern, J. (1990). Public policy: The Americans with disabilities act: How this new law will change your park and recreation agency. *Recreation...Access in the 90s, 1*(1), 1-5.

McGovern, J. (1991a). Public policy: Employment, leisure service agencies, and the ADA. *Recreation...Access in the 90s, 2*(1), 11-21.

McGovern, J. (1991b). Justice department publishes final rules on the Americans with Disabilities Act. *Parks and Recreation, 26*(11), 12-14.

McGovern, J. (1992). The Americans with disabilities act: How will this law be enforced and what is its impact on recreation programming? *Impact*, 21-23.

McLean, M., & Hanline, M. F. (1990). Providing early intervention services in integrated environments: Challenges and opportunities for the future. *Topics in Early Childhood Special Education, 10*(2), 62-77.

McQuillen, M. P. (1990). Introduction. In S. M. Rao (Ed.), *Neurobehavioral aspects of multiple sclerosis* (pp. 3-4), New York, NY: Oxford University Press, Inc.

Medgyesi, V. (1988). Media watch: How the press reports on disability issues. *Habilitation News, 8*(5), 10-11.

Merlo, A., Staniszewski, S. C., & Sarrett, S. (1990). *Accessibility: An overview.* Albertson, NY: National Center for Disability Services.

Michels, R. (1985, January 27). Greater research necessary into mental ills, addictions. *Sunday Journal-Star.*

Miller, E. (1991, July 1). The rabbi of roundball. *Sports Illustrated*, pp. 5-6.

Miller, H., Rynders, J. E., & Schleien, S. J. (1993). Drama: A medium to enhance social interaction between students with and without mental retardation. *Mental Retardation, 31*(4), 228-233.

Miracle Recreation Equipment Co. (1993). *A word about ADA*. Monett, MO.

Mirenda, P. (1985). Designing pictorial communication systems for physically able-bodied students with severe handicaps. *Augmentative and Alternative Communication, 1*, 58-64.

Misenti, M., Lucas, B., & Thompson, G. (1992). *Understanding brain injury: Neurologic rehabilitation*. Boston, MA: Headlines.

Mobily, K. E. (1989). Meaning of recreation and leisure among adolescents. *Leisure Studies, 8*(1), 11-23.

Mobily, K. E., Lemke, J. H., & Gisin, G. J. (1991). The idea of leisure repertoire. *Journal of Applied Gerontology, 10*, 208-223.

Mobily, K. E., Lemke, J. H., Ostiguy, L. J., Woodward, R. J., Griffee, T. J., Pickens, C. C. (1993). Leisure repertoire in a sample of Midwestern elderly: The case for exercise. *Journal of Therapeutic Recreation, 25*(1), 84-99.

Montagnes, J. A. (1976). Reality therapy approach to leisure counseling. *Journal of Leisurability, 3*, 37-45.

Montgomery, R. (1992, November). First encounters. *Parenting*, pp. 261-262.

Moore, J. Technology is not magic. *Exceptional Parent, 21*(7), 60-62.

Moss, K. (Ed.). (1993). *P.S. News, 5*(1).

Mount, B., & O'Brien, J. (1988). Person centered planning. In J. O'Brien & C. L. O'Brien (Eds.), *Framework for accomplishment* (pp. 1-4). Lithonia, GA: Responsive Systems Associates.

Mount, B., & Zwernik, K. (1988). *It's never too early, it's never too late: A booklet about personal future planning*. St. Paul, MN: Metropolitan Council.

Mundy, J., & Odum, L. (1979). *Leisure education: Theory and practice*. New York, NY: John Wiley & Sons.

Munson, W. W., Baker, S. B., & Lundegren, H. M. (1985). Strength training and leisure counseling as treatments for institutionalized juvenile delinquents. *Adapted Physical Activity Quarterly, 2*(1), 65-75.

Murphy, J. A. (1987). *How does a blind person get around?* New York, NY: American Foundation for the Blind, Inc.

Murphy, J. F. (1975). *Recreation and leisure service: A humanistic perspective.* Dubuque, IA: W. C. Brown.

Murphy, R. F. (1990). *The silent body.* New York, NY: W. W. Norton & Co.

Murray, C. (1988). *In pursuit of happiness and good government.* New York, NY: Simon and Schuster.

National Easter Seals Society. (1981). Portraying persons with disabilities in print. *Rehabilitation Literature, 42*, 284-285.

National Information Center for Children and Youth with Disabilities (NICHCY). (1991). *Spina bifida.* Washington, DC: Author.

Nelson, M. (1987, November, 20). Miss deaf Pennsylvania breaks barriers. *Bloomsburg Press-Enterprise.*

Neulinger, J. (1974). *The psychology of leisure.* Springfield, IL: Charles C. Thomas.

Newton, J. S., Horner, R. H., & Lund, L. (1991). Honoring activity preferences in individualized plan development: A descriptive analysis. *Journal of the Association of Severe Handicaps, 16*(4), 207-221.

Nietupski, J., Hamre-Nietupski, S., & Ayres, B. (1984). Review of task analytic leisure skill training efforts: Practitioner implications and future research needs. *Journal of the Association for Persons with Severe Handicaps, 9*(2), 88-97.

Nissen, S. J., & Newman, W. P. (1992). Factors influencing reintegration to normal living after amputation. *Archives of Physical Medicine and Rehabilitation, 73*, 548-551.

Novak, A., & Heal, L. (Eds.) (1980). *Integration of developmentally disabled individuals into the community.* Baltimore, MD: Paul Brookes Publishing.

O'Brien, J. (1988). *Personal futures planning.* Lithonia, GA: Responsive Systems Associates.

Odom, S., Hoyson, M., Jamieson, B., & Strain, P. (1985). Increasing handicapped preschoolers peer social interactions: Cross-setting and component analysis. *Journal of Applied Behavior Analysis, 18*, 3-16.

Odom, S., & McEvoy, M. (1988). Integration of young children with handicapped and nonhandicapped children: Mainstreaming versus integrated special education. In S. Odom & M. Karnes (Eds.), *Early interventions for infants and children with handicaps: An empirical base* (pp. 241-267). Baltimore, MD: Paul H. Brookes.

Oestreicher, M. (1990). Accessible recreation: 20 years behind the times. *Parks and Recreation Magazine, 25*(8), 52-55.

Olson, D. H., McCubbin, H. I., Barnes, H., Larsen, A., Muxem, M., & Wilson, M. (1983). *Families: What makes them work.* Beverly Hills, CA: Sage.

O'Morrow, G. S. (1980). *Therapeutic recreation: A helping profession.* Reston, VA: Reston.

Orlick, T. D., & Mosher, R. (1978). Extrinsic rewards and participant motivation in a sport related task. *International Journal of Sport Psychology, 9*, 27-39.

Overmier, B., & Seligman, M. (1967). Effects of inescapable shock upon subsequent escape and avoidance learning. *Journal of Comparative and Physiological Psychology, 63*, 28-33.

Overs, R. P., Taylor, S., & Adkins, C. (1974). Avocational counseling for the elderly. *Journal of Physical Education and Recreation, 48*(4), 44-45.

Paciorek, M. J. (1993). Technology only a part of the story as world records fall. *Palaestra, 9*(2), 14-17.

Parent, W. S. (1993). Quality of life and consumer choice. In P. Wehman (Ed.), *The ADA mandate for social change* (pp. 19-41). Baltimore, MD: Paul Brooks Publishing.

Parette, H., & Van Biervliet, A. (1991). School age children with disabilities: Technology implications foe counselors. *Elementary School Guidance and Counseling, 25*(3), 183-193.

Patrick, G. D. (1987). Improving attitudes toward disabled persons. *Adapted Physical Activity Quarterly, 4*(4), 316-325.

Perlman, I. (1987, March). To help the handicapped, talk to them. *Glamour*, p. 64

Perske, R. (Ed.). (1979). What it means to be a real advocate [Special Issue]. *Deficience Mentale/Mental Retardation, 29*(2), 15.

Peterson, C. A., & Gunn, S. L. (1984). *Therapeutic recreation program design: Principles and procedures (2nd ed.).* Englewood Cliffs, NJ: Prentice-Hall.

Petty, R. E., & Cacioppo, J. T. (1981). *Attitudes and persuasion: Classic and contemporary approaches.* Dubuque, IA: W. C. Brown.

Prentke Romich Company. (1992). *Changing Lives.* Wooster, OH: Author.

Project LIFE. (1988). *Project LIFE: Leisure is for everyone, training package.* Chapel Hill, NC: University of North Carolina at Chapel Hill.

Rag Time (1989, February). *TASH Newsletter, 15*, 6, 8.

Ray, M. T., Abery, B., DePaepe, P., Cameron, J., & Green, R. (1989). Linking lives. *Impact, 2*(3), 7, 17.

Ray, M. T., & Meidl, D. (1991). *Fun futures: Community recreation and developmental disabilities.* St. Paul, MN: SCOLA of Arc Ramsey County.

Rees, L., Spreen, O., & Harnadek, M. (1991). Do attitudes toward persons with handicaps really shift over time? *Mental Retardation, 29*(2), 81-86.

Research and Training Center on Independent Living. (1984). *Guidelines for reporting and writing about people with disabilities.* Lawrence, KA: Author.

Retzinger, J. (1990). Chair Image. *Spinal Network Extra*, p. 6.

Rice, H. G. (1992). Understanding shrinkage of the residual limb. *Amputee Foundation of Greater Atlanta, 1*(3), p. 2.

Rice, J. M. (1989). Decreasing osteoarthritis pain: A psychological case report with follow-up data. *The Clinical Journal of Pain, 5*(2), 183-188.

Richler, D. (1984). Access to community resources: The invisible barriers to integration. *Journal of Leisurability, 11*(2), 4-11.

Rizzo, T. L., & Vispoel, W. P. (1991). Physical educators' attributes and attitudes toward teaching students with handicaps. *Adapted Physical Activity Quarterly, 8*, 4-11.

Rizzo, T. L., & Vispoel, W. P. (1992). Changing attitudes about teaching students with handicaps. *Adapted Physical Activity Quarterly, 9*, 54-63.

Rizzo, T. L., & Wright, R. G. (1987). Secondary school physical educators' attitudes toward teaching students with handicaps. *American Corrective Therapy Journal, 41*(2), 52-55.

Rook, K. S. (1987). Social support versus companionship: Effects on life stress, loneliness, and evaluations by others. *Journal of Personality and Social Psychology, 52*, 1132-1147.

Roper, P. A. (1990). Special Olympics volunteers' perceptions of people with mental retardation. *Education and Training in Mental Retardation, 25*(2), 164-175.

Rosenberg, M. J., & Houland, C. I. (1960). Cognitive, affective, and behavioral components of attitudes. In C.Hovland & M. Rosenberg (Eds), *Attitude organization and change* (pp. 1-14). New Haven, CT: Yale University Press.

Rosenthal, R., & Jacobson, L. (1968). *Pygmalion in the classroom*. New York, NY: Holt, Rinehart, & Winston.

Ross, C. D. (1983). Leisure in the deinstitutionalization process: A vehicle for change. *Journal of Leisurability, 10*(1), 13-19.

Ross, C. D., & Van den Haag, E. (1957). *The fabric of society*. New York, NY: Harcourt Brace Jovanovich.

Ross, M. (1975). Salience of reward and intrinsic motivation. *Journal of Personality and Social Psychology, 32*, 245-254.

Rousey, A., Best, S., & Blacher, J. (1992). Mothers' and Fathers' perceptions of stress and coping with children who have severe disabilities. *American Journal on Mental Retardation, 97*(1), 99-109.

Rowe, J., & Stutts, R. M. (1987). Effects of practical type, experience, and gender on attitudes of undergraduate physical education majors toward disabled persons. *Adapted Physical Activity Quarterly, 4*, 268-277.

Rowitz, L. (1992). A family affair. *Mental Retardation, 30*(2), iii-iv.

Rowitz, L., & Stoneman, Z. (1990). Community first. *Mental Retardation*, 28(3), iii-iv.

Royal, C. (1992). The road to personal freedom. *OSERS: News In Print, 5*(2), 8-11.

Rusch, F. R., Chadsey-Rusch, J., White, D. M., & Gifford, J. L. (1985). Programs for severely retarded adults: Perspectives and methodologies. In D. Bricker & J. Filler (Eds.), *Severe mental retardation: From theory to practice*. Reston, VA: Council for Exceptional Children.

Rynders, J., & Schleien, S. (1991). *Together successfully: Creating recreational and educational programs that integrate people with and without disabilities*. Arlington, TX: Association for Retarded Citizens-United State, National 4-H, and the Institute on Community Integration, University of Minnesota.

Sable, J. (1992). Collaborating to create an integrated camping program: Design and evaluation. *Therapeutic Recreation Journal, 26*(3), 38-48.

Saetermoe, C., Wideman, K., & Borthwick-Duffy, S. (1991). Validation of the parenting style survey for parents of children with mental retardation. *Mental Retardation, 29*, 149-157.

Safilios-Rothschild, C. (1970). *The sociology and social psychology of disability and rehabilitation*. New York, NY: Random House.

Salisbury, C., & Evans, I. (1988). Comparison of parental involvement in regular and special education. *Journal of the Association for Persons with Severe Handicaps, 13*, 268-272.

Sanford, M. E., & Petajan, J. H. (1990). Effects of multiple sclerosis on daily living. In S. M. Rao (Ed.), *Neurobehavioral aspects of multiple sclerosis* (pp. 251-265). New York, NY: Oxford University Press, Inc.

Schalock, R. L., Keith, D. D., Hoffman, K., & Karan, O. C. (1989). Quality of life: Its measurement and use. *Mental Retardation, 27*, 25-31.

Schalock, R. L., Stark, J. A., Snell, M. E., Coutler, D. L., Polloway, E. A., Luckasson, R., Reiss, S., & Spitalnik, D. M. (1994). The changing conception of mental retardation: Implications for the field. *Mental Retardation, 32*(3), 181-193.

Schleien, S. J. (1993). Access and inclusion in community leisure services. *Parks and Recreation, 28*(4), 66-72.

Schleien, S. J., & Green, F. P. (1992). Three approaches for integrating persons with disabilities into community recreation. *Journal of Parks and Recreation Administration, 10*(2), 51-66.

Schleien, S. J., Olson, K., Rogers, N., & McLafferty, M. (1985). Integrating children with severe handicaps into recreation and physical education programs. *Journal of Park and Recreation Administration, 3*(1), 74-78.

Schleien, S. J., & Ray, M. T. (1988). *Community recreation and persons with disabilities: Strategies for integration*. Baltimore, MD: Paul H. Brookes.

Schleien, S. J., Ray, M. T., Soderman-Olson, M., & McMahon, K. T. (1987). Integrating children with moderate to severe cognitive deficits into a community museum program. *Education and Training in Mental Retardation, 22*(2), 112-120.

Schleien, S. J., & Werder, J. (1985). Perceived responsibilities of special recreation services in Minnesota. *Therapeutic Recreation Journal, 19*(3), 51-62.

Schwier, K. (1988, October). Respite not a luxury, its essential. *SACL Dialect*, 6, 14.

Seligman, M. (1975). *Helplessness: On depression, development, and death.* San Francisco, CA: W. H. Freeman.

Seligman, M., & Maier, S. (1967). Failure to escape traumatic shock. *Journal of Experimental Psychology, 74*, 1-9.

Shamir, B. (1988). Commitment and leisure. *Sociological Perspectives, 31*(2), 238-258.

Shamir, B. (1992). Some correlates of leisure identity salience: Three exploratory studies. *Journal of Leisure Research, 24*(4), 301-323.

Shapiro, J. P. (1993). *No pity: People with disabilities forging a new civil rights movement.* New York, NY: Times Books.

Shapiro, J. P. (1994). The mothers of invention. *U.S. News and World Report, 116* (1), 38-42.

Sharpton, W. R., & West, M. (1992). Severe and profound mental retardation. In P. J. McLaughlin & P. Wehman (Eds.), *Developmental disabilities: A handbook for best practices* (pp. 16-29). Stoneham, MA: Andover Medical Publishers.

Shary, J. M., & Iso-Ahola, S. E. (1989). Effects of a control-relevant intervention on nursing home residents' perceived competence and self esteem. *Therapeutic Recreation Journal, 23*(1), 7-16.

Shaver, J., Curtis, C., Jesunathadas, J., & Strong, C. (1987). *The modification of attitudes toward persons with handicaps: A comprehensive integrative review of research. Final report to the U.S. Dept. of Education, Office of Special Education and Rehabilitation Services (Project No. 023Ch50160, Grant No. 6008530210).* Logan, UT: Utah State University, Bureau of Research Service.

Shaw, S. M. (1992). Family leisure and leisure services. *Parks and Recreation, 27*(12), 13-16, 66.

Sherrid, P. (1988). The prison of paralysis, the freedom of words. *U.S. News & World Report*, p. 60.

Shivers, J. (1981). *Leisure and recreation concepts: A critical analysis.* Boston, MA: Allyn and Bacon.

Sibley, W. A. (1990). Diagnosis and course of multiple sclerosis. In S. M. Rao (Ed.), *Neurobehavioral aspects of multiple sclerosis* (pp. 5-14). New York, NY: Oxford University Press, Inc.

Siegel, B. (1991). Toward DSM-IV: A developmental approach to autistic disorder. In M. M. Konstantareas & J. H. Beitchman (Eds.), *The psychiatric clinics of North America: Pervasive developmental disorders,* (pp. 53-68). Philadelphia, PA: Harcourt Brace Jovanovich.

Singer, G. H. S., & Irvin, L. K. (1989). Family caregiving, stress, and support. In G. H. S. Singer & L. K. Irvin (Eds.), *Support for caregiving families: Enabling positive adaptation to disability* (pp. 3-25). Baltimore, MD: Paul H. Brookes.

Siperstein, G. N., Budoff, M., & Bak, J. J. (1980). Effects of the labels "mentally retarded" and "retard" on the social acceptability of mentally retarded children. *American Journal of Mental Deficiency, 84*, 596-601.

Skellenger, A., McEvoy, M., McConnell, S., & Odom, S. (1991). *Environmental arrangements intervention manual.* Unpublished manuscript, George Peabody College, Vanderbilt University, Nashville, TN.

Sloman, L. (1991). Use of medication in pervasive developmental disorders. In M. M. Konstantareas & J. H. Beitchman (Eds.), *The psychiatric clinics of North America: Pervasive developmental disorders* (pp. 165-182). Philadelphia, PA: Harcourt Brace Jovanovich.

Smith, J. (1988). Multiple Sclerosis. In S. Maddox (Ed.), *Spinal Network* (pp. 86-87). Boulder, CO: Spinal Network and Sam Maddox.

Smith, J. (1990, Winter). Computer voice activation: The future is nearly here. *Spinal Network Extra,* 47-48.

Smith, M. R. (1992). Semeiotics and the coverage of people with disabilities. *Disability Studies Quarterly, 12*(1), 1-4.

Smith, N. R., Kielhofer, G., & Watts, J. H. (1986). The relationship between volition, activity pattern, and life satisfaction in the elderly. *Journal of Occupational Therapy, 40*, 278-283.

Smith, R. (1993). Sport and physical activity for people with physical disabilities. *Parks and Recreation, 28*(2), 22-27.

Smith, S. A., & Yoshioka, C. F. (1992). Recreation functioning and depression in people with arthritis. *Journal of Therapeutic Recreation, 26*(4), 21-30.

Smull, M. W. (1992). Full inclusion and the value of students with severe disabilities. *AAMR News and Notes, 5*(6), 3.

Smull, M. W., & Donnehey, A. J. (1993). The challenges of the 90s: Increasing quality while reducing costs. In V. J. Bradley, J. Ashbough, & B. Bailey (Eds.), *Creating individual supports for people with developmental disabilities: A mandate for change at many levels.* Baltimore, MD: Paul H. Brookes.

Snell, M. E. (1988). Curriculum and methodology for individuals with severe disabilities. *Education and Training in Mental Retardation, 23*, 302-314.

Speigel-McGill, P., Bambara, L. M., Shores, R. E., & Fox, J. J. (1984). The effects of proximity on socially oriented behaviors of severely multiply handicapped children. *Education and Treatment of Children, 7*, 365-378.

Staff. (1989). Professionally speaking. *Evergreen Stroke Association, 11*(6), p. 10

Stainback, S., & Stainback, W. (1983). Influencing the attitudes of regular class teachers about the education of severely retarded students. *Education and Training of the Mentally Retarded, 17*(2), 88-92.

Stainback, S., Stainback, W., Strathe, M., & Dedrick, C. (1983). Preparing regular classroom teachers for the integration of severely handicapped students: An experimental study. *Education and Training of the Mentally Retarded*, 204-209.

Stainback, W., & Stainback, S. (1987). Facilitating friendships. *Education and Training in Mental Retardation, 22*, 18-25.

Stainback, W., Stainback, S., & Jaben, T. (1981). Providing opportunities for interaction between severely handicapped and nonhandicapped students. *Teaching Exceptional Children, 13*, 72-75.

Stark, J. (1992). Presidential address 1992: A professional and personal perspective on families. *Mental Retardation, 30*(5), 247-254.

Stark, J., & Goldsburg, T. (1990). Quality of life from childhood to adulthood. In R. Schalock (Ed.), *Quality of life.* Washington, DC: American Association on Mental Retardation.

Stewart, C. C. (1988). Modification of student attitudes toward disabled peers. *Adapted Physical Activity Quarterly, 5*, 44-48.

Storey, K., Stern, R., & Parker, R. (1991). A comparison of attitudes toward typical recreational activities versus the Special Olympics. *Education and Training in Mental Retardation, 25*, 94-99.

Strohmer, D. C., Grand, S. A., & Purcell, M. J. (1984). Attitudes toward persons with a disability: An examination of demographic factors, social context, and specific disability. *Rehabilitation Psychology, 29*(3), 131-145.

Strully, J. & Strully, C. (1985). Teach your children. *The Canadian Journal of Mental Retardation, 35*(4), 3-11.

Terrill, C. F. (1992). What's in a name? *AAMR: News and Notes, 5*(5), 8.

The results are in! (1986, March/April). *The Disability Rag*, p. 33.

Thompson, A. (1991). Class shows picture of life with disability. *The Daily Collegian,* November 13th, 4.

Thompson, A., & Vierno, P. (1991, November 13). Wheelchairs change way people react. *The Daily Collegian*, p. 4.

Thurman, K. S., & Lewis, M. (1979). Children's response to differences: Some possible implications for mainstreaming. *Exceptional Children, 45*(6), 468-469.

Tinsley, H. E. A., & Tinsley, D. J. (1982). A holistic model of leisure counseling. *Journal of Leisure Research, 2*, 100-116.

Tinsley, H. E. A., & Tinsley, D. J. (1986). A theory of the attributes, benefits, and causes of leisure experience. *Leisure Sciences, 8*, 1-45.

Torres, I., & Corn, A. L. (1990). *When you have a visually handicapped child in your classroom: Suggestions for teachers (2nd edition)*. New York, NY: American Foundation for the Blind.

Treavor-Roper, P. D., & Curran, P. V. (1984). *The eye and its disorders (2nd ed.).* Oxford, UK: Blackwell Scientific Publications.

Tripp, A., & Sherrill, C. (1991). Attitude theories of relevance to adapted physical education. *Adapted Physical Activity Quarterly, 8*, 12-27.

Turkington, C., & Sussman, A. E. (1992). *The encyclopedia of deafness and hearing disorders.* New York, NY: Facts On File, Inc.

Turnbull, A. P., & Behr, S. K. (1986, May). *Positive contributions that persons with mental retardation make to their families.* Paper presented at the annual meeting of the American Association on Mental Deficiency, Denver, CO.

Turnbull, A. P., & Summers, J. A. (1985, April). *From parent involvement to family support: Evolution to revolution.* Paper presented at the Down Syndrome State of the Art Conference, Boston, MA.

Ulrich, M. (1986). Life guards and life lines. *Parent to Parent, 9*(6), 6-7.

Ulrich, M. (1987). And crown thy good with brotherhood. *Parent to Parent, 10*(8), 1-3.

Ulrich, M. (1989). Tony and Aaron: A mother's hopes for sons. *Impact, 2*(3), 14.

Ulrich, M. (1991). Evaluating evaluation: A fictional play. In L. M. Meyer, C. A. Peck, & L. Brown (Eds.), *Critical issues in the lives of people with severe disabilities.* Baltimore, MD: Paul H. Brookes.

Uomoto, J. M., & Brockway, J. A. (1992). Anger management training for brain injured patients and their family members. *Archives of Physical Medicine Rehabilitation, 73*, 674-679.

U.S. Architectural & Transportation Barriers Compliance Board. (1992). Equal access to meetings, information. *Access America, 2*(2), 10.

U.S. Department of Justice, Office of Attorney General. (1991). Nondiscrimination on the basis of disability by public accommodations and commercial facilities; Final Rule. *Federal Register. No. 28 CFR 36*, Washington, DC: U.S. Government Printing Office.

Vallerand, R. J., Gauvin, L. I., & Halliwell, W. R. (1986). Negative effects of competition on children's intrinsic motivation. *Journal of Social Psychology, 126*, 649-657.

Van Andel, G. E., & Austin, D. (1984). Physical fitness and the mentally handicapped. A review of the literature. *Adapted Physical Activities Quarterly, 3*, 207-220.

Vandercook, T., York, J., & Forest, M. (1989). The McGill Action Planning System (MAPS): A strategy for building the vision. *Journal of the Association for Persons with Severe Handicaps, 14*(3), 205-215.

Vanderheiden, G., & Lloyd, L. L. (1986). Communication systems and their components. In S. W. Blackstone & D. M. Bruskin (Eds.), *Augmentative communication: An introduction* (pp. 49-162). Rockville, MD: American Speech-Language-Hearing Association.

Vanderheiden, G., & Yoder, D. E. (1986). Overview. In S. W. Blackstone & D. M. Bruskin (Eds.), *Augmentative communication: An introduction* (pp. 1-28). Rockville, MD: American Speech-Language-Hearing Association.

Veilleux, F., Saint-Hilaire, J. M., Giard, N., Turmel, A., Bernier, G. P., Rouleau, I., Mercier, M., & Bouvier, G. (1992). Seizures of the human medial frontal lobe. In P. Chauvel, A. Delgado-Escueta, E. Halgren, & J. Bancaud (Eds.), *Advances in neurology, Vol. 57. Frontal lobe seizures and epilepsies*. New York, NY: Raven Press.

Veno, D. (1986). Wild mountains and errant attitudes: Taming them requires mainstreamed planning. *Disabled U.S.A., 1-2,* 13-14.

Vernon-Levett, P. (1991). Head injuries in children. *Critical Care Nursing Clinics of North America, 3*(3), 411-421.

Voelkl, J. E., & Birkel, R. C. (1988). Application of the experience sampling method to assess clients' daily experiences. *Therapeutic Recreation Journal, 22*(3), 23-33.

Voeltz, L. M., Wuerch, B. B., & Wilcox, B. (1982). Leisure and recreation: Preparation for independence, integration and self-fulfillment. In B. Wilcox & G. T. Bellamy (Eds.), *Design of high school programs for severely handicapped students* (pp. 175-209). Baltimore, MD: Paul H. Brookes.

Wade, M. G., & Hoover, J. H. (1985). Mental retardation as a constraint on leisure. In M. G. Wade (Ed.), *Constraints on leisure* (pp. 83-110). Springfield, IL: Charles C. Thomas.

Wallach, F. (1991). A partnership that's saving kids. *Parks and Recreation, 26*(10), 52-54.

Ward, M. J. (1988). The many facets of self-determination. National Information Center for Children and Youth with Disabilities: *Transition Summary, 5*, 2-3.

Wassman, K. B., & Iso-Ahola, S. E. (1985). The relationship between recreation participation and depression in psychiatric patients. *Therapeutic Recreation Journal, 13*(3), 63-70.

Webster's New Collegiate Dictionary. (1977). Springfield, MA: G. & C. Merriam.

Wehman, P. (1993). *The ADA mandate for social change*. Baltimore, MD: Paul H. Brookes.

Wehman, P., & Schleien, S. (1981). *Leisure programs for handicapped persons: Adaptations techniques, and curriculum*. Austin, TX: Pro-Ed.

Wehmeyer, M. I. (1994). Perception of self-determination and psychological empowerment of adolescents with mental retardation. *Education and Training in Mental Retardation, 29*(1), 9-21.

Weinberg, N. (1978). Modifying social stereotypes of the physically disabled. *Rehabilitation Counseling Bulletin, 22*, 114-124.

Weinberg, R. S., & Ragan, J. (1979). Effects of competition, success/failure, and sex on intrinsic motivation. *Research Quarterly, 50*, 503-510.

Weirs, P. (1988, October 28). Integrated recreation activities set for today. *The Daily Collegian*, p. 8.

West, M., & Parent, W. S. (1992). Consumer choice and empowerment in supported employment services: Issues and strategies. *The Journal of the Association for Persons with Severe Handicaps, 17*(1), 47-52.

Wikler, L., Wasow, M., & Hatfield, E. (1983, July-August). Seeking strengths in families of developmentally disabled children. *Social Work*, pp. 331-315.

Wilcox, M. J. (1993). Partner-based prelinguistic intervention: A preliminary report. *OSERS News in Print, 5*(4), 4-9.

Williams, R. (1991). Choices, communication, and control—A call for expanding them in the lives of people with severe disabilities. In L. H. Meyer, C. A. Peck, & L. Brown (Eds.), *Critical issues in the lives of people with severe disabilities* (pp. 543-544). Baltimore, MD: Paul H. Brookes.

Witt, P. A., Ellis, G., & Niles, S. H. (1984). Leisure counseling with special populations. In T. E. Dowd (Ed.), *Leisure counseling: Concepts and applications* (pp. 198-213). Springfield, IL: Charles C. Thomas.

Wolfensberger, W. (1972). *Normalization: The principle of normalization in human services.* Toronto, ON: National Institute on Mental Retardation.

Wolfensberger, W. (1977). *A multi-component advocacy/protection scheme. Law and mental retardation: A monograph series.* Toronto, ON: Canadian Association for the Mentally Retarded.

Wolfensberger, W. (1983). Social role valorization: A proposed new term for the principle of normalization. *Mental Retardation, 21*(6), 235-239.

Wolfensberger, W. (1989). Bill F.: Signs of the times read from the life of one mentally retarded man. *Mental Retardation, 27*(6), 369-373.

Wolfensberger, W., & Thomas, S. (1983). *PASSING (Program Analysis of Service Systems' Implementation of Normalization Goals: Normalization Criteria and Ratings Manual) (2nd ed.).* Toronto, ON: National Institute on Mental Retardation.

Woodrich, D. L., & Joy, J. E. (1986). *Multi-disciplinary assessment of children with learning disabilities and mental retardation.* Baltimore, MD: Paul H. Brookes.

Wortman, C., & Brehm, J. (1975). Responses to uncontrollable outcomes: An integration of reactance theory and the learned helplessness model. In L. Berkowitz (Ed.), *Advances in experimental social psychology, Vol. 8.* New York, NY: Academic Press.

Wright, B. A. (1988). Attitudes and the fundamental negative bias: Conditions and corrections. In H. E. Yuker (Ed.), *Attitudes toward people with disabilities* (pp. 3-21). New York, NY: Springer.

Wuerch, B. B., & Voeltz, L. M. (1982). *Longitudinal leisure skills for severely handicapped learners: The Ho'onanea curriculum component.* Baltimore, MD: Paul H. Brookes.

Yessick, J. T. (1991). *The relationship between leisure dispositions and well-being in middle-aged adults.* Unpublished doctoral dissertation, University of Utah, Salt Lake City.

York, J. (1994). A shared agenda for educational change. *Newsletter: The Association for Persons with Severe Handicaps 20*(2), 10-11.

Young, L. W. (1990). Being temporarily disabled is an eye-opening experience. *Centre Daily Times.*

Yuker, H. E. (1977). *Attitudes of the general public toward handicapped individuals (Awareness Papers).* Washington, DC: White House Conference on Handicapped Individuals.

Yuker, H. E. (1988). *Attitudes toward persons with disabilities.* New York, NY: Springer Publishing Company.

Zertuche, C. (1993). From the field-fantasy. *Parks and Recreation, 28*(4), 8, 10-11, 90.

Zigler, E., & Butterfield, E. C. (1968). Motivational aspects of changes in IQ test performance of culturally deprived nursery school children. *Child Development, 39*, 1-14.

Zoerink, D. A. (1988). Effects of a short-term leisure education program upon the leisure functioning of young people with spina bifida. *Therapeutic Recreation Journal, 22*(3), 44-52.

Author Index

A

B

C

D

E

F

G

H

I

J

K

L

M

R

S

Y

Z

Subject Index

A

B

C

D

E

F

G

H

I

J

L

M

N

O

P

Q

R

S

T

U

V

W

Other Books From Venture Publishing

The Activity Gourmet
by Peggy Powers
Adventure Education
edited by John C. Miles and Simon Priest
Assessment: The Cornerstone of Activity Programs
by Ruth Perschbacher
Behavior Modification in Therapeutic Recreation: An Introductory Learning Manual
by John Dattilo and William D. Murphy
Benefits of Leisure
edited by B. L. Driver, Perry J. Brown and George L. Peterson
Beyond Bingo: Innovative Programs for the New Senior
by Sal Arrigo, Jr., Ann Lewis and Hank Mattimore
The Community Tourism Industry Imperative—The Necessity, The Opportunities, Its Potential
by Uel Blank
Dimensions of Choice: A Qualitative Approach to Recreation, Parks, and Leisure Research
by Karla A. Henderson
Evaluation of Therapeutic Recreation Through Quality Assurance
edited by Bob Riley
The Evolution of Leisure: Historical and Philosophical Perspectives
by Thomas Goodale and Geoffrey Godbey
The Game Finder—A Leader's Guide to Great Activities
by Annette C. Moore
Great Special Events and Activities
by Annie Morton, Angie Prosser and Sue Spangler
Internships in Recreation and Leisure Services: A Practical Guide for Students
by Edward E. Seagle, Jr., Ralph W. Smith and Lola M. Dalton
Introduction to Leisure Services—7th Edition
by H. Douglas Sessoms and Karla A. Henderson
Leadership and Administration of Outdoor Pursuits, Second Edition
by Phyllis Ford and James Blanchard
Leisure And Family Fun (LAFF)
by Mary Atteberry-Rogers
The Leisure Diagnostic Battery: Users Manual and Sample Forms
by Peter A. Witt and Gary Ellis
Leisure Diagnostic Battery Computer Software
by Gary Ellis and Peter A. Witt

Leisure Education: A Manual of Activities and Resources
by Norma J. Stumbo and Steven R. Thompson
Leisure Education II: More Activities and Resources
by Norma J. Stumbo
Leisure Education: Program Materials for Persons with Developmental Disabilities
by Kenneth F. Joswiak
Leisure Education Program Planning: A Systematic Approach
by John Dattilo and William D. Murphy
Leisure in Your Life: An Exploration, Fourth Edition
by Geoffrey Godbey
A Leisure of One's Own: A Feminist Perspective on Women's Leisure
by Karla Henderson, M. Deborah Bialeschki, Susan M. Shaw and Valeria J. Freysinger
Leisure Services in Canada: An Introduction
by Mark S. Searle and Russell E. Brayley
Marketing for Parks, Recreation, and Leisure
by Ellen L. O'Sullivan
Outdoor Recreation Management: Theory and Application, Third Edition
by Alan Jubenville and Ben Twight
Planning Parks for People
by John Hultsman, Richard L. Cottrell and Wendy Zales Hultsman
Private and Commercial Recreation
edited by Arlin Epperson
The Process of Recreation Programming Theory and Technique, Third Edition
by Patricia Farrell and Herberta M. Lundegren
Quality Management: Applications for Therapeutic Recreation
edited by Bob Riley
Recreation and Leisure: Issues in an Era of Change, Third Edition
edited by Thomas Goodale and Peter A. Witt
Recreation Economic Decisions: Comparing Benefits and Costs
by Richard G. Walsh
Recreation Programming and Activities for Older Adults
by Jerold E. Elliott and Judith A. Sorg-Elliott
Research in Therapeutic Recreation: Concepts and Methods
edited by Marjorie J. Malkin and Christine Z. Howe
Risk Management in Therapeutic Recreation: A Component of Quality Assurance
by Judith Voelkl
A Social History of Leisure Since 1600
by Gary Cross

The Sociology of Leisure
by John R. Kelly and Geoffrey Godbey
A Study Guide for National Certification in Therapeutic Recreation
by Gerald O'Morrow and Ron Reynolds
Therapeutic Recreation: Cases and Exercises
by Barbara C. Wilhite and M. Jean Keller
Therapeutic Recreation Protocol for Treatment of Substance Addictions
by Rozanne W. Faulkner
A Training Manual for Americans With Disabilities Act Compliance in Parks and Recreation Settings
by Carol Stensrud
Understanding Leisure and Recreation: Mapping the Past, Charting the Future
edited by Edgar L. Jackson and Thomas L. Burton

Venture Publishing, Inc.
1999 Cato Avenue
State College, PA 16801
Phone (814) 234-4561 or FAX (814) 234-1651